Concise Medical Textbooks

Psychiatry

Concise Medical Textbooks

Antimicrobial Chemotherapy
D. Greenwood

Biochemistry
S. P. Datta and J. H. Ottaway

Cardiology
D. G. Julian

Community Health, Preventive Medicine and Social Services
J. B. Meredith Davies

Dermatology
J. S. Pegum and Harvey Baker

Embryology
M. B. L. Craigmyle and R. Presley

Gastroenterology
Ian A. D. Bouchier

Introduction to General Practice
Michael Drury and Robin Hull

Medical Microbiology
C. G. A. Thomas

Obstetrics and Gynaecology
R. W. Taylor and M. G. Brush

Ophthalmology
Kenneth Wybar

Paediatrics
John Apley

Pathology
J. R. Tighe

Pharmacology
R. G. Penn

Psychiatry
Sir William Trethowan and Andrew Sims

Renal Medicine
Roger Gabriel

Respiratory Medicine
David C. Flenley

Sociology as Applied to Medicine
Donald L. Patrick and Graham Scambler

Fifth Edition

Psychiatry

Sir William Trethowan CBE,
MA MB (Cantab), DSc (Hon.), FRCP, FRACP,
FRCPsych., FRANZCP (Hon.)
Emeritus Professor of Psychiatry
University of Birmingham

A. C. P. Sims
MA, MD (Cantab), DRCOG, FRCPsych.
Professor of Psychiatry,
University of Leeds

Baillière Tindall, London

Published by Baillière Tindall,
1 St Anne's Road, Eastbourne BN21 3UN

© 1983 Baillière Tindall

First published 1964
Fourth edition 1979
ELBS edition 1979
Fifth edition 1983

ISBN 0 7020 1021 9

Typeset by Wyvern Typesetting Ltd, Bristol

Printed in Great Britain at The Pitman Press, Bath

British Library Cataloguing in Publication Data

Trethowan, *Sir* William
    Psychiatry.—5th ed.—(Concise medical textbook)
    1. Psychiatry
    I. Title   II. Sims, A.C.P.
    616.89   RC454
    ISBN 0–7020–1021–9

Contents

The illustration on the front cover was painted by a depressed patient with anorexia nervosa and appears to be her impression both of an avenue of trees and of a view into her own oesophagus. The reproduction is by kind permission of the Curator, the Guttman–Maclay Collection, the Institute of Psychiatry.

Preface

It is sad to have to report that since the last edition of this book was published, its original author, Professor E. W. Anderson, Emeritus Professor of Psychiatry at the University of Manchester, has died. As there can be no doubt about his considerable influence upon British psychiatry it is appropriate to reiterate here something of what was said about this in the Preface to the previous edition of this book.

Professor Anderson's major contributions to clinical psychiatry were derived not only from his own extensive experience as a clinician and teacher, but from his knowledge of German psychiatry gained during a lengthy period of postgraduate study in that country immediately prior to World War II. This led him to become one of the foremost exponents of phenomenology in the United Kingdom. Indeed, the phenomenological approach as espoused by Anderson and by many of his pupils can be regarded as a welcome corrective to the somewhat milk-and-water Meyerian approach which characterized British psychiatry in the immediate postwar years, and which has proved not to have stood the test of time.

As with previous editions, the fundamental philosophy upon which this book is based is that psychiatry rests firmly on clinical observation rather than upon hazy theoretical speculations. It also encompasses the notion that an appreciation of the nature of clinical phenomena requires a detailed knowledge of phenomenological psychopathology, having sufficient regard to the minutiae of the symptoms and signs of mental illness. At the same time attention towards some of the more dynamic aspects of mental life has not been neglected, especially where these seem to foster empathy with patients' problems by leading to a better understanding of their content.

The Fifth Edition sees the co-option of a new author—Professor Andrew Sims of Leeds. The reason for this is that the senior author is shortly retiring from active clinical practice and from the Chair of Psychiatry at Birmingham and, indeed, by the time this edition sees the light of day, will already have done so. It is also hoped that the co-option of Professor Sims will ensure continuity and uphold the tradition with which this book is associated, especially as, before taking up his Chair in Leeds, Professor Sims worked both in the University Department at Birmingham and at one time in that at Manchester.

While I myself remain for the time being the book's principal author and responsible in the main for its contents, Andrew Sims has injected into its pages much which is new and up to date. Thus he has been responsible for extensive revision of those chapters dealing with emotional and neurotic disorders, with the general result that there is now a great deal more emphasis placed on the behavioural aspects of these conditions than heretofore.

Among other innovations, an attempt has been made in Chapter 5 to correlate the classification of mental disorders used in this book, and which is based largely on the *International Classification of Diseases* (ICD 9), with diagnostic practices in North America as based on the third edition of the American Psychiatric Association's *Diagnostic* and *Statistical Manual of Mental Disorders* (DSM III), a not altogether easy task as some of the differences in diagnostic nomenclature are considerable.

Nearly all chapters have been extensively revised and some entirely rewritten. Their sequence has also been altered to some extent to what is hoped will be found to be a rather more logical pattern. Owing to the need to include new material without, insofar as is possible, increasing the overall length of the book, several chapters have been shortened or have had some of their original content replaced. Chapter 10 on *Epilepsy* and Chapter 17 on *Disturbances of Sexual Behaviour*, written originally with considerable help from Dr T. A. Betts, have been likewise revised. A new chapter entitled *The Psychiatry of Old Age* has been included, this being a matter of continually growing concern. The chapter on *Child and Adolescent Psychiatry* has been extensively rewritten with the help of Dr Ian Berg with, once again, a much stronger behavioural approach to the treatment of the disturbed child. In addition to separate chapters on psychological and physical treatments, a third chapter on *Social Treatment* has now been included, incorporating both new material and some of that dealing with the social aspects of mental illness to be found in previous editions.

Finally, the concluding chapter on *Psychiatry and the Law* has been rewritten by Professor R. S. Bluglass, Honorary Professor of Forensic Psychiatry at Birmingham, so as to incorporate the provisions of the new Mental Health Act which is due to become operational on 30 September 1983, and, in this respect at least, making the Fifth Edition of this book as up to date as possible.

Achieving this end has entailed many hours of hard work, not the least part of which has been the typing and retyping of the manuscript by Mrs June Dugan and Mrs Monika O'Connor. We have very considerable cause to be most grateful to both of them.

November 1982   W. H. Trethowan

1

Introduction

Psychiatry comprises the recognition, prevention, diagnosis and treatment of illnesses of which the principal manifestations are mental. Some of these disorders are apparently of psychological origin; while in others there may be some more or less obvious physical cause, the symptoms are, again, predominantly mental. Although psychiatry has only relatively recently become an established specialty, it has, during the last half-century, grown to be one of the largest branches of medicine. It has had a long fight to establish itself as a medical discipline—a constant struggle against fear, ignorance and prejudice. Only now, following a fairly radical change of attitude by both the public and the caring professions, does the battle appear to have been won.

There are several reasons why psychiatry has been slow to achieve maturity. Firstly, there are still many who find it difficult to reconcile mental symptoms with illness, tending to attribute these to moral shortcomings or weakness of character. Secondly, mental disorders differ totally from physical diseases in that in many of them there is no easily demonstrable morbid basis, or obvious physical invalidism. Thirdly, superstitious notions about what is essentially *mental* in nature have not yet entirely vanished. Indeed, fear of mental illness, being widespread, has led to a persistent tendency to look askance upon those who are mentally ill. Finally, despite modern advances in treatment, much mental illness regrettably remains chronic, so that those who suffer tend to be seen as condemned to lifelong social incapacity, and looked on as 'second-rate citizens'. All these factors have tended to induce a negative attitude towards both psychiatry and its patients.

There are also 'antipsychiatric' attitudes, which can be identified. One is that psychiatry is seen by some as no more than a matter of common sense. If this really were so, then it must be said that common sense must surely be a very uncommon quality! It has also been suggested, because the results of psychiatric treatment are so poor, that the subject is hardly worthy of attention. But this is clearly bound up with unrealistic expectations of cure. Because psychiatrists may not be able to *cure* their patients, it seems to some that they should be regarded as having failed altogether. How justified is this belief? Many mental illnesses are insidious in onset and run a prolonged and chronic course. Are they, therefore, any less curable than a number of chronic physical disorders, such as rheumatoid arthritis, chronic bronchitis and emphysema, diabetes, psoriasis and many other disabling disorders? While many of these illnesses can be relieved, they cannot be cured. Is not the same as true of many psychiatric disorders? Thus, although diabetes can now be adequately controlled, it is rarely, if ever, curable. The same might be said of schizophrenia.

Antipsychiatric attitudes are also unfortunately to be found among psychiatrists themselves; such as the belief that ultimately when all is known, mental disorders will be fully explicable in mechanistic terms and, by the same token, remediable by some sort of biochemical adjustment. This has clearly led some to neglect psychological and environmental factors in treatment and to place undue reliance on drugs and other physical measures. Conversely, and at the opposite extreme, there are those who cling to the notion that virtually all types of mental abnormality will, in due course, be completely explicable in terms of upbringing or early environmental experiences, and that any form of physical treatment, especially that requiring some degree of compulsion, must be regarded as an insult to human dignity. This and other conflicts of opinion have led to a polarization of psychiatry into *organic* and *psychodynamic* schools. Recently, however, renewed interest in descriptive and phenomenological psychopathology has led to growing eclecticism and a coming together of opposing viewpoints, together with increasing realization that mental disorders can only be properly understood and managed when account is taken of a much wider range of factors—genetic, constitutional, biochemical and other physical influences—along with psychological, environmental and social influences including those which govern conditioned responses of various kinds.

In line with this there has been considerable discussion in recent years of models appropriate to psychiatry. Some would espouse a *medical* or *organic* model, seeing psychiatric disorders as fully akin to other medical conditions. Others would regard a *psychological* model as more appropriate; while a third group prefer a *social* model, putting the family foremost. The truth probably is that while one or other of these models may be the most appropriate to any particular case, not all can be given the same weight even where an eclectic attitude is considered desirable. What is called for is flexibility.

History of psychiatry

The history of psychiatry falls into several fairly distinct epochs, the first of these, which is usually referred to as the *prescientific* or *superstitious* era, ranges over many centuries. Following this, an increase in scientific knowledge which affected the whole of medicine in the United Kingdom and Europe occurred. This also included psychiatry and gave rise to a new understanding of mental disorders. Tracing these advances back over several centuries, it may be seen how the emergence of so many new ideas culminated in the establishment of psychoanalysis and related psychodynamic schools and, more recently, in growing eclecticism, both in the United Kingdom and elsewhere.

The prescientific era

Although scattered references to mental illness were made by the early Egyptians and the ancient Hebrews, the true history of psychiatry seems to have begun with the Greeks. Up until then mental illness appears to have been seen as of supernatural origin or as a gift of the gods. In ancient Greece such superstitious views were questioned by Hippocrates (460–375 BC), who taught that the brain is the seat of the mind and, in particular, that epilepsy, then regarded as the 'sacred disease', had a natural origin. His teaching on the temperaments as well as his classification of mental disorders into mania, melancholia and phrenitis still find echoes in the present day.

Some other early Greek and Roman physicians advocated a humane approach to the mentally disordered. Thus Asclepiades (*c.* 150 BC) considered music and baths as valuable treatments and insisted that the mentally ill should not be confined in the dark but treated in well-lit places—a lesson only recently learned in treating delirious patients. Arateus of Cappadocia (*c.* AD 30–90), who also opposed coercive and cruel treatment, gave excellent descriptions of melancholia and mania, and even seems to have recognized the kind of mental deterioration which is characteristic of schizophrenia. He too was much against coercive and cruel treatment of the mentally ill.

But, with the collapse of the Roman Empire, and following the death of Galen (AD 200), much which can now be seen as enlightened vanished into obscurity so that a new demonological era began. Thus the belief that mental disorder was due to demoniacal possession or was a result of witchcraft dominated the Middle Ages from the eleventh century onwards, so that for some three centuries or more treatment fell into the hands of priests and exorcists. The doctrines of the time, together with mass suggestibility as manifested, for example, by the dancing manias, almost certainly contributed to the belief that demoniacal possession, or bewitchment, was responsible for certain psychopathological phenomena, those resulting from hysterical conversion reactions and also possibly of other kinds. However, to maintain, as some have done, that witchcraft, heresy and mental illness became fused into one, and that on this account many mentally ill persons perished at the hands of the Inquisition, is probably an overstatement. There is, indeed, considerable evidence that those who were truly mad were often seen as such and not merely as possessed or bewitched. The *Malleus Maleficarum*, for instance, contains few if any examples of cases of persons who can be recognized as suffering from psychoses.

Despite this, the attitude in Christendom towards the mentally ill was undoubtedly barbarous and contrasts with that of Islam, witnessed by the establishment of mental hospitals in Turkey and other Mohammedan countries long before such asylums were founded in Europe. However, there were exceptions, such as the establishment, in 1377, of St Mary of Bethlehem Hospital in London.

The scientific era

Before the firm establishment of psychiatry as a medical discipline in Germany, dawn broke in England as early as the seventeenth century. Thomas Sydenham (1624–89), showing a typically English empiricism in his writings on hysteria, clearly recognized the part played by emotion in the genesis of this disorder. John Haslam (1764–1844), Apothecary to Bethlehem, also stands out as a first-rate clinical observer and one of the foremost psychiatrists of his day; his writings won international recognition. About the same time, a figure of comparable stature emerged in Revolutionary France: Philippe Pinel (1745–1826). Pinel emphasized clinical observations and *inter alia* psychological factors in the aetiology of mental disorder and its corollary, the 'moral' treatment of the mentally ill, although it is chiefly as a philanthropist that he has gone down in history. His gesture in liberating 50 patients from their chains at the Bicêtre during the Revolution is linked inseparably with his name. His pupil Esquirol (1772–1840) made an even greater contribution to psychiatric knowledge. Esquirol, an outstanding clinical observer, emphasized the necessity of basic statistics concerning patients, and it is to him we owe the definitions of hallucination and illusion which have stood to this day. Rightly, he must be regarded as one of the founders of modern psychiatry.

In the early years of the nineteenth century in England, the most outstanding figure was J. C. Prichard (1786–1848), to whom belongs the credit of describing those abnormal personalities with antisocial tendencies (now described as *psychopathic*), to whose disorder he gave the name of 'moral insanity'. Yet the most far-reaching English contribution at this time, possibly partly under the impetus of Pinel, lay in the introduction of more humane methods in the treatment of the mentally sick associated with the names of William Tuke (1732–1822), the founder of the York Retreat, which was opened in 1796, and with John Conolly (1794–1866), who within a period of three months totally abolished mechanical restraint at Hanwell, then England's largest mental hospital, in which he followed Edward Charlesworth (1783–1853) and Robert Gardiner Hill (1811–78) who had done the same at Lincoln, although on a smaller scale and over a longer period of time. These men were products of the great English humanitarian tradition whose influence helped to make the institutional care of the mentally ill in the British Isles second to none in the world.

The somatic approach

In Germany the long and bitter struggle between the speculative philosopher and the inductive empiricist was finally and decisively settled in favour of the latter. The turning point was in 1845 when Wilhelm Griesinger (1817–68) published his textbook of psychiatry, in which he clearly stated that 'mental diseases are brain diseases'. This outlook was entirely materialistic: thus the causes of mental illness were to be sought in cerebral lesions, the search for which was pursued with unremitting zeal. Griesinger stressed that the individual *symptom* for which a specific cerebral localization was sought was, however, a symptom of a *unitary psychosis*, by which was meant a single mental illness manifesting itself in different forms. Organic psychosis, particularly *general paralysis* (GPI), was taken as a model. However, as this naïve approach soon proved useless to explain most common mental illnesses it was, in the end, abandoned, despite a valiant attempt to maintain this languishing somatic orientation by Morel (1809–73) who, under the influence of darwinian theories, put forward his *degeneration hypothesis*. According to this, tainted stock showed progressive deterioration through the generations from mild mental disturbance to idiocy. Likewise, Lombroso (1836–1909) tried to relate crime to mental disorder and to identify the criminal by physical 'stigmata' of degeneration.

The clinical descriptive approach

The first to break the organicist deadlock of Griesinger and his school was Kahlbaum (1828–99), who recognized independent forms of mental illness as *disease entities*. It was on this basis that Emil Kraepelin (1856–1926) undertook his epoch-making work of differentiating and classifying the various clinical forms of psychiatric illness, his classification soon being adopted the world over and which still forms the essential basis of many modern attempts at classification.

Kraepelin demanded that in order to establish a disease entity, certain conditions must be fulfilled, such as causes, symptomatology, course, outcome and pathological findings. The mental disorder that seemed to satisfy all these criteria was once again *general paralysis*. In the large majority of cases, however, not all these criteria could be satisfied. Kraepelin was forced, therefore, in the absence of tangible pathological evidence, to fall back on purely psychological symptoms. By a meticulously careful study of clinical phenomena and the course and outcome of various illnesses, he succeeded in differentiating manic-depressive psychosis, paranoia, and dementia praecox, later in 1911, styled schizophrenia by E. Bleuler (1857–1939). Kraepelin's achievements constitute a landmark in the history of psychiatry. Although his work has had many critics, particularly on the score of the rigidity of his disease entities, this criticism is not entirely just, since Kraepelin was one of the most objective and least prejudiced of investigators and well aware of the provisional nature of his categories.

Although the careful clinical descriptive approach of German psychiatry contributed greatly to the understanding of the psychopathology of the psychoses, their treatment underwent no radical change until, in 1917, Wagner-Jauregg introduced the treatment of general paralysis by malaria. In 1933, von Meduna started to treat schizophrenia by inducing epileptic convulsions, using camphor and other drugs, a treatment later found to be more valuable in affective disorders than in schizophrenia. In 1937, convulsive therapy was greatly refined by Cerletti and Bini, who achieved the same results by electrical means. In 1936, Moniz introduced prefrontal leucotomy and, in 1938, Sakel the treatment of schizophrenia by deep insulin coma—now, since the advent of modern psychotropic drugs, superseded.

The psychodynamic approach

The history of psychodynamics and many of today's concepts of abnormal emotional reactions stem from Mesmer (1743–1815) and the 'discovery' of *animal magnetism*. Mesmer was a charlatan—a 'psychological sans-culotte' as Zilboorg called him—who, like others of his kind, discovered something which, although he himself did not realize its true nature, had far-reaching consequences. Out of the controversy which soon surrounded animal magnetism and its originator, arose the concept of *mesmerism*, or *hypnotism* as it later came to be called. Continuing experiments during the nineteenth century by Braid and Elliotson in England and by Liebeault, Bernheim and Charcot in France, gradually gave rise to a new concept of mental disorder in which the belief arose that mental processes which were largely hidden or *unconscious* could produce symptoms or exert an effect upon behaviour. This culminated in the work of Sigmund Freud (1856–1939), one of the most radical and challenging figures in the history of psychiatry. In 1885, Freud visited Paris to observe Charcot's experiments on hypnosis at the Sâlpetrière. Returning to Vienna and starting in private practice, Freud began by using hypnosis but soon abandoned it in favour of *free association*, the method which gave birth to *psychoanalysis*.

It is impossible as yet to assess the significance of Freud's contributions, not merely to psychiatry, but to present-day thought, to literature and the arts. It can be said, however, that his teaching has profoundly altered psychiatric thinking, even among those who do not accept his views. Freud's influence was particularly strong in the United States and by no means negligible in the United Kingdom, particularly during and just after World War I, when his teachings gave enormous impetus to the study of the neuroses and to the development of psychotherapy.

The Freudian school of psychoanalysis soon produced a number of offshoots. The most prominent of these is undoubtedly that of Carl Jung (1875–1961) whose school of *analytical psychology* is best known for the concepts of archetypes, the 'collective' or 'racial unconscious', and for the division of personalities into 'introverts' and 'extraverts'. Freud and Jung seemed to have parted company as a result of Jung's non-acceptance of Freud's theories of infantile sexuality. Others who broke away or who developed their own extensions of Freud's original doctrines include Alfred Adler (1870–1937), best remembered for his concept of the *inferiority complex*, Sullivan (1892–1949) who considered that mental illness was largely derived from disturbed interpersonal relationships, and Melanie Klein (1882–1960) who developed some rather remarkable theories concerning hostile and aggressive impulses in childhood leading to unbearable feelings of guilt.

Freud's psychodynamic concepts also exerted a considerable effect on Adolf Meyer (1866–1950), a Swiss, who spent most of his working life in the United States and who also had a considerable influence on Anglo-American psychiatry. Meyer, who was especially critical of Kraepelin, endeavoured in his *psychobiological* approach to escape from a rigid diagnostic framework and to see each individual as a unique whole, to assess the diverse factors leading to his illness, to evaluate the favourable factors making for possible adjustment and to base treatment upon these.

Psychiatry today

Other than advances in treatment brought about by drugs, which may well turn out to have been overvalued, most advances which have occurred since World War II have been in the social field. Dogmatic attitudes and assertions are, however, much less common than they were. Psychiatry has not only become more eclectic in its outlook, but has begun to exhibit a greater degree of humility in the face of continuing ignorance of certain fundamental problems which have so far proved obstinately resistant to solution. Many contributions which come from other disciplines have also been well received: anthropology, sociology, psychology and philosophy.

From philosophy are derived the important contributions of Karl Jaspers (1883–1967) whose psychopathology is basically represented in this book, and the various schools of existential analysis which in its many variants forms a worldwide trend, although the value of this approach remains debatable. Recently it would seem that it is from biochemistry that perhaps the most promising advances may be expected, although positive gains even in this field are still relatively slight. But whatever advances may be made in whatever sphere, it seems highly likely that psychopathology will remain the essential basis of psychiatry and the psychiatrist's essential tool.

Inevitably in a discipline like psychiatry, where knowledge of the causes of the majority of the disorders which fall within its purview is lacking, theories, opinions and conjectures abound. Thus as each attack on a fundamental problem fails, or proves inadequate, eager searches for new lines of approach must be made. As has already been shown, these have brought about many swings of the pendulum of psychiatric thinking. These swings have perhaps been more frequent in recent years. However, there still remains an important and not insubstantial body of factual knowledge.

Perhaps the most striking of all recent developments has been the return to *behaviourism* and the application of concepts derived from *learning theory* to the formation of psychiatric disorders and in particular to abnormal emotional reactions. This revival of what was initially derived from Pavlov (1849–1936), whose work on conditioning opened a new chapter on treatment, is now generally known as behaviour therapy, the techniques of which have been developed by Watson and Skinner, who have demonstrated the value of *operant conditioning*, and by Wolpe who has demonstrated the value of *reciprocal inhibition* in the treatment of complex as well as simple neurotic states. In view of the waxing and waning of therapeutic enthusiasms which still so strongly characterize psychiatry, it is perhaps still too early to pass judgement on the final value of behaviour therapy. Nevertheless there seems little reason to doubt that its place in the total range of treatments is secure (see Chapter 22).

Apart from such things, the present trend seems to be away from *clinical psychiatry* as it affects individual patients, towards broader, more general social considerations. These include epidemiological enquiries into the incidence and prevalence of mental illness and into the possible significance of environmental factors. Such studies are destined, no doubt, not only to lead to an increase in knowledge, but to lead to changes both of clinical and administrative significance. The possibility of a 'breakthrough' in the biochemical field has already been mentioned. However, there is an ever-present danger that too great absorption in such matters may lead to a neglect of clinical aspects of the subject in which there are still so many problems to be solved. Whatever discoveries may be made in biochemical or other related disciplines, it is extremely doubtful whether the clinical or psychopathological aspects of mental illness will ever, in any way, diminish in importance.

Further reading

Hunter, R. and Macalpine, I. (1963) *Three Hundred Years of Psychiatry, 1535–1860*. London: Oxford University Press.
Zilboorg, G. and Henry, G. W. (1941) *A History of Medical Psychology*. London: George Allen & Unwin.

2

Psychopathology

Just as a knowledge of pathology is fundamental to the understanding of physical disease, so is a knowledge of psychopathology fundamental to the understanding of psychiatry. However, this analogy cannot be taken too far. Physiopathology deals with macroscopic and microscopic alterations in the structure of bodily organs brought about by disease and also with disturbances of function as reflected, for example, by abnormalities of body chemistry. In contrast, psychopathology is concerned primarily with mental happenings, even though these may in some instances be due to lesions within the central nervous system or to various kinds of biochemical or metabolic derangement. However, psychopathology, too, has its macroscopic and microscopic aspects; the former consisting of the exhibition and interpretation of grossly abnormal behaviour, the latter of an appreciation by empathetic examination of the minutiae of mental processes and the nature of subjective experience.

Currently the term *psychopathology* seems to have acquired two somewhat separate meanings, *phenomenological* and *psychodynamic*. As defined by Karl Jaspers, who can be considered as the leader of the phenomenological school, *phenomenology* means, in effect, *living into* the patient, putting oneself into his or her person in order to understand as intimately and in as much detail as possible the nature of the subject's mental experience. It also means portraying in words the nature of the experience as subtly and as accurately as possible while, at the same time, defining it in appropriate technical terms and differentiating it from other kinds of experience. This is an empirical procedure which takes place at a conscious level.

Concepts of psychopathology are constantly evolving and tend to change with the growth of knowledge in other allied fields. Thus with the advent of *psychoanalysis*, a dynamic concept of mental life evolved originally by Freud, *psychopathology* came to be equated in the minds of many with *psychodynamics*. Although Freud never denied a constitutional or biological basis for mental illness, psychoanalytic theories are essentially those which try to relate past psychological events to the present-day development of symptoms.

While psychodynamic interpretations may make the content of symptoms meaningful, such interpretations must be regarded as something which may lead to greater *understanding* rather than providing a basic *explanation*. While these two words tend to be used in the English language as if they were synonymous, Jaspers stresses the distinction. By *understanding* he means the natural acceptance of the development of one psychic state out of another as a logical or comprehensible event. Thus an insulted person becomes angry. This is psychologically understandable to all normal people in our culture. However, there are some who do not become angry when insulted. To understand this, knowledge of the subject's background is necessary: his moral, religious and social attitudes; his special character; his intelligence; in short, all those factors, personal and environmental, which contribute to his personality and allow the observer to appreciate why, when insulted, he does not react as most other people do. This is psychological understanding or understanding by empathy. The process is subjective. In contrast, *explanation* is much more objective in that it correlates certain frequently recurring, tangible, observable facts so that rules can be established, such as, for example, the frequent correlation between cerebral toxaemia and delirium. *Explanation*, furthermore, has a predictive value which *understanding* does not.

Likewise, an awareness of the difference between *form* and *content* is fundamental to an understanding of psychopathology. Thus hallucinations are, to those who experience them, just as real as perceptions. Hallucinations are, for example, prominent in delirious states, in which they are commonly visual. The *content* of a hallucination is that which the sufferer believes he sees such as a hideously distorted face, a menacing animal or a gruesome scene. The content of a hallucination does not, however, bear a direct relationship to the nature of the phenomenon, that is, to the *form* which it takes; that it is visual and not auditory or tactile; that it is not a delusion or some completely different kind of symptom. Furthermore, neither form nor content *explains* the other. The content of a hallucination or of any similar symptom must of course be derived from the patient's mental life. He can only experience a hallucination, however distorted, of something already known to him. It is impossible to conceive of anyone's experiencing a hallucination of some object not merely forgotten but previously completely unknown. Thus if a subject has a visual hallucination of a snake, it must be assumed that there exists in his mind a concept of snakes and of their nature, and the capacity to imagine what snakes look like. However, this has nothing to do with the reason for the hallucination occurring in the first place or for the form it takes. In the case of delirium, it is caused by an organic disturbance of brain function which in turn may be brought about by a wide variety of pathological states—febrile infections, toxic influences, and so on.

To take another example, a patient suffering from a major depressive illness may dwell on all sorts of morbid or gloomy possibilities, some of which may achieve delusional strength. While there is growing evidence in some cases at least that his state of depression may be the result of some biochemical process which affects whatever homeostatic mechanism it is that normally controls mood, it is because his mood is lowered that he starts to dwell on depressing thoughts. Once again the exact content of these thoughts must be derived from his previous experience and from his psychic life. He may, for example, show bitter and exaggerated self-reproach over some past minor act of wrongdoing. This may be so trivial and may have happened to long ago that although the sufferer unwaveringly ascribes his depressed state of mind to it, it will be obvious to the observer that it must be an effect, not a cause. Indeed, because of his depressed state of mind it is more than likely that without the one experience to set off such bitter self-blame, the patient would have found another to take its place, for who are there amongst us who cannot find some regrettable incident in our past lives with which to reproach ourselves if needs be?

In considering anxiety and other reactions, form and content may be drawn a little closer to one another. Thus a patient with specific *monophobia* of cats may develop anxiety symptoms, leading him to take evasive action only if a cat draws near. It may be assumed that his phobia is due to adverse conditioning resulting from some past unfortunate experience in which cats played a part. Yet, even this seemingly adequate formulation leaves too much unexplained. Why, for example, did he so readily become adversely conditioned whereas others exposed to similar influences may have escaped their effects? When more generalized and less specific phobic states are considered, such as *agoraphobia*, a completer explanation becomes proportionately more difficult to achieve.

One may agree, therefore, with Jaspers that mental disorders cannot be explained in terms of psychopathology alone. Certain mechanisms lying outside awareness must be invoked. Unfortunately knowledge of many of these is still very scanty. They include all those factors covered by the term *inborn disposition (anlage)*, a term which not only covers hereditary endowment but includes characteristics of all kinds acquired by the subject in the course of interaction with his environment. However, the mind although important is only one manifestation of human life. To *explain* the symptoms of mental disorder it is necessary to know much more about the interrelation of brain function with mental processes, but we are a long way from that. Indeed there are grounds for believing that however refined knowledge of neurophysiology or brain function becomes, it will never prove possible to translate content of mind into physical terms, or consider it as anything other than mental.

Apart from this, there is clearly much more to be learned about mental processes. Advances in neurophysiology have led to the construction of electronic models which imitate mental processes, normal and abnormal, from which certain deductions may possibly be made as to their nature. Cybernetics is also an actively growing field although its application to clinical psychiatry is as yet limited. The procedures used by behaviourist psychologists to produce 'experimental neuroses' in animals represent a similar approach to those human experiments in which 'model psychoses' may be induced by certain drugs. These 'models', far from replacing psychopathology as a basic science for psychiatry, have brought to it something of a renaissance. For instance, to make a meaningful electronic model of the mechanisms involved in memory, it is necessary to be familiar with the variety of phenomena associated with memory and with the range of pathological abnormalities which have been observed and described in studying memory disorders. In the case of a 'model' psychosis, the investigator must observe the psychopathological phenomena produced by the drugs and determine their similarity or otherwise to the symptoms of well-known clinical syndromes. It is the study of psychopathology which supplies this important information.

Psychiatric symptoms

This chapter deals with the principal symptoms, together with the mechanisms which underlie them, from which those with a wide variety of psychiatric disorders may suffer. Some others will be further considered in subsequent chapters under the heading of those conditions to which they are especially relevant. Here, however, they are considered collectively, although grouped for convenience according to the way in which they appear to be related to one another.

Disturbances of consciousness

Consciousness is a state of mind which refers to the nature of a subject's mental experience at any given moment in time. If he is said to be conscious, this implies that he is more or less aware of himself and his environment; if unconscious, then he is not. If his consciousness is *clouded*, then his awareness of himself and his environment must necessarily be incomplete, according to the degree of his level of consciousness and the manner in which this may fluctuate. Note, however, that this use of the term *conscious* differs from that in which the subject may state that he is 'aware of something' meaning that he has some particular idea in mind. Whereas the former refers to his *state* of consciousness, the latter refers to the *content* of his consciousness. Note also that while a subject's state of consciousness may obviously have a striking effect upon its content, in that he may not become so readily aware of environmental events as he otherwise might do were he fully conscious, the same perhaps is not nearly so true the other way round. The exception, however, may be that if he is preoccupied intensely enough with a certain idea, he may be less inclined to become aware of environmental stimuli which might otherwise engage his attention. Under this circumstance it is appropriate to speak of *narrowing* of consciousness as against *clouding*. It would seem possible to draw an analogy here with a camera which, if out of focus, produces only a blurred image of the whole field, as against a camera sharply focused on a particular object largely to the exclusion of its surroundings.

Although affecting all psychic functions, alterations in the level of consciousness become most obvious in relation to *object awareness*. That is because even in the fully conscious subject, object awareness has only a relatively narrow range, so that at any one time it is only possible to pay attention to a relatively few objects while maintaining only a dimmer awareness of the rest which remain at the fringe of consciousness.

In terms of content, therefore, what is conscious—that is to say, 'in mind' at any particular moment of time—is like the tip of an iceberg. In terms of the state of consciousness the rest of the iceberg may be included, in that this consists of a large store of a great many other things any of which the subject could more or less immediately become aware of, were his attention drawn to them by some appropriate stimulus. Thus in a normal state of consciousness and unless fully concentrating to the exclusion of all else on some particular idea, the content of consciousness is likely to be constantly changing especially where environmental happenings continually obtrude and the more so when they evoke anxiety, pain and other unacceptable feelings which may demand resolution as speedily as possible.

The quality of consciousness changes from moment to moment; it becomes lowered when the subject is fatigued so that he is generally less alert, but narrowed and intensified in danger, so that he concentrates particularly upon whatever is threatening him to the exclusion of all that is irrelevant. The range of consciousness also diminishes with age, while showing great variation from one person to another. Under pathological conditions it is not only the range and acuteness of consciousness which are disturbed but other mental functions as well.

Torpor

The term *torpor* refers to a state of pathological drowsiness in which mental activity demands the greatest effort. Attention can be aroused only with great difficulty; perceptions are slow, laboured and incomplete. The range of consciousness is diminished, imagination is reduced in content and clarity, drive disappears and there is a gross reduction of emotional response. The flow of mental events is slowed down to the point of extinction so that the patient is always ready to fall asleep.

Torpor must be distinguished from *stupor*, as may occur in severely retarded depressive states, in catatonic schizophrenia and in some other conditions. Although in severe stupor some clouding of consciousness may be apparent, this is not due to any organic cause nor is it associated with the disturbance in memory and degree of subsequent amnesia which characterize torpor.

Delirium

Milder forms of delirium, often referred to as confusional states, resemble torpor in that consciousness is clouded but instead of inactivity, motor restlessness occurs. Delirium is like a bad dream, with disintegration of conceptual thinking and, in severer cases, illusions, hallucinations—especially visual ones—and delusions. Perception of the external world is fragmentary, fleeting and distorted. Incoherence may dominate the clinical picture together with an emotional disturbance which may lead the sufferer to become greatly disturbed, even terrified, so that unless restrained he may go berserk. If his attention can be gained at all, this is usually only momentary. Even without formal testing, which is usually impossible to carry out, he may be observed to be grossly disorientated. Indeed, he may so mistake his surroundings as to believe he has been incarcerated in prison and that those around him are threatening his life. As his delirium deepens, torpor may supervene, followed, if unrelieved, by coma.

Even in a state of deep torpor, motor restlessness may persist so that the patient may clutch or pick at the bedclothes (*carphologia*) or sweep away imaginary objects.

Oneiroid states

The term *oneiroid* means dreamlike. While oneiroid states are in many ways similar to delirium, the sufferer's inner experiences are less fragmented. Indeed, the experience of a patient in an oneiroid state which may last days or weeks is fairly coherent and may even be scenic in character.

Such conditions bear some resemblance to *twilight states*, although they are more likely to be of toxic origin or an early symptom of acute schizophrenia, in which event the term *oneirophrenia* may be used.

Twilight states

Twilight states can be divided into several groups. In the first, object awareness is so narrowed that the patient remains aware of only part of his surroundings, the rest of the world being shut out. Thus a punch-drunk boxer, although barely conscious, may continue to fight. He may even lay effective blows but, being only partly aware of his situation, may be unable to take effective action whereby to defend himself from his opponent's onslaught. The condition is usually transient, although accompanied by amnesia.

Epileptic twilight states.   Twilight states may occur in temporal lobe epilepsy in which, during an attack, the patient may carry out some relatively complex activity such as walking along a crowded street or, more dangerously, driving his car. Suddenly the attack ceases leaving the subject wondering how he came to be where he is. Again there is usually complete amnesia for the episode. Occasionally epileptic states are of much longer duration and unless terminated may last several days or weeks.

Panic attacks. Other twilight states are due not so much to narrowing of object awareness but to incomplete or lopsided understanding by the patient of his situation. This may occur because of an overwhelming affective state such as terror or panic. Under these circumstances customary attitudes and inhibitions may fall into abeyance, leading the patient to behave in an unaccustomed, sometimes physically aggressive or even murderous manner. Once again such states are usually followed by complete amnesia. Some are liable therefore to become of forensic importance.

Dissociative twilight states. These, which are also known as *hysterical twilight states,* are the outcome of a ready tendency whereby some subjects dissociate, leading them to behave automatically without apparently any conscious awareness of doing so. The simplest example is sleep-walking (*somnambulism*). Another example is the twilight state or trance which may be induced by hypnosis and in which there is rapport only with the hypnotist. Although it is commonly believed that only he can command the subject to awake, the latter, left to his own devices, usually does so spontaneously after a time. The relationship between the subject and hypnotist is characterized by a powerful emotional contact which takes the place of the wish-fulfilment aspects of the hysterical twilight state.

The dynamic unconscious

Although the notion that the content of mind of which the patient is seemingly not conscious can nevertheless exert an effect on behaviour preceded, by many years, Freud's formulation of the so-called *unconscious*, this nevertheless is a fundamental tenet of psychoanalysis. It is easy to cite examples. Who, for instance, can truthfully say that he never failed to keep an appointment that he really did not wish to keep? Or mistook the time or perhaps took the wrong bus? Another subject who has to write an unpleasant letter finds that in some mysterious way he has mislaid his fountain pen. How often does a slip of the tongue reveal with startling frankness what the speaker really feels: feelings which perhaps he had clearly hoped to conceal?

Freud drew attention to many of these kinds of mistakes, pointing out that they were by no means accidental but influenced by motives of which the subject was not fully aware or did not want to be made aware.

Whereas *conscious* means directly present in awareness—here and now, at this very moment—*unconscious,* in the Freudian and *dynamic* sense, refers to all other mental processes which could with greater or lesser difficulty be brought into awareness under appropriate circumstances or are near enough to becoming conscious to be able to exert an effect on behaviour (*preconscious*).

Disorders of perception

Perception is a psychological process whereby sensation from any source and entering consciousness via any channel acquires meaning. A small brown object, having a certain shape, seen sitting on a bough and heard emitting a warbling sound, is a bird. Normally there can be no doubt about it! Recognition is so certain and instantaneous as almost to bypass conscious awareness. Likewise, a pain felt in the sole of the foot while walking barefooted across a floor is instantaneously perceived as being due to some sharp foreign body: a piece of glass possibly, or an upturned drawing pin; the exact source of the sensory stimulus being soon established via visual and other sensory pathways. Whereas perceptual disorders may sometimes be an outcome of a distortion of sensory input—a phantom limb is a good example—most such disturbances have really very little to do with sensory input channels. This is because the subject either has insight into his malfunction or soon gains this so that he accommodates himself to his distorted sensory experience. Thus, the fortification spectra which herald an attack of migraine are soon recognized by the sufferer for what they really are. Although they could be construed as hallucinatory, they are not customarily regarded as such. In contrast, most disorders of perception are associated with absence of insight and if externally engendered, to a failure to interpret correctly the *meaning* of sensory stimuli.

Perception must be distinguished from *imagery*. In both the observer is 'faced' with an object, something separate from himself. When perceived, the object *exists* tangibly, it is *real*. When imagined, it is pictorial and subjective. When perceived an object appears in *outer* space; when imagined it appears in subjective *inner* space, 'in the mind's eye', as it were. Perceptions are constant and independent of the will, whereas images have to be continuously re-created, a process entirely dependent on the will to do so.

Alterations of perception

Changes in intensity.   Ordinary noises may seem deafening: the mere closing of a door may sound like a shot; the ticking of a clock inordinately loud. Such changes may occur in organic or delirious states, after head injury or during a 'hangover'. In states of torpor or in severe depression the contrary may occur so that the world may appear dimmer, everything seems to taste stale or insipid, and so on.

Changes in quality.   Otherwise quite ordinary colours may suddenly seem intense, so that scenes and objects assume a new degree of beauty and exert a fresh fascination. Even objects seen in the peripheral field may become extremely vivid and obtrude on the subject's attention. Such experiences have been described by those under the influence of drugs such as mescaline or LSD-25 or as occurring in certain states of exaltation or ecstasy (see p. 31).

Alternatively perception may become strange and unreal. A patient may complain that everything around him appears indistinct as if in a fog or distant as if seen through the wrong end of a telescope. Voices may be heard as if they come from far away. Such experiences tend to be associated with other *depersonalization* phenomena (see p. 30).

Some changes in the quality of perception may involve more than the mere sensory stimulus, but a disturbance of empathy also. Thus a subject finds that he can no longer *feel* himself into others; they may seem to him to be dead or unreal. Alternatively an *intensification of empathy* can occur, so that the subject feels himself overwhelmed by the emotional experiences of others. Paranoid patients may experience *distorted empathy* so that aspects of the behaviour of persons with whom they are in contact, their gestures, chance remarks and so on are perceived as having a meaning which would certainly not be apparent to normal subjects.

Abnormal concomitant perceptions. Abnormal concomitant perceptions are among the many bizarre perceptions which schizophrenics may experience. Thus, for example, every time he hears someone talking, a schizophrenic may feel something pushing against his chest. He hears voices but only when an aeroplane flies overhead. Someone looks in his direction and he feels 'electricity' passing through his body. Here a normal percept is associated simultaneously with a hallucination, this being known as a *functional hallucination*.

Under the influence of drugs such as lysergic acid or mescaline, *synergistic* perceptions may occur. Thus a sudden loud sound produces the sensation of a flash of light, and vice versa.

False perceptions

There are two principal groups of false perceptions, *illusions* and *hallucinations*, of which the latter are the most important. An *illusion* is a false perception of a real object. Whereas an external object is usually present, its nature or meaning is misperceived. In the case of hallucination no external object is present. While the sensory aspect of the perceptual experience is missing—although to the patient this does not seem to be so—nevertheless and in the case of *true* hallucinations, whatever object he hallucinates seems to him to be completely real. It is fully projected and has complete corporeality. His hallucinatory experience therefore is as vivid to him as if the object which he hallucinates were actually present.

Illusions. In their simplest form illusions are due to *inattention*; failure to spot misprints is a common example. Where, however, attention is grossly impaired as a result of *clouding of consciousness* in a delirious state, misinterpretations of the environment are extremely common and tend to occur together with hallucinations. Thus a patient with *delirium tremens* may mistake his bedside bars for those of a prison cell, viewing with terror his nursing attendants as gaolers who threaten to do him harm.

Another type of illusion (*affect illusion*) may occur under the influence of strong emotion or may be mood determined. Thus a person afraid while walking in the dark may perceive half-hidden shrubs as minatory figures which threaten to attack him. Those with intense depression may misinterpret the squeal of tyres of a passing car as the tortured screams of their loved ones.

Illusions must be distinguished from *mistaken intellectual judgements*, such as when a piece of crystal is believed by one without expertise in such matters to be a diamond.

Illusion of doubles. The illusion of doubles (*Capgras syndrome*) is a condition which is usually found in schizophrenia and in which the patient insists that a relative or friend, although a perfect likeness, is not the person he or she appears to be, but an imposter. The condition may extend to include animals, such as the family dog, or objects, such as a letter, where the patient, for example, while agreeing that the handwriting is precisely similar to that of his wife, will nevertheless insist that it is a forgery. Although included here for the sake of completeness, this symptom should more properly be regarded as a delusion rather than a true illusion.

Hallucinations. Hallucinations are not brought about by misinterpretations of sensory perception as are illusions, but occur side by side with ordinary sense perceptions which criterion differentiates them from dream images. Hallucinations can be classified in several ways:

1. *Elementary.* Elementary hallucinations include flashes, bangs, etc. and are probably due to excitation of more peripheral structures such as sensory end organs. Alternatively, somewhat more complex geometric coloured patterns, such as may be produced by mescaline or lysergic acid, may possibly emanate from the visual cortex.

2. *Complex.* Examples such as conversations, faces or variety of scenes and sensations are probably due to a much more widespread degree of cerebral involvement, notably of the temporal lobes but of other structures also.

Hallucinations may also be classified according to the particular sensory modality in which they occur: visual, auditory, tactile, olfactory, kinaesthetic, etc. This has some diagnostic importance. For example, whereas auditory hallucinations are particularly common in schizophrenia, visual hallucinations are relatively rare, except in the early stages and where the onset of the disorder is acute. If, therefore, visual hallucinations are prominent, an organic cause should always be suspected. Again, olfactory hallucinations are a common feature of temporal lobe epilepsy (*uncinate attacks*). However, hallucinations of almost any kind can occur in this condition. Moreover, olfactory hallucinations are by no means uncommon in schizophrenia, although they may often only be elicited if direct enquiry is made.

In as much as he is able to describe them, a patient's organically determined hallucinations appear to have very much more of the quality of ordinary perceptions than those of the schizophrenic. Indeed, what characterizes schizophrenic hallucinations—of whatever kind—is their bizarre quality, and also the fact that many schizophrenics seem to realize that their hallucinatory experiences are of a personal nature and in some way intended for them alone. Because of this they may not appear to be at all surprised to learn that others do not share their experiences. Schizophrenic patients, furthermore, tend often to be somewhat secretive about their hallucinations and often deny having them, even when their behaviour obviously indicates otherwise. The bizarre nature of schizophrenic hallucinations may be exemplified by the patient who stated that 'he could see a rat coming out of the back of his neck' (*extracampine hallucination*, that is, one occurring out of the normal perceptual field) or another who maintained that he could hear a voice coming from a neighbouring town.

True hallucinations cannot be *explained* in psychological terms alone. Although their *content* may often reveal something of the patient's personality and inner preoccupations, the fact that this reveals itself in the *form* of a hallucination and not in some other way is, in itself, an insufficient explanation. While the psychodynamic notion that hallucinations are due to dissociation, so that a portion of the patient's mind is split off and projected so as to reappear, for example, as a hallucinatory voice, may have some validity in understanding the occurrence of pseudohallucinations (*see below*), it would seem more likely that the basis of true hallucinations—whether of organic or schizophrenic origin—must be sought in morbid alterations of brain function.

3. *Lilliputian hallucinations.* These according to Leroy, consist of 'a vision of small people, men and women of minute and slightly variable height . . . mobile, coloured and generally multiple'. They are rare and usually of arteriosclerotic, toxic or epileptic origin. Lilliputian hallucinations in which miniature people are seen against a normally sized background have to be distinguished from *micropsia* where normal environments are seen in miniature.

4. *Pseudohallucinations.* Pseudohallucinations are a phenomenon to which some would not wish to grant the status of a psychopathological entity. Nevertheless, they differ in several important respects from true hallucinations and, when recognized for what they are, have considerable implications for diagnosis.

Pseudohallucinations were first described by Kandinsky, later by Karl Jaspers and more recently by Sedman who defined them as a special form of imagery. They are not fully projected as are true hallucinations, but appear in inner subjective space in the 'mind's eye'. Pseudohallucinations differ, however, from imagery in that they may to some degree be projected in front of the subject and often occur in vivid sensory detail. They cannot, like images, be evoked or changed voluntarily and the subject's attitude towards them is passive or receptive.

Pseudohallucinations are usually described as occurring only in hearing and sight. Only very rarely are other sensory modalities such as touch involved. Pseudohallucinations may also occur simultaneously in more than one modality and in a connected fashion. Thus the ghostly figure which utters words which the subject hears is a pseudohallucinatory experience. Whereas true hallucinations may occur simultaneously in several sensory modalities, the content of one type of hallucination is in no way congruent with that of another occurring at the same time.

Perhaps what best demarcates and distinguishes pseudo- from true hallucinations most of all is the fact that they appear to be bound up very much with the psychological state of the sufferer and thus are readily susceptible to psychodynamic interpretation. Pseudohallucinations may occur in any form of mental illness, but are thought to be especially characteristic in patients with hysterical disorders often having an admixture of obsessional trends. They are often significantly bound up with the patient's current situation and are common, for example, in bereavement reactions where the widow may see her dead husband sitting in his favourite chair by the fireside, perhaps also hearing him speak to her. Here there is an obvious element of wish fulfilment. Such experiences have also often been described in religious writings and may have an apocalyptic character.

5. *Hypnagogic hallucinations.* Many quite normal people are affected by hypnagogic hallucinations while at the point of dropping off to sleep (*hypnagogic state*) or when gradually awakening (*hypnopompic state*). Such hallucinations are particularly liable to occur in *narcolepsy* in which condition the subject may spend much of the night in a half-waking, half-sleeping state. Except in the latter instance when they may be elaborate, most hypnagogic hallucinations are of a relatively elementary kind—hearing a bell ring, a knock on the door, or one's name called out. These experiences are sudden, clear and projected. They usually wake the subject at once to full consciousness so that their true nature is almost immediately recognized. In themselves they are of no pathological significance.

False bodily perceptions

False bodily perceptions include certain instances of false awareness not mediated by the special sense organs. Thus during a hypnagogic state a subject may feel as if a part of his body is growing enormously in size.

Very rarely and in clear consciousness a patient may describe a feeling of another person just behind him or sitting by his side. He may be able to locate the 'person' accurately, even describing him and his actions in detail: 'Every time I get up, he gets up.' This experience may be elaborated to a feeling by the patient that he has a double (*doppelgänger*) and is occasionally associated with the experience of a hallucination of the self (*autoscopic hallucination*). A patient with temporal lobe epilepsy, constantly felt as if someone completely resembling herself was sitting close beside her on her left. If anyone else tried to sit there she felt considerable discomfort. When she had a seizure this began with an autoscopic hallucination of herself as seen from above.

Similar experiences having a different quality have been reported occasionally by those under great physical and mental stress; for example, two airmen shot down at sea had an irresistible awareness of the presence of a third person with them in their rubber dinghy.

Abnormal imagery

The most important aspect of abnormal imagery belongs to memory; images representing former perceptions which have been experienced in the past and conjured up when these are recalled. As all memories are slightly falsified, these images do not coincide exactly with the previously experienced perceptions which underlie them. These falsifications, however, have to be distinguished from *memory hallucinations*, such as schizophrenics may experience, leading them to claim that certain things have happened to them in the past which in actual fact have not. Features characteristic of memory hallucinations are: an awareness of remembering something previously forgotten; a feeling by the subject that he must have been in a state of altered consciousness such as having been 'hypnotized' or 'drugged' when the 'remembered' event happened; or a feeling that he must, at the time, have been 'a person without a will'. Thus a patient sitting in a restaurant remembered seeing a woman opposite looking at him. He stated: 'She must have hypnotized me.'

Ego disorders

The ego is an empirical concept. It was re-defined by Freud as that part of the mind which organizes perception and copes with reality. In effect it constitutes the self. Thus ego awareness, as against object awareness, is awareness of oneself as against all those external things which a person is aware are not part of him. This separation of self and environment is not present at birth but seems gradually to come into being during the first five years of life as the growing child begins to learn both about himself and the world around. The growth of self-awareness and object awareness proceed therefore in parallel, the establishment of one kind of awareness being dependent on the other.

The self or ego can however be divided into two: an active aware part—the observer as it were—defined as *I* and a passive observed part, defined as *me*. It is *I* also who observes the difference between *me* and *not me*, the boundary between the two or between the self and environment being referred to as the *ego-boundary*. *Me* of course includes the concept of *my-ness* and all that belongs to *me* together with *my body*, the concept of which depends upon the adequacy of the body image. It may be noted moreover that the ego-boundary is not absolutely hard and fast. It can extend to include clothing, providing this is well worn or familiar, also tools, and in the hands of a competent driver, even his car, which he temporarily incorporates as part of himself and his body image when driving it. Nevertheless, it is recognized at least from the intellectual point of view that although these clothes, this tool, this automobile are *mine* and *belong to me*, they do not actually do so to the same degree as *my* face, *my* hand or any other part of *my* body.

In summary, therefore, the normal individual is aware of his existence and separate identity, so that all that he thinks and does and experiences is accompanied at the same time by awareness of the *I-ness* and *my-ness* of his behaviour, of his unity at any given moment in time and of being an individual having a continuing identity. Thus he is aware that he is (more or less) the same person as he was yesterday, last week and so on. Note also that the *I* of any passing movement becomes the *me* of the next, giving rise to a sense of continuity in time.

Only in altered states of consciousness such as in falling asleep is this structure loosened. However, changes in any one or more aspects of ego stability may occur in several psychotic states, for example in delirium where a loss of the sense of *I-ness* and *my-ness* occurs. In states of clear consciousness breaking of the ego-boundary leading to loss of awareness of self or confusion of self-identity is virtually pathognomic of schizophrenia. However, there are some other forms of ego disorder to be considered, of which the three main types are *depersonalization*, *derealization* and *ecstasy states*, and some other striking conditions as well, such as *déjà* and *jamais vu* which may occur as part of a temporal lobe epileptic attack or in schizophrenia.

Depersonalization

In depersonalization the patient's perception of the external world seems changed. Although his surroundings are recognized as essentially unchanged, they seem in some way to have lost the quality of reality. Sometimes this change is experienced by the subject in himself, so that his body seems unreal; he feels himself to be like a puppet or automaton, his psychic life, thoughts, memories, seem 'as if' they were not his own, yet he knows quite well that they are his. The experience of change in the outer world is known as *derealization* whereas the feeling of unreality of the self is called *depersonalization*. Sometimes the latter term is used to cover both states. Each may exist independently although they are often combined. The syndrome is *non-specific* and may occur in most forms of mental illness. It occurs most commonly in depressive states mostly in young people, particularly young women, and in obsessional disorder, particularly those forms characterized by much rumination and by hypochondriasis. Sometimes it seems to occur by itself and when this happens the term *depersonalization syndrome* may be appropriate. Whether it ever actually does occur in isolation from another more basic disturbance is, perhaps, doubtful. Often it emerges that the patient has had a depression, the more florid symptoms of which have disappeared, or are very little in evidence.

The subject often states that the disorder came on suddenly— something snapped in his head (sometimes called a *psycholeptic* attack) and depersonalization occurred. The clinical phenomena may take many forms, but in essence the experience is constant: 'I don't feel the same'; 'everything seems unreal' ('things outside'; 'my body'). Sometimes patients pinch themselves to convince themselves they really exist, and will often contrast their morbid state with their previous normality. Depersonalized patients will often say that they can no longer experience emotion and are cut off from their own feelings. This experience often induces severe anguish, particularly when they make comparisons with their former unconcerned acceptance of their normality. The condition may last for years, with only very rare intermissions, or it may be transient in certain psychoses, as in severe depression and also certain atypical illnesses. Depressives may complain of being 'cut off' from their families or, if religious, from God. Thus depersonalization forms a fertile ground from which delusion-like ideas spring, such as being deserted by God. The cause and cure of the phenomenon remain unknown.

Many theories have been propounded to explain depersonalization, but none is satisfactory. Mayer-Gross suggested a preformed cerebral mechanism, others have suggested an emotional anomaly. It has been viewed psychodynamically as a defence mechanism, a need to escape from oneself, but this seems more than a little implausible, especially in view of the highly unpleasant nature of the condition. Depersonalization phenomena may also arise in the normal individual under certain conditions, in fatigue and in the weakness and langour following convalescence from physical illness.

Ecstasy states

The characteristic features of ecstasy states are firstly, a feeling of intense joy, associated with a deep tranquillity; secondly, an alteration of the ego of which the 'boundaries' seem to dissolve, merging the individual with the cosmos or with God; thirdly, a disorder of perception; and lastly, feelings such as that the riddle of the Universe is solved or no longer exists. Ecstasy states have been described by individuals of all races and cultures and at all times in history, notably by mystics such as St Teresa of Avila, by Buddhist Ascetics and Islamic Sufis, also by numerous other unusual individuals, such as the poet Wordsworth.

The condition, which is, however, rather rare, may possibly also occur as a feature of manic–depressive illness of cyclothymic type during a swing from depression to mania. Some, however, would not agree with this, having regard to the fact that the experience of ecstasy seems to leave a permanent mark on the subject's personality.

Delusions

Delusions are not only of the greatest theoretical and practical importance in psychiatry, but are regarded, by laymen and by lawyers in particular, as those symptoms most characteristic of mental derangement. Nevertheless, their psychopathology is still a controversial matter.

Delusions can be defined as '*Reality judgements which are unacceptable to other people of the same age, class, education and race as the person who expresses them, and which cannot be changed by logical argument or the presentation of evidence to the contrary.*' A simpler definition is that a delusion is '*a false belief, inappropriate to the socio-cultural background of he who holds it and which cannot be corrected by an appeal to reason*'. Neither of these definitions is wholly adequate; indeed, it can hardly be expected that any definition will be sufficient to cover the complexity of the problem. One reason for this lies in the difficulty of defining *reality*, this being something which is in part culturally determined and dependent on an ever-changing social pattern.

Breaking down these definitions of delusions into their component parts it will be seen that there are four elements to be considered.

1. The overwhelming conviction or 'incomparable subjective certainty' which surrounds a delusional judgement.

2. Its incongruity in the face of logical argument and all reasonable evidence as to its falsity.

3. The erroneous nature of its content. (*Note.* This, however, is not invariable. A man may have a delusion of his wife's infidelity although he may have no evidence that she is actually being unfaithful to him. Nevertheless she may be being so, despite his not knowing about it. In this sense, therefore, some delusions are occasionally 'true'.)

4. A delusional judgement is individual, other than in the case of *folie à deux* when the same false belief may be shared by two (and sometimes more) subjects. Otherwise delusions are not shared by peers of similar cultural background, race, religion and educational achievement. What is implied here is that if a primitive jungle-dweller believes that his misfortunes are due to sorcery or to some taboo which has been broken, such beliefs cannot be considered as truly delusional as they are appropriate to the socio-cultural setting in which he dwells. However, quite a different view would probably be taken of a similar belief expressed by a well-educated man living in Westernized suburbia.

Classification of delusions

As there appears to be some confusion in the way terms appertaining to delusions of various kinds tend to be used by different authors, it should be explained that here they are divided into *primary*, sometimes called *autochthonous delusions* or *delusions proper*, and *secondary delusions* including *delusions of explanation* and those which are determined by mood and other factors.

Primary delusions. In primary delusions an entirely new meaning is given to some other completely unrelated psychological event. They consist in essence of a *disturbance of symbolization* at an essentially personal level. Thus a subject sees a bus approaching with the word 'Newcastle' on the driver's cab. This at once tells him that his neighbours are plotting to kill him by setting fire to his house. Sometimes the ideational content is not clear although the patient *knows* that an event has some very special significance for him.

A primary delusion is, by definition, incomprehensible from the start. Although some have tried to explain its emergence as being due to personality factors or underlying emotionally toned attitudes, all these seem to ignore the fundamental characteristics of the phenomenon, treating primary delusions as if they were secondary delusions of explanation. In contrast, Jaspers and other phenomenologists hold that *delusions proper* are primary pathological phenomena, not understandable in psychological terms and arising out of the disease *process* which is most characteristic of schizophrenia and which contains the very essence of the delusional experience as such.

But despite the sudden emergence of a primary delusion certain antecedents may be evident. In some cases the very first stage may consist of a peculiar and virtually indescribable experience in which the patient begins to feel that everything has suddenly taken on a new and sinister meaning without his being able to say just what this is. This state is known as a *delusional atmosphere* or *delusional mood (wahnstimmung)* although it is not a mood in the more usual sense. The next stage is the emergence of a *delusional perception* or *misinterpretation* which occurs as the patient begins to read new meaning into familiar objects and situations. Thus the vase of flowers standing on the table in the bay-window of the front parlour being yellow indicates to him that all the world is aware of his cowardice—he is at once convinced of it.

The theory has been put forward that as all thinking is thinking of meanings and all perceptions convey meanings, it is the meaningful part of thinking or perception which is disordered when delusions arise, not the thought nor the perception themselves. Thus a patient may see causal relationships between events and between events and himself without good reason, such relationships being highly subjective.

In other instances the primary delusional state does not arise out of a disorder of meaning which relates to external objects or events but from inner sources. Thus in the case of *delusional imagination* or *memory*, the subject suddenly conceives a special significance in certain images. He may, for example, suddenly believe he is the illegitimate son of some exalted person. A memory that a member of the Royal Family once glanced in his direction a few years ago on some public occasion confirms this belief absolutely. Alternatively he may become suddenly aware of cataclysmic events without any concrete or definite notion of their occurrence. Thus he knows that the end of the world has suddenly come or that a town many miles away has been destroyed by an earthquake. It is likely, once again, that such *delusional awareness* is compounded from inner visions and fantasies.

Secondary delusions.   Secondary delusions or delusions of explanation may arise out of the primary delusional state as when a patient develops the idea that all his queer feelings can be put down to being bewitched or to the machinations of the British Broadcasting Company who are influencing his thoughts via the medium of television or something of that kind. Alternatively they may be mood determined (*holothymic*) in origin so that if depressed he may believe himself to be the wickedest person in the whole world and in league with the Devil or, if elated, believe himself to be all-powerful, a millionaire perhaps or even one of the Holy Trinity. Other delusions of explanation may be evoked by somatic sensations of one kind or another so that the patient becomes convinced his abdominal gurgles indicate cancer or some frightful disease.

Incorrigibility of delusions

Where a secondary delusion of explanation follows upon a primary delusional state this probably leads to a lessening of anxiety on the basis that any explanation, even an erroneous one, is better than none. Thus the patient who develops a delusional belief that the strange electric sensations in the back of his neck are due to wireless waves emanating from the local radio station may paradoxically obtain some comfort from this knowledge in believing that he has discovered some tangible reason for feeling the way he does. Firm secondary delusional formation probably therefore has a re-integrative effect and furthermore possibly explains why those schizophrenics with well-established unchanging paranoid delusions show a much better preservation of personality than those with hebephrenia in whom delusions are less firmly fixed and constantly changing.

Even with delusions occurring with clouding of consciousness the patient tries to order his thoughts and test his delusions, but in such states this process is not as evident as it is in clear consciousness. This sifting of the evidence and testing one's belief occurs in normal thinking and constitutes an event which is psychologically understandable. However, Jaspers holds that in delusional thinking this process of sifting the evidence is of a different order and not psychologically understandable. It is rooted in a personality change inherent in the illness itself and cannot be further analysed. The retention of the morbid idea to which the patient clings with unshakeable conviction is, in the face of all evidence to the contrary—as seen by others—perhaps the most striking characteristic of delusions. Despite this, such patients often do not behave as if they really believed their delusions were true. The patient who believes herself 'royal' scrubs the floor. This *double orientation* suggests that the delusion is to the patient a symbol for something quite different. This is further supported by the experience that delusions often change in one and the same patient, whereas a delusional attitude remains unaltered.

Other theories about the origin of delusions
The theories of the phenomenological schools so far presented rest on the assumption that the primary delusion or delusion proper is the result of an as yet undiscovered somatic process, and not understandable in purely psychological terms—a view not universally held. Three differing views will be briefly mentioned.

Freud considered that delusions were psychogenic in origin and the result of 'psychic mechanisms' such as projection, introjection, etc. Thus he saw delusions of persecution as being due to repressed homosexuality. This view, however, while throwing interesting light on the content of the delusion, fails to explain the occurrence of the phenomenon of delusion. Psychoanalysis has shown repressed homosexuality to occur in quite different syndromes which do not show delusions.

Bleuler tried to bridge this difficulty by accepting the assumption of the schizophrenic somatic *process*, explaining that the primary effect of this process was a loosening of the associational framework, making it possible for delusions to be formed under the overwhelming pressure of powerful affects, comparable in this respect to the experiences of normal people in similar emotional situations. Thus slight exaggerations and distortions can become pathological. Here the differences between primary delusions and secondary delusions as earlier defined become obscured.

Kretschmer, while accepting the phenomenologist's view of 'process' schizophrenia, believed that delusions were the result of certain abnormal personality developments and were thus psychologically understandable in the framework of these abnormal personalities. This arises in patients suffering from 'sensitive delusions of reference' (*Sensitiver Beziehungswahn*) as a result of tensions emanating from inner complexes. Because many, although not all, of these patients later develop process symptoms of schizophrenia, Kretschmer's distinction is not generally accepted, so that many currently regard this as an attenuated form of schizophrenia rather than a personality disorder.

Overvalued ideas

Overvalued ideas must be clearly differentiated from delusions and obsessions. They are convictions which arise from a strong affect comprehensible in the light of the personality and the life history of the individual who holds the conviction. The idea is one which so dominates the subject that he must pursue it at all times however inappropriately. Overvalued ideas are found among fanatics—a kind of personality deviation. They can be personal or individual such as a 'chip on the shoulder', or of social, religious or political content, as with many a speaker at Speakers' Corner, Hyde Park. To distinguish an overvalued idea from a monideistic delusion can sometimes be difficult.

Compulsive phenomena

Compulsion is a state in which a subject cannot rid his mind of certain contents of consciousness, although recognizing these as absurd or, at least, as dominating consciousness persistently and without logical reason. The word *compulsion* implies that while the subject strives to rid himself of his unwelcome ideas he finds that his endeavours arouse so much anxiety that in the end he has to give in. It is essential to avoid confusion between compulsion and passivity feelings with delusions of influence. It is precisely the patient's resistance which differentiates the two. A compulsion is felt as something alien at the very moment it occurs. As opposed to passivity feelings which are accepted by the ego (*ego-participation*) there is, in the case of compulsion, *ego-repudiation*, although at the same time the subject does not regard his unwelcome ideas as due to some alien influence. Compulsions can therefore only arise in the presence of an awareness of control and choice in the psychic life.

Compulsive phenomena can be divided into two main categories.

1. Those in the wider sense of the word, where content is less important and the feeling of subjective compulsion is the most prominent feature. Thus an image, an idea, a memory, a question can come into the mind again and again. Hence it may prove impossible to get rid of an irritating snatch of melody no matter how hard one tries. Instead of a single thought there may be whole trains of thought which intrude, such as urges to count everything, to spell out all names seen, or to ruminate endlessly about the meaning of life, the injustice of the world, and so on, and so on, and so on! Such compulsions bear a close relationship to overvalued ideas, both being common in compulsive or anankastic personalities (see Chapter 15).

2. Compulsions in the narrower sense of the word, where the alien character of the content, which is nevertheless strongly affectively toned, is much more prominent. In this group we find compulsive affects, strange moods—apparently unmotivated—against which a subject fights

without success; compulsions to consider something as true, the impossibility of which is at the same time also seen; and lastly, compulsive urges which are in total contradiction to a patient's real desires (consciously at least), such as a sudden compulsion to break a shop window, assault a stranger in the street or harm his children.

Obsessional ideas

Obsessional ideas are characterized by the fact that the patient oscillates between a belief and the knowledge that they are untrue: 'What if . . .?' Here there is a conflict between conviction and knowledge of the opposite being true, which is very different in quality from ordinary doubt, or from ordinary conviction. For example, a girl is fondled for the first time by a boyfriend. Afterwards she worries because she feels she might be pregnant. Whereas she knows sexual intercourse has not taken place, the idea keeps coming back all the time; 'I am not sure, I am always in doubt'. When reassured by the doctor she stops importuning, but the next day starts to worry again: 'Maybe he only wanted to be kind.' Normal doubt is characterized by a weighing against each other of the opposing reasons with arrival finally at a psychologically unitary judgement. In obsessional doubt there is at the same time conviction and knowledge that the contrary is true. These two opposing views vie continually with each other, but neither ever gains complete ascendance. In normal doubt when the correctness or falsity of a content cannot be decided, conviction and adherence to one or other may be held in abeyance and any final decision postponed until more evidence becomes available.

Compulsive urges

Any urge which occurs may give rise to a conflict of motives. If the urge leads to some kind of action, the outcome of the conflict will give either the feeling of assertion of the ego or the feeling of the ego having been overpowered. This is normal. If, however, the urge is felt to be alien or absurd, this is to be regarded as a compulsive act. If such urges are relatively harmless, like checking, washing, or similar rituals, the subject normally gives in. If they are dangerous, like murderous impulses, urges to attack people, or to set fire to things, the subject almost invariably opposes them successfully.

Compulsive urges and acts are often understandable as consequences of obsessional phenomena. Thus a person who feels that the kitchen is contaminated with bacteria is compelled to sprinkle it with disinfectant. *Compulsive rituals* are those in which the action is intended—magically— to forestall a disaster, such as the example of a patient who felt compelled to read all the newspapers every day so as to prevent murders from happening. Where, as is likely, the aim can never be achieved, this is ascribed to lack of exactness in executing the rituals. Thus expanded, more papers must be read and re-read in order to make sure. It is not long before the situation becomes so out of hand that the subject is completely submerged. Yet to resist his urges arouses so much anxiety that he is compelled to give in, even though he fully recognizes the absurdity and uselessness of his behaviour. The whole wretched business can be summed up in the phrase: 'Making sure of making sure!'

Phobias

Phobias used to be regarded as negative compulsions in which those affected feel compelled to avoid something, often a very ordinary activity, in order not to arouse anxiety. A more up-to-date view is that phobic anxiety is anxiety attached to a specific object or situation. Thus a patient may have a phobia of thunder, of cats, of heights, of going outdoors. Such fears are of endless variety. Some occur singly, others are multiple. In many cases, conditioning plays a part; in others it is thought that anxiety may have become displaced from its original source and newly attached to an object or situation which did not previously occasion it.

Whatever their basis, phobias certainly lead to compulsive or near compulsive alterations of behaviour, usually of a negative kind. Thus a patient with a phobia of heights may not be able to climb upstairs beyond the second floor. An agoraphobic may not be able to move more than a few yards from her front door. Another unable to stay in a closed room also cannot board a bus or travel in a railway carriage. Her usual explanation is that she fears she may panic and be unable to alight quickly enough, or may not be able to leave the house, because she fears she may faint. At the same time she knows that these anxieties are really groundless, and tries hard to fight them, but without success. Phobias sometimes occur along with other compulsive phenomena, but are more often found as isolated symptoms. Many sufferers learn to live with them and never seek medical advice, although since behaviour therapies have achieved some success, many more are now doing so.

Clinical significance of compulsive phenomena. Compulsive phenomena occur in obsessional disorders, in which they may reach such a degree of intensity so as to become almost totally disabling (see Chapter 15). They may also be symptomatic of a schizophrenic or manic–depressive illness. Sometimes, particularly in the early phases of these psychoses, obsessional symptoms so dominate the clinical picture that they actually obscure the psychotic nature of the illness. Compulsive phenomena also occur in patients with organic cerebral lesions and have also been described in cases of cerebral tumour, head injury, temporal lobe epilepsy and in postencephalitic states where they can be particularly severe.

Disorders of feeling

It is essential to differentiate two types of disorder of feeling: those which although abnormally intense are nevertheless psychologically understandable in terms of the experiences which have brought them about; and those which are not understandable, but can only be explained in terms of extrapsychic causes such as psychotic episodes or are the result of alterations in bodily function or due to some systematic physical illness.

An example of the first type is the depression which follows bereavement which persists for longer than expected owing to there having been a previously abnormal emotional relationship between the bereaved and the deceased. An example of the second type may be a mood change arising primarily from some kind of biochemical fluctuation adversely affecting the central nervous system, but which is subjectively explained by the sufferer as due to his own inadequacies.

Changes in bodily feeling

Changes in bodily feeling which normally contribute to the basis of a subject's total emotional state are frequently deranged in psychoses and in personality disorders. Lowering of vitality, for example, constitutes the central feature of endogenous or primary depressive illnesses. The painful feelings which so characteristically accompany depression may be localized in the limbs, forehead, chest, abdomen or almost anywhere. Such symptoms so dominate the clinical picture of depression as to lead frequently to wrong diagnosis.

Changes in feelings of competence and self-reliance

Although not continuously conscious of it, most normal people have a sufficient degree of awareness of their own competence in everyday situations as to give them self-confidence in their actions. However, in depressive illnesses an overwhelming feeling of inadequacy is so common as to lead the sufferer to declare his uselessness; to state that he cannot make up his mind; that he is incompetent, clumsy, that his memory and intellect are failing, and, if pressed, that all is lost.

Apathy

Apathy reflects an absence of feeling. In extreme cases, as may arise in psychotic states, the subject becomes quite indifferent to anything—pleasant or unpleasant—which may happen. There is no drive to act. He may state that he feels empty, like a camera, seeing all but registering nothing. Those who feel this way may neglect themselves, failing to eat or even seeming not to mind painful injuries.

Loss of feeling

Loss of feeling occurs most strikingly in states of *depersonalization* (see p. 30), in personality disorders, in depression, and also in schizophrenia—

anhedonia: in which experiences which most people would consider pleasurable give no joy whatsoever. Apart from this there may be a painful awareness of loss of feeling. Those affected may complain that they no longer have any feelings of affection for their loved ones, that they have lost their *joie de vivre* and all enthusiasm for matters normally of interest. Since they complain bitterly about all this, it is obvious that the power to feel which they fear is lost is paradoxically still present.

Changes in the emotional tone accompanying perceptions
Since all perceptions evoke feeling tone, this may be altered according to circumstances. In functional psychoses and in toxic states, or in drug-induced model psychoses, changes in feeling tone may be marked. The colours of flowers may seem luminous and of great beauty; a familiar piece of furniture may suddenly become a threatening object; a radio programme may suddenly sound sinister and so on; yet perception remains unaltered.

Likewise, in swings from depression to elation there may be a sudden change in feeling tone from black despair in depression, where all may appear bathed in gloom, to a state approaching and sometimes reaching ecstasy in mania, where all may appear to be coloured by joy and a sense of 'at-oneness' with the environment.

'Free-floating' emotions
Emotional changes brought about by other than psychologically understandable events are those where patients may feel a need to search for an explanation in order to understand why they feel as they do. Failing this they tend to rationalize. Sometimes, however, they have sufficient insight to realize that their feelings are not due to any particular experience, but to endogenous factors beyond control. Thus patients with organic brain syndromes such as cerebral arteriosclerosis and who may be tearful may say apologetically 'I don't really feel like crying but I can't help it.'

Complex elaborations arising from free-floating emotions
Sometimes free-floating emotions may give rise to a new and intense emotional state, such as a feeling of clairvoyance, a feeling of ultimate revelation, a feeling of infiniteness or a state of grace. Alternatively, feelings of imminent danger together with a sense of panic may occur.

Disorders of thinking

In considering thought and its disorders, it is necessary once again to distinguish carefully between the processes of thought and its content. If the thought process is abnormal, its content is almost certain to be abnormal also. The converse, however, is not necessarily true, for where thought processes are normal their content can still be highly deviant, although perhaps in quite a different sense.

When analysing thought processes it is also necessary to distinguish between *goal awareness* which is subjectively experienced: the successful selection of relevant problem-solving associations, which are objectively demonstrable; and the *determining tendency*, a theoretical postulate invoked to explain the mechanism of thought and which relates to consciousness of goal-awareness. Apart from this it must be remembered that affect and emotion not only govern the speed and quality of thinking, but play a major part in determining the direction which thinking may take; and in the distortions of judgement which may follow.

Conceptual thinking

Concepts are synthesized from elements which consist of images, emotions and sensations which may be either simple or complex. By a process of association these elements become fused into meaningful wholes and together with others into still larger wholes or concepts, which when sufficiently developed lead to the ability to employ symbols and think abstractly. Loss of this power is a common casualty in mental illness. Thus the *categorical function*, that is, the power to think in categories or universals, is reduced, leading to an impairment of 'abstract' thinking which is then replaced by *concrete* thought. This can be demonstrated by various tests such as asking the subject to interpret metaphors or proverbs. Thus if when asked to interpret the proverb: 'People in glass houses shouldn't throw stones', the reply comes: 'Because it would break the glass', this can be regarded as an example of concreteness of thought. This kind of disturbance occurs in the mentally handicapped, in whom the power to think abstractly never develops, with organic brain lesions or in schizophrenia, in which it is lost.

Dereistic thinking

Dereistic thinking is that form of thinking which is not directed towards reality situations. It is of considerable importance in psychiatry, occurring markedly as it does in dreams, fantasy and fairy tales as well as in a variety of morbid states. Dereistic thinking is determined by affectively and instinctually set goals. Its outstanding feature is its disregard of contradictions of reality. But although prominent in schizophrenia, it is doubtful how far it goes in explaining the various phenomena of schizophrenic thought disorder.

Some degree of fantasy is a necessary component of all thinking, especially in creative thought where the boundary line between it and nebulous dereistic thinking may be hard to draw. Perhaps the most outstanding example of dereistic thinking is *pseudologia phantastica* where patients like James Thurber's 'Walter Mitty' act out their unreal romances in the real world. While knowing quite well that they have abandoned a firm footing in reality, they continue to spin their yarns with increasing zest. It is as useless to ask them whether they 'believe' in their fantasy role as it is to ask children at play whether they really believe they are 'Mothers and Fathers', 'Teachers' or 'Cowboys and Indians'.

Speed of thought

Acceleration of thinking.   Pressure of thought characteristically occurs in manic states giving rise to *flight of ideas*. Here, while the association of ideas is greatly facilitated, it is determined nevertheless by superficial aspects of what the subject sees and hears. Distractability is the keynote; thus the manic patient tends repeatedly to fly off at a tangent, being diverted into another stream of associations by no more than a chance word or some other quite irrelevant extraneous stimulus. Rhyming, punning and clang associations are common. The flow of associations is largely passive; there is diminution of the determining tendency so that the goal is constantly changing. Sometimes ideas flow so fast and the pressure to express them verbally is so strong, that severe incoherence is the result.

Retardation.   Retardation is the polar opposite of acceleration of thinking and occurs in association with depression. The stream of thought is slowed so that instead of many associations, however superficial or trivial, there is a poverty of thought amounting at times to *monideism* and preoccupation with one, usually painful, topic. The stream of thought may be likened to a river of glue which in the case of depressive stupor reaches stagnation. This condition needs to be distinguished from schizophrenic *blocking* (see p. 43). As in flight of ideas, the determining tendency is diminished. Psychomotor retardation may also affect other activities such as movements or speech, although this is not invariable. Distractability is minimal.

In *mixed states* in which both manic and depressed features may be simultaneously present, a patient who seems both agitated and retarded and who appears to have poverty of thoughts and an inability to utter these, may later explain that at the time his thoughts were racing. If this happens in association with elation rather than depression, the term *manic stupor* may be appropriate.

Perseveration

Perseveration may be defined as the persistence of behaviour and thought after they have ceased to be relevant, analogous perhaps to playing a worn gramophone record which may lead the stylus to become stuck in a groove. Examples are often found in patients with brain damage. A pen is shown and named correctly. The patient is then shown a knife, he calls it a pen; he is then shown a cigarette lighter, and he calls this a pen also. There is a diminished capacity to shift. A hint of this symptom is found in states of fatigue. Perseveration must be differentiated from catatonic stereotypy. The point of difference is that stereotypies are active while perseveration is passive. The causes of both are unknown.

Circumstantiality

The inability to separate the important from the unimportant can be due to lack of intelligence and therefore is often found in mentally handicapped patients. It occurs, however, in other conditions, notably in those who are brain damaged. Once started, such people are not to be interrupted in their narration. Not a single circumstance or detail is spared the listener, nor can the wood be seen for the trees. The constant repetition of some tale of woe in complete and never-changing form is sometimes referred to as *global perseveration*.

Incoherence

Incoherence is a form of thought disorder characterized by fragmentation of the thought stream, loss of essential connections, fleetingness and blurring of concepts which cannot be retained. Fusion of words with parts of other words occurs. The final product may be largely meaningless, even nonsensical (*word salad*). A diminution of attention is a fundamental factor, often the result of impairment of consciousness. Incoherence is characteristic of toxic confusional states, deliria and acute organic states of all kinds. It can also occur to a lesser degree in states of fatigue.

Schizophrenic thought disorder

The principal types of schizophrenic thought disorder are as follows.

Sharing of thoughts with others. This is a common schizophrenic experience which should probably be included amongst the ego disorders. It usually gives rise to a secondary delusion of explanation that some *telepathic* influence is at work.

Thought withdrawal. Here the subject may complain that his thoughts are drained away or sucked out of his head. This is often accompanied by bizarre delusional elaborations; also closely linked with ego disorder. Both thought withdrawal and sharing are of high diagnostic value in schizophrenia.

Thought blocking. This is a sudden cessation of thought. The patient feels his mind has become blank; his thoughts have stopped. Although it is said that if the symptom is very severe it may lead to a state of catatonic stupor, it is doubtful whether stupor is really brought about by the same mechanism as blocking. As the symptom is often very similar to the *absences* of petit mal, differentiation may be difficult. Likewise, a normal person may suddenly lose his train of thought. This, however, cannot properly be regarded as blocking for when reminded of what he was talking about he is usually able to resume his discourse without difficulty.

Écho de la pensée (thought resonance).   This term describes thoughts heard aloud and is a borderline symptom between thought disorder and hallucination. The patient hears his thoughts almost like a whisper but recognizes that they are his own thoughts, so the projective quality of hallucination is not entirely present.

Crowding of thoughts.   This can be regarded as the opposite of thought block. The patient feels as if compelled to think. Likewise, the content of his thoughts may strike him as much richer than normal.

Nebulosity or indefinite thought.   This may be described in diverse ways: 'My thoughts are not crystal clear'; 'They feel like cotton wool', and so on. Any topic may be continuously discussed without, however, conclusions being reached. The symptom when unsuspected may frustrate the doctor who is trying to obtain a coherent history. The patient may say that his 'thoughts are falling over one another'; 'I no longer have my thought processes in hand'. Experiences such as these may be concealed behind the harmless-sounding complaint of 'loss of concentration'. This frequent complaint must therefore always be carefully investigated.

Talking past the point.   This is not so much a different subjective experience from some of the symptoms described above but their outcome. The effect on the patient's ability to converse and to reach satisfactory conclusions is such that he never, as it were, 'hits the bull's eye' but is always 'off centre'. Thought disorders are often difficult to detect or to demonstrate clearly in an unstructured clinical interview, but such clinical tests as the interpretation of stories, proverbs and the definitions of differences and similarities are sometimes helpful.

Paralogy.   This is a form of talking past the point which may occur in schizophrenia, but which also occurs in a similar form in hysterical pseudodementia. Here the patient gives approximate answers, e.g. $2+2=5$, or when shown an apple calls it a banana. His answer indicates pretty clearly that he knows the correct answer, which is suppressed. A similar disturbance is found sometimes in the *buffoonery syndrome* of hebephrenia.

Experimental work in the field of schizophrenic thought disorder is usually aimed at demonstrating similarities and dissimilarities with other forms of thinking, such as that found in children, in emotional disturbances, in brain-damaged persons and in dreams or fatigue states. As in organic states, schizophrenic thinking is characterized by concreteness, and the power to think symbolically is commonly impaired (*desymbolization*). There is also a tendency towards *palaeological thought* which may be overinclusive in as much as the patient may identify a part with the whole so that an associative link may become an identifying link. Yet another feature is *omnipotence of thought* in which a patient believes that events occur because he or some other person or some other thing personified has thought them and thereby willed them to happen.

Further aspects and examples of schizophrenic thought disorder are discussed in Chapter 7.

Disorders of memory

Four distinct elements in memory can be distinguished (the four 'R's').

1. *Registration*, the ability to add new material to the store of memories.
2. *Retentiveness*, the ability to store knowledge which can be called to consciousness.
3. *Recall*, the ability to bring definite memories to consciousness at any chosen moment and under appropriate conditions.
4. *Recognition*, a feeling of familiarity which accompanies memories.

Disturbance of any one of these elements may give rise to memory disorders all of which differ from each other. Memory should not be viewed too mechanically. The contents of memory are always subject to the influence of emotion, this making it anything but a mechanical filing system. Memories are constantly selected in deposition as well as in recall, and emotion may suppress, change, distort or induce false memories. In all memories there is an affect-determined 'falsification' which may vary from trivial to substantial (i.e. memories may be modified according to how the subject *feels* about them). If a series of pictures of relatively indifferent content are given to a number of persons who are asked to recall what they have seen some time later, the results vary enormously. If this is so with memories of relatively indifferent content, distortion will clearly be even more marked with emotionally loaded memories.

Another memory disorder is the experience of *déjà vu*. This is particularly striking if, as in schizophrenia, the patient has lost reality judgement. He may feel that he knows the hospital to which he has come for the first time and be convinced that he has been there before. *Déjà vu* and its opposite, *jamais vu*, in which familiar surroundings or faces suddenly appear new and strange, may also be symptomatic of a temporal lobe seizure. These kinds of false memories which may be termed *paramnesia* have already been mentioned in passing under the heading of ego disorders (see p. 29), to which category they may more properly belong.

Other false memories, phenomenologically of quite a different order from *confabulations*, are *pathological lies*, which may come almost to be believed by the liar himself, or *delusional misinterpretations* of past events. For example, because an acquaintance failed to greet the patient yesterday, this means that he must know that he is of royal descent. Confabulations are changing, loosely held false memories, which are common in organic syndromes and in particular in Korsakow's psychosis. Here they seem to be fantasied, in order to fill gaps in a failing memory ('*despairing confabulations*'). Such confabulations can be influenced by the examiner. They may also occur in schizophrenia (*memory hallucinations*).

Amnesia

Amnesia may be due to failure of various memory elements.

1. In states of gross disturbance of the sensorium, as for instance in a severe delirium, little or nothing is registered so that little or nothing can be retained or recalled. There is no real memory.

2. Perception may have been intact but retention may be disturbed so that lasting memories are not established. This is sometimes found in lesions of the diencephalon. If a patient is asked a short question and can reply immediately, he may be able to give a correct answer, but a few minutes later will have forgotten the question altogether.

3. Sometimes events which have been registered in the normal way are destroyed by trauma. This occurs in the retrograde amnesia following head injury which, although usually only of a few minutes' duration, may extend over several days and occasionally even weeks prior to the injury.

4. Sometimes both grasp and retention are intact and memories do exist but cannot be recalled. That they do exist can be shown when the subject is subsequently able to recall them under hypnosis or by abreaction. This type of amnesia may occur in hysteria or other abnormal emotional reactions and may appertain to certain selected events only or refer to virtually the whole of the subject's previous life. Several types of amnesia may all be present at the same time, thus in retrograde amnesia partial recovery of memories may be facilitated by hypnosis.

Disturbances which occur in clear states of consciousness

Disturbances in grasp.   A patient's memory for past events may seem intact but new things can no longer be learned, possibly because he cannot mentally hold on to (i.e. grasp) them securely or for long enough for them to enter his memory store. Such a disturbance occurring in clear consciousness may be a sequel of carbon-monoxide poisoning. It may be due to syphilis of the central nervous system or alcoholism (*Korsakow's syndrome*). The condition is thought to be associated with lesions in the mamillary bodies or in the mamillo-thalamic tracts.

Disturbances in retentiveness. While the store of memories constantly increases, it also normally undergoes erosion. Thus we forget in the course of time things which we remembered before. This normal process can be enhanced greatly by ageing or other progressive pathological changes in the brain. Even the language store may suffer from loss of words. It is interesting that concrete names go first whereas abstract parts of speech such as conjunctions are retained longer. More recent memories tend to be the soonest lost; those older are better remembered. However, this pattern is less well established than once thought. Furthermore, many apparently better retained earlier memories may be no more than trivial ones. Foreign languages learned later in life are affected more than the mother tongue, although this is not invariable.

Disturbances in recall. Disturbances in recall may also be a feature of advancing age or an expression of on-coming brain failure. What is evident in the first instance is increasing slowness rather than total loss of recall. The subject's emotional state may also interfere with the process such as in the case of normal people when in a state of nervousness during an examination. In others inability to recall often refers to certain complex events which are of emotional significance. Disturbance of memory often appears to exist in hebephrenic patients who do not answer to the point, in patients who suffer from depression who are constantly preoccupied by their complaints and in manic patients who lack the power to concentrate on a topic of conversation.

Falsification of memory

Falsification is a normal attribute of memory, which can be morbidly exaggerated. There can also be morbid falsifications of memory of a different character.

1. In *pseudologia phantastica*, or *pathological lying*, the person who lies seems at the time of lying not to be entirely aware of what is truth and what is made up. Under strong affect, and in the case of those with personality disorders, memories of past events may be grossly distorted. Thus a self-righteous person vividly remembers how some other person put him in the wrong while he himself ignores his own shortcomings.

2. In *paranoid states* patients often present their persecutory complaints in the form of memories. Such memories may suddenly take on new meanings. Thus the subject suddenly realizes now that the man whom he met last year and who winked at him wanted to show him he was being watched. It did not strike him at the time, but now he remembers it clearly. This can be construed as a delayed delusional percept.

3. In severe cases of memory loss caused by organic lesions patients may fill in the gaps on the spur of the moment by *confabulation* (see p. 46).

4. A person who may remember something correctly may be unsure whether it really happened or whether he merely dreamt it. Such a memory may exist out of any context or without any associated background memories. This experience may occur transitorily in normal persons but can also occur in a severe and persistent form in *Korsakow's syndrome*.

Further reading

Fish, F. (1967) Symptoms and signs in psychiatry. In: Hamilton, M. (ed.) *Clinical Psychopathology*, revised reprint 1974. Bristol: John Wright.

Jaspers, K. (1962) *General Psychopathology*, translated by J. Hoenig and M. Hamilton, 7th edn. Manchester: Manchester University Press.

Kräupl Taylor, F. (1966) *Psychopathology, Its Causes and Symptoms*. London: Butterworths.

3

Psychiatric Interviewing

A psychiatrist's technique is largely contained in his ability to obtain information from his patients. Interviewing skill is to him as manual dexterity is to the surgeon. However, the purpose of a psychiatric interview is not merely to elicit evidence of mental abnormality, but also to establish a relationship conducive to the instigation of whatever treatment may be recommended. Essentially it is a procedure calling for considerable understanding; not only of what questions should be asked and how to ask them but how the manner of asking may govern the quality of the replies which the patient may give.

A good case history, if it does not arrive at the whole truth, narrows possibilities, facilitates differential diagnosis and, thereby, enables the construction of a working hypothesis of the nature of the patient's problem. Ideally this formulation, as it is customarily called, seeks to answer three questions: *'What is the nature of the patient's illness? Why did he become ill in the way he did?* and *Why did he become ill when he did?*' Because a single interview rarely allows such a totally comprehensive formulation to be made, it should nevertheless pave the way towards further exploration. Thus a single interview is rarely ever complete in itself. Apart from such considerations, case history-taking should never be allowed to become one sided so that the interviewer asks questions and the patient merely gives answers. Indeed, at the appropriate juncture, the patient should always be given an opportunity to ask questions especially as these often tend to throw further light on the problem, sometimes more so than information gleaned from any previously given answers. Even when, as sometimes happens, the doctor makes an almost instantaneously correct guess—for there are disorders which can be diagnosed instantly—he would still be wise to listen to what his patient has to say. There are still too many persons who, after seeing their doctor, depart unsatisfied either because they feel that their complaints were brushed aside or too lightly treated or because they wished to ask some question, vital to them, but were given no chance to do so.

The implication here is that even the very first interview with a new patient should be considered not only as diagnostic, but therapeutic also. However, whether it also fulfils the latter purpose will depend on the interviewer's realization of this potential, the success of his efforts to establish rapport with his patient and giving him ample opportunity for therapeutic interaction.

Apart from this the only basic difference between a psychiatric and any other kind of interview lies in the nature of the questions the interviewer is permitted to ask; thus many of the matters touched upon will be of a highly personal nature and not appropriate to interviews of other kinds. However, even before a psychiatrist can put such questions he may need to convince his patient that by partaking in what must sometimes inevitably be an embarrassing or even a distressing procedure, he can be expected to obtain some benefit thereby. In most cases cooperation is not difficult to obtain as the approach of a patient to his doctor tends to be coloured by the hope that the doctor, by virtue of his skill and experience, will have the answer to the problem. He is likely, therefore, to do what the doctor asks of him. Non-cooperation is usually the result of undue anxiety, defensiveness, delusional beliefs or a complete failure by the patient to understand his situation, who the doctor is, why he is there, what it is all about and so on.

The type of psychiatric interview required will depend to a large extent upon the nature of the problem. If the patient is obviously grossly demented, this speedily becomes an observable fact, to be dealt with according to degree and the nature of attendant circumstances. If he is psychotic, suffering perhaps from a schizophrenic illness, a detailed elicitation and evaluation of symptoms may be needed to arrive at the correct diagnosis. In those subjects whose disorders apparently depend to a much greater degree upon interpersonal, environmental or other difficulties, a different type of approach may be needed.

A psychiatric interview consists of much more than mere verbal communication, indeed content is not always of paramount importance. Verbal communication is also vocal communication, in that there is much to be gleaned not only from the words which are uttered but from intonation, hesitancy of speech, and manner of enunciation. Non-verbal, non-vocal communication has also to be considered; thus facial expression, gesture, avoidance of eye gaze and other types of accompanying behaviour all add further meaning to the words which are uttered. Sometimes what is *not* said is of crucial importance and on occasions silence can be remarkably revealing.

The interviewer is not just an observer, nor is he merely a recording machine, although ability to be a good listener is a prime requirement. For the interview to proceed smoothly it is almost invariably necessary for him to become to some degree personally, though not emotionally, involved. By the use of an empathetic approach he tries to understand how his subject feels by imagining how he himself would feel in the same situation. Sullivan called this process *participant observation*. However, the interviewer in partaking inevitably adds something to the situation which derives from himself. This must be closely watched and simultaneously analysed, for while any inference based upon the interviewer's feelings about the patient and his problem may be of great value in directing the interview towards a profitable outcome, it can also distort material and lead to false conclusions. Where then, in the interviewer's mind, some inference occurs, this must be regarded not as a fact but as a hypothesis which needs to be tested to ascertain whether it is correct or should be modified. This process spills over from one part of the interview to another and from one interview to the next.

The interviewer's task is therefore not only to listen to the patient and observe his behaviour but also to examine what he himself says and does. Thus in any interview there are at least two persons to be heard and two to be observed, both as individuals and in terms of their interaction.

No patient can be expected under the most elementary circumstances, to give without help all the information required, simply because he is not aware of all that the psychiatrist needs to know. He must therefore be taught as the interview progresses how he can best help in the discovery of the basic nature of his problem. This strikes at the very core of psychiatric interviewing; considerable skill being required to guide the patient along profitable lines without, at the same time, being so directive as to distort the meaning of what he says. Herein lies the fault of leading questions. Leading questions suggest answers which are not necessarily in accord with the facts or may lead to undue simplification which does not do the facts justice. Further distortion may occur as a result of the patient wishing to please the interviewer by giving answers which, consciously or not, he believes the interviewer may wish to hear.

Despite this, leading questions need not be avoided altogether. They are, however, generally best used only after an interview has been in progress for some time and then mainly to clarify matters left open or unsettled. They may be of value in ruling out quickly certain negative possibilities or matters which, if discussed at length, could turn out to be time wasting and irrelevant. Leading questions may also be used to test inferences already made and in this way come very near to being interpretations which offer the patient a chance of acceptance or rejection as the case may be.

One other disadvantage of leading questions is that they tend to evoke conventional answers. Thus if a doctor asks a patient: '*Are you happily married?*' the answer is likely to be in the affirmative. Few people who are unhappily married care to admit this to a relative stranger, be he a doctor or anyone else, early in the procedings. Rephrasing the question in the form of an invitation: '*Tell me about your marriage*' is more likely to produce relevant information for if the patient starts to gloss over the facts, he may become sufficiently uneasy to blurt out at least some of the truth. In any event conventional answers are always suspect; for, as Sullivan said, the more conventional a person's statements are, the more doubtful is it that they give you any idea of what he really means.

This points to the need for a positive consideration of the kinds of questions an interviewer should ask. Ideally before he asks any question whatsoever he should be absolutely clear why he does so. Similarly, when the answer comes, he should ask himself whether what he has heard has an unequivocal meaning or whether the answer given could mean something different from what is immediately apparent. It is surprising how often people say exactly the opposite of what they mean but without deliberately lying. If there is doubt in the interviewer's mind as to the exact meaning of what he has heard, he will need to resort to further interrogation to obtain clarification. In this way a psychiatric interview tends to be punctuated by episodes of questioning in order that the interviewer may become as sure as possible that he really does understand what he is told. This has the secondary effect of helping the patient by enabling him to formulate more clearly what is in his own mind. By having to put his troubles as clearly as possible into words he may start, often for the very first time, to find out how he really feels about the various problems which beset him. This 'to and fro' between doctor and patient is familiar as a feedback process made all the more necessary where difficulties in communication exist.

Interviewing the patient

Setting the scene

A psychiatric interview falls into several parts. The first should be directed at putting the patient at ease and should never be neglected or hurried. Indeed the beginning of an interview may govern the whole of its subsequent success. It needs some experience to strike a satisfactory blend between formality and informality. The interviewer also needs to feel confident in his role; if he is insecure or lacks confidence, he may react by becoming unduly pompous or formal. This may put off the patient who has, like everyone else, been exposed to pomposity on other occasions. An unduly formal attitude may lead the patient to feel that the psychiatrist is unlikely to be sympathetic to his difficulties, as a result of which he may find himself unable to be forthcoming. At the opposite pole, if the interviewer assumes an air of undue informality, he runs the risk of appearing casual or disinterested. Just as a patient usually comes for consultation with a preconceived notion that he is likely to obtain help, so may this preconception be damaged if the psychiatrist's attitude and behaviour do not coincide closely enough with the image the patient may have conceived of him before they met. It should also not be forgotten that although a psychiatric interview usually has a purpose which is implicit in the mind of patient and doctor, it is still initially a meeting between two strangers and carries with it the tendency which colours all such meetings to 'fence for position', a process whereby those involved endeavour to identify one another. By the same token *transference*, which, in essence, means that the feelings of both patient and psychiatrist for one another may be coloured by feelings derived from earlier relationships with others, is a phenomenon which may be present right from the start of an interview and may modify or, if negative, interfere with the establishment of a satisfactory doctor–patient relationship.

Apart from the obvious assumption of an air of sympathetic interest, getting an interview off to a good start may be enhanced by several kinds of manoeuvre. Where the psychiatrist has some foreknowledge of the patient's problem, such as may have been gleaned from a referral letter, to refer to this may be a useful opening gambit. It may also provide an opportunity for amendment right at the beginning of any data which may have become distorted in its passage towards the psychiatrist. In difficult cases it may be permissible, providing that there is at least some information to hand, for the interviewer to suggest to the patient that he knows more about the problem than he really does. This, however, should only be done with great caution. If, as sometimes happens, prior information is completely lacking and the patient fails to respond to an open invitation to proceed, the interviewer may have to fall back upon a more general gambit which, in effect, may consist of a tentative interpretation of the reasons for such hesitation. Here sound intuition may be required. It may not merely be that the patient is embarrassed by the prospect of having to give an account of himself, but he may, in fact, be much more unwilling to be interviewed than is at first apparent. There are several reasons for this which need to be borne in mind.

In the case of some psychotic patients, complete lack of insight may lead them to believe that there is nothing wrong at all. Alternatively those who are suspicious and deluded may suspect a trap. Some patients who present at interview only at the instigation of their relatives or as a result of pressure by some other person may transfer their resentment at this circumstance on to the psychiatrist. This is quite common among disturbed adolescents who may be among the most difficult of all patients with whom to make a satisfactory rapport initially. Again, the patient who believes his symptoms are due to some physical cause may resent having been referred to a psychiatrist either because he feels it to be a futile waste of time or because he infers from the referral that others think his symptoms are merely imaginary. This situation can be made worse if the referring doctor omits to tell the patient that it is a psychiatrist to whom he has been referred, using perhaps the euphemism 'nerve specialist' or something seemingly even more innocuous. By the time the patient arrives in the psychiatrist's consulting room he may have little doubt whom he is to see and, feeling he has been deceived, is likely to project his indignation upon the luckless psychiatrist.

There are many other possibilities and probably no specific ways of dealing with any or all of them. However, as a general rule, as soon as the psychiatrist becomes aware of some trouble of this kind—the sooner the better—he should bring the matter into open discussion. To a hostile patient, it is often wise to say '*I can see that you are unhappy*' or '*Perhaps you are wondering why you were asked to see a psychiatrist? Many people do.*' The phrase 'many people do' is an example of generalization, a very useful tactic for reducing anxiety by making the patient feel that he is not so very abnormal in feeling the way he does; that others share his feelings, and so on. It is also sometimes important to give the patient some idea of what a psychiatrist is and does. Even today many people have fantasies about psychiatrists ranging in nature from regarding them at one end of the scale as quacks, to suspecting, at the other, that they have quite remarkable, if not actually supernatural, powers. It is wise for the psychiatrist to identify himself in the patient's eyes as a doctor concerned with both physical and psychological ailments but perhaps having some special experience in the evaluation of the latter. If the patient is convinced that his symptoms are purely physical and that mind plays no part in them whatsoever, then the psychiatrist should indicate that he respects this view while perhaps providing an illustration of just how psychological experiences can produce physical symptoms, stressing at the same time that such symptoms are by no means inaginary. The common example of just missing being run over and reaching the opposite pavement breathless, palpitating and with a host of other disagreeable physical symptoms with which all are familiar but which are obviously the outcome of sudden acute anxiety, may be useful.

It not uncommonly turns out that the patient resents the psychiatrist either because he feels ashamed at being unable to control his emotions or because he equates being sent to a psychiatrist with the possibility which exists either in his own mind or he believes exists in the minds of others that he is going insane and may be committed or something of that kind. This too may need an airing, for until it has been aired, no reassurance is possible.

The presenting complaint

Assuming that the preliminaries have passed off successfully, the interviewer may invite the patient to proceed by asking a question, such as: '*What can I do for you?*' or, if the interviewer has already shown that he knows something of the problem: '*I wonder if you would care to tell me more about it*'. In psychiatry this kind of question is much more appropriate than the old-fashioned and stilted: '*Of what are you complaining?*' which almost seems to reduce the status of the patient to that of supplicant.

Presenting complaints do not always provide an immediate clue to their basis, nor do they necessarily bear directly upon the patient's real problem. Often the presenting complaint is merely a *ticket of admission* which serves the purpose of bringing patient and doctor together. This, perhaps, is often truer of the first contact between a patient and his family doctor, where clarification of the presenting problem may lead to its being recognized as psychiatric, so that psychiatric referral then follows. However, the psychiatrist may also be confronted with problems which present once or even twice removed from their real nature.

A complaint of headache is a good example of a common symptom having many different causes. While occasionally the cause is some local lesion, in the majority of cases its origin is more obscure. If the cause is not organic it may be an expression of a difficulty in living. In short, although the patient comes to the doctor complaining of headaches and demanding relief, careful elucidation of the facts may indicate that the real trouble is that he does not get on with his mother or wife, or perhaps dislikes his job or has been passed over for promotion. A difficulty arises here in as much as the patient who has a headache as an accompaniment, for instance, to an attack of fever is not at all surprised. The patient, however, who has a headache because he does not get on with his wife, may not only not perceive the link between these events but may be positively unwilling to do so. If this is so his complaint may be said to be *ego-defensive*, in that although it causes him discomfort it nonetheless protects him from the anxiety which might otherwise be evoked by having to face up to his real difficulties. Many emotional and psychosomatic symptoms come into this category. They require considerable elucidation and, even when their ego-defensive nature is perceived, it is probably unwise for the therapist, except under exceptional circumstances, to attack them directly. Indeed it is because such symptoms are so often defensive that it is imperative that no attempt should be made to demolish them until the psychiatrist is confident that he can give the patient something better to put in their place.

Detailed inquiry

Sullivan defined detailed inquiry as that part of the psychiatric interview which is given over to clarifying and improving early approximations of understanding. Once started, many patients are able to give a fairly comprehensive account of their symptoms and sometimes also of underlying or related difficulties. Then, after a time, they come to a halt. At this juncture the psychiatrist may need to indulge in a short period of questioning in order to elicit further details. However, before doing so more information may often be obtained by prompting alone. This may vary from making non-verbal sounds to indicate attention and interest or uttering short phrases such as '*I see*' or '*I understand*' to more active encouragement such as repeating the patient's last few words, possibly with a slight upward inflection, or saying: '*Please go on*', or: '*Could you tell me more about that.*' Those patients who say relatively little may need active encouragement; those who are garrulous or whose discourse wanders may call for more active intervention—both in order to save time and to prevent both psychiatrist and patient from becoming lost. Much of the skill in interviewing lies in the psychiatrist's ability to manipulate the level of the patient's anxiety, keeping this sufficiently high to lend impetus to the proceedings but not letting matters get so far out of hand that a block occurs. Anxiety may be raised by being provocative, looking as if surprised, and by staring directly at the patient. In contrast it may be lowered by making sympathetic noises or general statements, such as: '*I think a lot of people feel that way*', or: '*I can appreciate how you must have felt*', and sometimes by looking away from the patient.

When the patient has concluded his initial account it is usually wise to ask whether there are any other matters troubling him which he has not recounted. This occasionally pays surprising dividends.

It is also useful at this stage to carry out a brief review, asking about the presence or absence of certain symptoms which the patient may not have mentioned. Apart from headaches, indigestion, bowel habits and other somatic symptoms, a detailed inquiry about sleep should be made. In women the menstrual pattern should also be investigated although it may be preferable to leave this until the time comes to investigate the patient's sexual habits.

Family history

Following a preliminary elucidation of what seems to be the presenting problem the interviewer should turn to the investigation of background factors. This usually starts with the family history.

From a factual point of view family histories are often highly unreliable. However, it may not be the facts which are the most important, with the obvious exception of genetically determined disorders, but feelings—how the patient feels about members of his family and his relationship with them. Many find questions about their families difficult to answer. Asked '*What sort of man was your father?*' they may, for example, reply: 'Do you mean how tall was he?' or mention some other physical characteristic. Even when the question is put in such a way as to promote discussion of interpersonal relationships within the family circle, it may be difficult initially to obtain a satisfactory account. Whereas a patient may willingly give an account of his mother's or father's age, state of health or occupation, it may prove much more difficult for him to describe his relationship with them. This is frequently due to conflicts over loyalty which arise as soon as he starts to discuss the matter.

If he overstresses their faults he may feel he is letting them down. This may lead him to do the opposite. If, on the other hand, he expresses antagonism to them he may, at the same time, feel unsure where the fault really lies—with him or them. After all, he may think, they reared him; they brought him up; surely he owes them something? There are also those who would deny reality and who paint a wish-fulfilling picture of home and parents in such idyllic terms that the interviewer's suspicions cannot fail to be aroused. Others may be wary of confessing how they really feel because they fear that their confidence may be broken and that the psychiatrist may convey their private feelings to parents, spouse or whoever is the significant person under discussion.

On becoming aware of such difficulties the psychiatrist should immediately bring the matter up, saying: *'I can see you may be a bit worried about telling me this'*, or: *'Perhaps you feel you oughtn't to talk this way.'* At the same time an assurance may be given that all such information will be fully safeguarded. Sometimes a patient may request such an assurance before proceeding further. To this the psychiatrist may reply: *'What goes on here is entirely between ourselves. We both know you have these feelings, but it is important for you to be able to tell me about them.'*

In passing, the interviewer should be aware that any description by a patient of his relatives or friends, given to a third party, will be distorted by how the patient feels about the person of whom he is talking. Sullivan called this *parataxic distortion*. This mechanism explains the surprise often felt when the person under discussion is later encountered for the first time and found to differ not inconsiderably from the image of him built up in the interviewer's mind during the patient's initial description.

In addition to the patient's feelings about his family, the main facts which need to be known are age, state of health and, if relevant, cause of death of parents; number of siblings and their state of mental and physical health together with their rank order of birth. Inquiry about the mental health of more distant relatives more often tends to draw a blank than to be useful. It should, however, never be neglected although if the results are negative, this cannot be taken at face value. The concealment of 'skeletons in the cupboard' even among members of a single family can be astounding!

Personal history

The personal history should consist of a summarized biography of the patient's life from birth onwards. Usually little information of value about the first five years can be gleaned at first hand, apart from the odd *screen memory* which usually consists of a static visual impression of an episode or two which the patient believes he can remember. Such early memories tend, however, to be elaborated; it is difficult to distinguish what a subject has been told from what he believes was a first-hand experience. A history of the earliest years of a patient's life must, therefore, if it is to be at all reliable, be gleaned from parents or someone who knew the patient well at the time. Certain information relating to the circumstances of the patient's birth, his early development and so-called milestones, may be of great importance in the investigation of mentally handicapped or brain-damaged patients. In those with personality disorders a history of separation in infancy from one or both parents should be sought.

Most persons are better able to recall much more of their lives after the age of five, although some still appear to be almost totally amnesic until adolescence. In such cases it may often be correctly inferred that childhood was so unhappy a time as to be best forgotten. However, even when earlier years are remembered, feelings are, once again, often more important than facts. Thus it may matter little where a patient went to school or even, within limits, how well or badly he did. What matters more is whether he enjoyed it, how he got on with his schoolmates, whether he was away much of the time and if so, why; was he popular or not, a leader or a follower; was his life made a misery by teasing or bullying, was he given a nickname and if so, what was it? So it is throughout childhood; while achievement or failure to achieve is not necessarily in itself insignificant, it is the feelings which surround them which may be more important still, not only the subject's own feelings but the feelings of those close to him.

In adult life some account should be taken of later educational attainments and occupational history. Once again, what is important is how the patient feels about his progress. If his record of attainment is only modest, is he relatively content that it should be so or bitter and frustrated? If the latter, does he blame himself, lack of opportunity or does he blame others?

A detailed and chronological account of the patient's previous physical and mental health, accidents, operations, births, miscarriages, hospital admissions, and other such possibly relevant events should also be included. The nature of previous treatments should be discovered; who carried them out and where? Such information should, in due course, be checked by the inspection of letters, specialists' reports and case-notes obtained from other hospitals where the patient may have been treated.

Sex and marriage

If the interview is proceeding smoothly and the rapport between interviewer and patient seems to be sound, attention may be turned to the patient's sexual history. If, for some reason, there are signs that he is unwilling to discuss this, the matter may be deferred until he shows himself readier to do so. Alternatively the psychiatrist may prefer to indicate to the patient that he appreciates the discussion of such highly personal matters may be a source of embarrassment, inquiring at the same time why this is so. Usually if the psychiatrist can talk calmly on the importance of a discussion about sex and without himself showing any embarrassment, the patient's cooperation will be obtained. Once again generalizations may help, for example, *'I often find that this is something which people find it difficult to talk about'*—thus making the patient feel he is not so very peculiar or in some way an odd man out.

What the interviewer needs to know first of all is how the patient came to learn about sexual matters and from whom. Did his parents tell him or did he pick up information at school? In the case of women, inquiry should be made as to the date of the menarche and whether they were adequately prepared for this event. Was sex talked about at home or was the subject tabooed? When did the patient start to masturbate? How often? Were there any accompanying fantasies? If so, what were they? Was much guilt attached to masturbation and if so did the patient try to overcome it? How? Such questions should not, however, be put peremptorily but slipped in one after another in a reasonably subtle but encouraging manner. It is very important whatever the interviewer may feel about the patient's behaviour, sexual or otherwise, that he should not allow moral issues to colour any comments he may feel obliged to make.

A history of seduction in childhood may be important and should be sought; also of sex play between children and adolescents, such as mutual masturbation. Were there any episodes of homosexual behaviour? In adult life and later adolescence, account should be taken of both heterosexual and homosexual relationships and their outcome.

The marital history must include not only sexual details but an account of the overall relationship between husband and wife. Once again conflicts over loyalty sometimes interfere with obtaining a clear picture. If the doctor becomes aware at the outset that he is about to be confronted with what is primarily a marital problem, he may do well to interview both partners together. As such joint interviews are potentially explosive they may call for the utmost skill in handling, although such skill may be amply repaid. Joint marital interviewing is not, however, for beginners.

An account of marital sex life calls first for an inquiry into the degree of sexual sophistication which both partners brought with them into the marital situation. Were either or both virgins at the time of marriage? Did premarital intercourse occur and if so with whom? Since marriage, how frequently does sexual intercourse take place? When and where does it usually occur? Are the attending circumstances satisfactory? What methods of contraception, if any, are preferred? Does the wife fear pregnancy? Do both partners obtain satisfaction? Is there any evidence of any unusual sexual behaviour?

A word of warning is called for. Many women and some men will maintain that their sex lives are satisfactory when further investigation reveals that this is clearly not so. There are two reasons for this. The first is that those who have unsatisfactory sex lives may find this difficult to admit, for to do so makes them feel inferior or inadequate. The second—and this applies to women especially—is that they may not be too sure what is to be expected from sex. It is not infrequent, therefore, to find that a woman who says that her sex life is satisfactory has in fact never actually experienced orgasm so that the word has no real meaning for her. Unless questions about this are sufficiently pressed the whole truth may never come to light.

Obviously, it is important to inquire about children. If there are none, why not? Is this by choice or accidental? How many children are there? How old? What sex? Were they all planned and wanted? What is their relationship to either parent and to each other? What is their state of health? Have there been difficulties in rearing? Do the parents agree on matters of child handling or discipline? Are any or all of the children a focus of parental conflict? It should be understood of course that questions about these matters should not be posed so directly as they are put here, where they are intended as a check-list.

Personality assessment

During the interview the interviewer, in addition to listening and trying to understand what he is being told, will also be continuously engaged in assessing the patient's personality and the way in which this may colour his condition. He should ask himself: 'What manner of person is this who confronts me?' In trying to answer this question the interviewer relies upon his experience and judgement, comparing the patient he is interviewing with others he has seen. In doing so he must have regard to the fact that some impressions of the patient's personality will be coloured by feelings derived from the interviewer's past relationships with various significant figures in his own life situation, of whom he may be unconsciously reminded by some aspect of the patient's personality (*counter transference*). This should lead him to examine any seemingly prejudicial attitudes he feels towards the patient with a view to negating these and making his assessment of the patient's personality as objective as he can.

A definite change in personality brought about by illness, unless extremely gross and obvious, can rarely be satisfactorily assessed without resort to an account given by someone who knew the patient both before and after the event. Even when there has been no definite change in personality, few are able to give an adequate account of their own character or temperament. Despite this, such a question as '*How would your best friend describe you?*' may occasionally be useful. Alternatively questions such as: '*Are you easily moved to anger?*' '*Are you unduly sensitive to criticism?*' may throw some light on personality traits. Also useful is some discussion of attitudes to current affairs, politics, religion or moral issues, but always with regard to the proviso that if the interviewer finds himself in disagreement (or undue agreement) with such views as may be expressed, he does not allow this to colour his own feelings towards the patient.

The obtaining of further information depends on a wide variety of individual circumstances. It is, however, often necessary to compromise at that point where sufficient background information is available to allow the interviewer to relate what is relevant to the patient's presenting problem. This process consists in essence of an interpretation of the patient's symptoms and difficulties in terms of what is known of his life situation. Even then, and in order that an adequate diagnostic formulation can be undertaken, it may still be necessary, especially in patients with psychotic or organically determined mental illness, to carry out a more formal examination of the current mental state. This is dealt with in Chapter 4.

Interviewing relatives

After interviewing the patient and sometimes, depending on the nature of the problem, even before doing so, it is nearly always necessary to interview one or more of his closer relatives. Apart from any relevant information they may be able to give, their concern for the patient may need attention. Likewise their cooperation in treatment will often be required.

Interviewing relatives is of particular importance in gaining information about background factors and those appertaining to the patient's earlier years. Where children and adolescents are concerned matters can hardly progress without an independent account of the patient's problems. Likewise, in the case of those who are grossly psychotic, confused, demented or for some reason unable or unwilling to cooperate, the psychiatrist may have to rely heavily on such information as can be obtained from secondary sources. In the case of in-patients, information derived from observations made by nursing staff is obviously important.

When interviewing relatives it must be borne in mind that their account of the patient can sometimes be grossly distorted owing to their own prejudices or abnormal attitudes towards the patient and his illness, sometimes to the point where the psychiatrist may begin to wonder who really is the patient! Occasionally a relative may share the same delusions as the patient (*folie à deux*). Relatives may also minimize or exaggerate the patient's complaints to a degree which can try patience and judgement to the utmost. They may also offer advice as to how and where the patient should be treated; on some occasions they may urge the psychiatrist to adopt a punitive attitude by requesting that the patient should be told firmly to 'snap out of it', or commanded to 'pull himself together'!

The patient being all too aware of such attitudes—indeed he will already have been well and truly exposed to them—may, for his part, be uneasy at the possibility that confidential matters he may have revealed during interview will be passed on by the psychiatrist, however unwittingly. On this account he may jib at the prospect of his relatives being seen at all. The psychiatrist on learning about this should seize the opportunity to reassure the patient by indicating that he is aware of the hazards inherent in the situation and by suggesting that he is well able to deal with any confidential issues which may arise.

As in the case of marital problems, where it may be wise to see husband and wife together, so may the same be true of certain family problems where, with the agreement of all concerned, several family members may be interviewed simultaneously. Some preliminary contact with whoever it is who appears to be the focal point of the family disturbance is, however, likely to be necessary.

Occasionally information needs to be obtained from those who are not relatives of the patient. These may include friends, probation officers, other social workers, schoolteachers, employers and so on. Usually such contacts do not give rise to difficulties providing the patient understands their purpose and is able to express his agreement. If, however, he is psychotic or out of touch and unable to do so, the psychiatrist may have to proceed nonetheless, having first assured himself that what may appear to be at least a technical breach of confidentiality, is likely to be in the patient's best interests.

Further reading

Sullivan, H. S. (1955) *The Psychiatric Interview*. London: Tavistock.

4

Examination of the Mental State

The examination of a psychiatric patient's mental state can be regarded as analogous to the physical examination of a patient suffering from a medical or surgical disorder. Although in any particular case, one may produce diagnostic information of greater relevance than the other, there are many instances in which any such assessment will necessarily be incomplete unless both the subject's mental and physical states are examined on the same occasion.

In medical training, high value is given to skill in eliciting and interpreting physical signs. In recent years, however, the value of this has become somewhat eroded, although not altogether displaced, by a growing number of laboratory and other investigations which reflect the complexity of modern medicine and changes in the patterns of disease. The same cannot yet be said of psychiatry. Mental examination together with skill in interviewing still remain the psychiatrist's principal stock in trade for, apart from certain organic disorders having a more or less direct effect on brain function, laboratory investigations have relatively little to offer as diagnostic aids. Furthermore, and despite early promises, psychological test procedures seem still to have little more to offer.

Assessment of current mental state

Interpretations of behaviour

Behaviour and facial expressions are of great importance and can convey valuable diagnostic information. Posture, gesture, general demeanour—even a handshake—may provide valuable clues to the subject's underlying personality and current state of mind.

Activity
Slow movements, relative immobility, poverty of gesture and facial expression, downcast eyes and infrequent blinking, may be indicative of *psychomotor retardation*. In contrast, rocking to and fro, wringing of the hands and knitting of fingers, restlessness and a tense and fearful appearance are all suggestive of acute *agitation*. Overactivity and

inability to sit still, accompanied by an untoward air of elation or irritability together with over-talkativeness, are the hallmarks of *hypomania*. Queer postures, bizarre grimaces, odd repetitive manner-isms and other stereotyped behaviour point to a diagnosis of *schizophrenia*. Fatuity, obvious disarray, lack of attention to personal hygiene and general appearance, fly-buttons undone, spilt food on clothing and general self-neglect are indicative of *dementia*. A patient who restlessly paces the waiting room or whose feet, when seated, continually tread the floor is likely to be suffering from the extrapyra-midal side-effects of neuroleptic drugs (*tasikinesia* or *akathisia*). Likewise, constant chewing movements are a sign of *tardive dyskinesia*. While all these for the most part are fairly obvious signs, there is much also to be learned from observing more minor alterations in activity and general behaviour.

Eye-gaze or its avoidance may be important, particularly where a half as against the whole truth is about to be told. A woman who, while recounting her woes, constantly twiddles her wedding ring may well turn out to have marital problems. Paranoid patients often exhibit a certain characteristic stiffness of manner which, while indicating a need to impress their delusional beliefs on others, reveals at the same time their basic lack of belief in themselves. The catalogue of such minor behavioural signs is extensive and an enthusiast could well spend a lifetime studying it.

Consciousness

Impairment or clouding of consciousness is the central feature of all delirious and confusional states. Determining the level of consciousness is, therefore, important, although rapid fluctuations can make this a difficult task. Observe whether the subject is fully alert, dulled or more or less inaccessible. How aware is he of his surroundings? Does he know where he is, when it is and why he is where he is? How does his current state of awareness govern his response to relatively straightforward questions?

Speech

Like other behaviour, speech may be retarded or accelerated, varying from virtual silence in stupor to incoherence in excitement. In manic patients: *volubility*, *distractability* and *flight of ideas* may be evident, sometimes with rhyming or punning (*clang associations*). In depression: replies may be slow in coming and, when they do come, limited to a few words. Thus speech may be *laconic*, and with little or no elaborations of such answers as may be given. In schizophrenia: *blocking, derailment of thought* and *bizarre associations, circumstantiality, general woolliness* and *neologisms*, which in severe cases may lead to such incoherence as to justify the term *word salad*, may be evident. In those with organic dementia, difficulty in articulation may give rise to *dysarthria*, a phenomenon also seen in some forms of chronic drug intoxication, notably with barbiturates. Various types of *aphasia* may also be encountered together with *stammering*, *lalling* (babyish articulation), *logoclonus* (perseverative repetition of the last syllable of a word or of a sentence) etc.

The affective state

In assessing a patient's affective state, direct inquiry is likely to be needed. Thus it may be necessary to ask him how he feels in himself; whether, if he is aware of being ill, he believes he will recover; or whether he feels the outlook is hopeless; whether he has *morbid thoughts* of dying and in particular if he is contemplating suicide. In contrast, if he appears elated, he may be asked if he feels that nothing at all is wrong, at least with himself! Or, does he confess only to feelings of apathy and indifference? It should also be determined, either from him or from his relatives, whether his presenting mood is constant, variable or labile, or whether if seemingly stable it has recently undergone a noticeable change. It should also be observed whether what he says about his affective state is consistent with his behaviour or whether seemingly incongruous.

Obsession or delusion?

Sooner or later certain dominant preoccupations are likely to emerge. If a subject feels under some kind of contraint and must check and recheck his actions or if useless thoughts distract him in a repetitive fashion, it is likely that he is suffering from obsessions. The clue here is that while he recognizes his thoughts and ideas are useless and unwanted and would like to be rid of them, he nonetheless still accepts them as his own. Thus he never believes that the ideas which so greatly trouble him have been planted in his mind by some outside agency as others, who are truly deluded, may do.

While obsessionalism is characterized by doubt, the hallmark of delusions is certainty. Thus, however grotesque a delusional notion may seem, to the sufferer there can be no doubt whatsoever of its truth. This is why a delusion will be found to be unshakeable even in the face of completely logical and contrary argument. Many patients with delusions dissemble and although holding to their beliefs with complete constancy may not admit their presence. Thus the elucidation of delusions often requires tact and subtlety and a guarded and oblique approach.

Ideas of reference may often be elicited by asking a patient how *sensitive* he is to the attitudes and remarks of others. Pressed, he may admit to being the subject of gossip among neighbours or workmates. He is aware, when he approaches, that others look significantly towards him or away or at one another: when they sniff or cough or make some gesture or a guarded half-heard remark, he is convinced that this has some meaning in regard to himself. He believes perhaps that there are allusions made to him or to things he has done in the newspapers, radio or television. He attributes some of his queer psychic and bodily sensations to outside influences. He feels as if in a trance, under a hypnotic spell, under the influence of electrical or radio waves, telepathy or drugs (*passivity experiences*). While the variation is endless, the theme is constant.

In depressive illnesses, especially those of later life, delusional ideas of cancer or of bowels blocked or turned to stone are not uncommon (*nihilistic delusions*). The patient may believe he is wasting or rotting away or even that he is actually dead (*Cotard's syndrome*). Such *hypochondriacal delusions* are especially bizarre in schizophrenia. Thus a delusional belief of change in sex is by no means rare. Hypochondriacal delusions apart, depressed patients may also entertain delusions of blame, guilt and self-reproach. Delusions of poverty are common. Elated manic or schizophrenic patients may believe they are endowed with Messianic powers or are of royal blood. Those with latent perverted sexual tendencies may begin to feel that others accuse them unjustifiably or look upon them askance. Spinsters sometimes believe that some eminent person is in love with them and believe themselves persecuted on this account (*erotomania*).

Perceptual disorders

Illusions are misperceptions which originate in external sensory stimuli. While a normal person under an illusion makes further investigations until the matter is clarified, in morbid mental states an illusory experience may, in contrast, be accepted as reality. Thus a severely depressed patient hearing the squeal of tyres of a car cornering too fast may accept unquestioningly that the noise he hears is the screaming of his loved ones being tortured. Here mood is the determining factor. In other cases impairment of consciousness is the prime mover. Thus illusions are a common feature of delirious states.

Hallucinations are perceptions which occur in the absence of any external stimulus. They occur in normal people only in the half-sleeping (*hypnagogic*) or half-waking (*hypnopompic*) state. As the experience of these hallucinations usually leads to an immediate return to full consciousness, insight into their subjective nature is the rule. Hearing one's name called out, a rap on the door or a ring of the bell are among the most common.

As with delusions, asking about hallucinations may call for an oblique approach. Even overtly psychotic patients sometimes seem to realize that hallucinations may indicate 'insanity' and will not admit to them. Thus the question: 'Do you hear voices?' may provoke a negative response, although, curiously enough, when it seems certain to the examiner from the patient's manner and attitude that he is experiencing auditory hallucinations, the direct question: 'What are the voices saying?' may produce an affirmative answer. Alternatively, questioning the patient as to whether he has had or is having any seemingly supernatural or other experiences for which he cannot account may produce valuable information. Having established the presence of hallucinations, then their content should be investigated. Whose voices are they and what do they say? Do they talk to the patient directly or refer to him in the third person? Do they talk directly to the patient or about him? Is what they say complimentary, malicious or, perhaps, obscene?

The same applies to hallucinations in other sense modalities. Has the subject any peculiar bodily sensations, tingling, feelings of cold or warmth, sensations of movement not under voluntary control; queer aches, pains or other sensations occurring without good reason? A feeling of insects crawling over the skin (*formication*) may occur in delirium and other organic brain states. Visions, almost exclusively *pseudohallucinations*, of the dead are not uncommon in recently bereaved persons. Otherwise, visual hallucinations are usually indicative of organic states and only occasionally occur in schizophrenia in its earlier and acuter stages.

It is important to inquire into the mode of development and occurrence of hallucinatory experiences. Do they occur only at night or by day also? Do they occur in a setting of clear consciousness or is there evidence of clouding? Are they fostered by other unconnected sensory stimuli such as a clock ticking, a dripping tap or the noise of an aeroplane flying overhead (*functional hallucinations*)? What is their effect upon the patient's general emotional state? Do they make him depressed or irritated or does he regard them with indifference? What is his own explanation of their occurrence?

Examination of the sensorium

If, following a fairly lengthy psychiatric interview, it is obvious to the examiner that the sensorium is intact, this part of the examination may be omitted or carried out in outline only. Nonetheless, failure to pursue the matter further may sometimes lead to what can be embarrassing surprises. Thus if there is any hint of disturbance of orientation, memory or other intellectual functions, these should be systematically examined. The following scheme has, subject to some variations, been found to work well in practice. It must be emphasized, however, that it is an unstandardized procedure and liable, therefore, to subjective judgement.

Orientation

'*What day is it today?*' '*Please give me the date in full.*' The subject should be able to give the day, month and year correctly. If he is two or three days out, this is not necessarily abnormal. Allowance must be made for those who have been in hospital for some time, during which one day becomes much like the next.

'*What is this place we are in?*' Fairly full details should be asked for. If the reply suggests any element of doubt, details of where the place of examination actually is in relation to the patient's normal dwelling should be requested.

Only very severely demented patients are, as a rule, truly disorientated in person, although it may sometimes appear that the subject is deluded into believing that he is not who he is known to be. Thus he may insist he is God or some other exalted person. This is not true disorientation of person but *double orientation*.

The accuracy of a patient's knowledge of himself can be further elicited by questioning him about his name, age, address and present circumstances. Apart from himself, he may well be found to be disorientated about those around him. Ask him, therefore: '*Who am I?*', '*Have we met before?*', '*Who are these other people (nurses, etc.)?*'

Memory

Memory involves registration, retention and recall, all of which should be tested. *Ziehen's test* is a sensitive indicator of registration or of retentive memory and easily applied. Ask: '*What is 8 and 7 added together?*'. Note the reply. Then ask the subject to carry out another task, usually to repeat after the examiner two sets of five given digits (e.g. 2–9–4–1–8; 3–7–1–6–5). Then ask: '*What was the little sum I gave you just now?*'. Even hesitation may be significant.

It is then usual to establish digit span. This is done by asking the patient to repeat five digits forwards after the examiner. If he does this correctly, proffer six and then seven. If he fails at any point or makes errors, repeat a different series of the same number of digits. If he fails again, one less is taken to be the digit span limit. If he succeeds on the second occasion, increase the number given by one more. A normal person of average intelligence should be able to reproduce seven digits in the same order as given with relative ease. Following this, the reverse digit span should be tested in much the same way. An illustration saves time. Say: '*For example: If I say 4–2–7, I want you to say 7–2–4*'. Start with three digits, then according to the patient's response, progress to four and then to five if he is able to cope with previous stages of the test. A normal person of average intelligence should be able to repeat at least five digits correctly in reverse order.

A useful test for longer term retention and recall is to give a fairly simple name and address and then ask the subject to repeat it after an interval of not greater than three to four minutes, during which some other mental task is undertaken. Having given the name and address, ask the patient to repeat it immediately so as to be sure he has grasped it correctly. Tell him he will be asked to recall it in a short while, then proceed to the secondary task.

Attention and concentration

Attention and concentration can be tested by the serial-sevens test, which may usefully be given after the name-and-address and before its recall. Tell the patient: *'I want you to take 7 from 100'*. Then, whatever his reply (93 or some other number) say: *'Will you please continue taking 7 away until you get right down to nought?'*. Note the number of mistakes and the time taken. A normal person should be allowed up to two minutes and up to two mistakes. This test, although difficult to accomplish if any degree of dementia is present, is most valuable when it reveals a tendency to perseverate. Thus some patients make repetitive mistakes, for example 93–88–83–78–73–68, and so on. If the test proves too difficult, ask him to name the months of the year in reverse order and, if incorrectly done, forwards also. The same may be done with the days of the week.

Another useful test is to tell the patient a short story or fable and then ask him to repeat it back and give its meaning. (The story of 'The Donkey with the Load of Salt' is a once much used example of such a test, now seemingly gone out of fashion.)

Nominal aphasia

Nominal aphasia, which is sometimes present in early cases of dementia, is often worth testing for. Correct testing may demonstrate that a subject, while knowing the nature and purpose of a common object, cannot give it its proper name. Thus an ashtray may be said to be 'A what you put your cigarette in.' The second feature of nominal aphasia is that if the patient is then given a number of choices including the correct name of the object, he almost invariably picks the correct one in preference to the others. Nominal aphasia is best demonstrated by asking the patient the names of the parts of an object. Thus, in showing a wristwatch the subject should be asked to name the dial, hands, winder, watchstrap, buckle, and so on.

In some patients with organic brain diseases, aphasia of other types may be present, also apraxia, dyslexia, acalculia, disorders of the body image, etc. These, although of interest, cannot be fully dealt with here. Appropriate neurological texts should be consulted for further details.

Mental arithmetic

Apart from the serial-sevens test, which some patients find impossible, more minor discrepancies in performance may be demonstrated by giving simple mental arithmetic tests. The identification and adding up of a small but random collection of coins is useful, following which the patient may be asked how much would be left if he had spent such-and-such an amount. Simple addition, subtraction, multiplication and division tests may be given, for example 14+17; 23−8; 4×13; how many 9s in 81, and so on. Subtraction is harder than addition; division harder than multiplication.

In all these tests and in the others already described, care should be taken not to press the brain-impaired patient too hard. If so, this may result in a *catastrophic reaction*, which may take the form of sudden emotional collapse by the patient with tears, distress, anger and refusal to cooperate further in the testing process.

General knowledge

Questions about current affairs are useful, such as those which have featured prominently in the newspapers during the last few days. Such questions also test retentive memory and, to a lesser degree, recall. Other questions may include the names of the head of state, leading government figures and their predecessors. Ask the patient to name six cities in England or elsewhere. Can he give the capitals of five or six or so of the world's major countries?

Tests for abstract thought

Abstract thought may be tested by asking the patient the difference between objects which have common properties which should be implied in his answer, for example a wall and a fence; a child and a dwarf; a king and a president. The answer to the *'child and a dwarf'* question that *'One will grow and the other won't'* is acceptable as this implies that while both are small in size, only in the child will this change. In contrast, the answer *'Children are small and dwarfs are ugly'* is not acceptable, as this does not imply any common association between the two. The interpretation of common metaphors or proverbs may also reveal a loss of the power of abstract thought. Thus he who interprets the common proverb: *'A rolling stone gathers no moss'* merely by replying that *'moss wouldn't stick to it if it was moving'* shows little or no understanding of its possible abstract meaning. Both those with organic brain failure and schizophrenia may give this kind or response. In addition, schizophrenic patients often tend to find some point of self-reference in proverbs given to them to interpret. This sometimes leads them to produce bizarre replies. But a word of warning is necessary. If tests such as these are to be meaningful, they must not be given in isolation, but only as part of a full mental examination.

Insight

The degree to which a patient is aware that he is suffering from mental illness or that a symptom such as hallucination is subjective and has no basis in reality is termed *insight*. Insight may fluctuate greatly even in the severest mental illnesses and in the same patient over a comparatively short period of time. Sometimes, even following recovery from a psychotic illness, insight is never fully gained into the nature of the experience undergone. In depressive illnesses patients frequently attempt to deny they are ill, maintaining that they are merely wicked, worthless and to blame for all that has occurred. Some, even while appreciating that they may be ill, may at the same time appear to be convinced that nothing can or should be done for them, and that the outlook is hopeless. It should also be remembered that the commonly made statement that patients with abnormal emotional reactions (neuroses) have insight while psychotic patients do not is not wholly true. In contrast, someone suffering a second or subsequent depressive illness may, by recalling his previous symptoms, become aware that he is being overtaken by something similar to what happened to him before.

Suicidal tendencies

Although already given passing mention, the need to investigate whether a patient is suicidal demands further emphasis. Inquiry into suicidal leanings should indeed *never be omitted*. Sometimes the matter is best approached obliquely by asking: *'Do you suffer from morbid thoughts?'*. Most patients interpret this in the sense of suicidal ideas. If doubt remains, ask: *'Have you felt like harming yourself in any way?'*. Most potentially suicidal patients will admit to suicidal thoughts: only a few dissemble. The advantage of the *'morbid thoughts'* question is if a patient takes offence at the suggestion that he may be suicidal when he is not, it can be explained to him that there are, of course, many other kinds of morbid thoughts.

Physical examination

If not already competently and recently carried out by another doctor, a thorough physical examination must be performed.

Physical examination is necessary, firstly, because it may help to relieve the patient of some of his more immediate anxiety; secondly, because satisfactory psychiatric treatment may be impossible if physical disease has not been excluded. Whoever carries out the examination must be careful not to implant in the patient's mind any hint that there may be something physically wrong when this indeed is not the case. Lamentable examples of this still come to notice all too frequently. Likewise, unnecessary investigations should be avoided because these tend to fix in the patient's mind the belief that he is suffering from something obscure which his doctors do not fully understand, which they cannot diagnose or which, he may become convinced, they are endeavouring to conceal from him.

Case records

The complexity of the material produced during a psychiatric interview and in the later more formal assessment of the patient's mental state necessitates the keeping of detailed records, at least of the initial interview and mental examination. Unfortunately, there are no real short cuts. Tape recording, while useful for research purposes, is valueless for routine case history, as it takes as long to replay and listen to the tape as to make the recording.

Some patients may become concerned or suspicious when the interviewer starts writing down what they say. If so, he should at once bring the matter into the open and refer to the need to obtain as exact and complete a record as possible primarily, it can be said, for the patient's sake. He should also emphasize the extremely private nature of psychiatric case records and the measures taken to preserve confidentiality. Sometimes when a very delicate matter emerges and the patient appears particularly uneasy at the possibility of its being written down, it may be wise for the interviewer to lay down his pen for a time. In subsequent interviews, after elucidation of the main problem and perhaps during the course of psychotherapy, it may be unnecessary to make any notes whatsoever during interview, but after the patient has left merely to record a brief précis of what seemed to be important.

One or two other points deserve mention. Often it is valuable to write down, *verbatim*, a patient's statements, particularly those concerning his relationship with others and his attitudes towards them. Such statements, especially if vivid, may in a few words convey more than half a page of description. Furthermore, if accurately transcribed, they lend objectivity to the case record in that they are examples of what the patient actually said at the time and not merely a subjective and sometimes mistaken interpretation of the meaning of what the patient said.

A very useful task for the inexperienced interviewer, although a somewhat formidable one, is to try to write down everything the patient says and everything he himself says, so that the case history comes in the end to resemble a play script. It is not recommended that this be done routinely, it being far too tedious a procedure, but occasionally and in suitable cases as part of the learning process. It is useful practice if the interviewer has to write down his own questions and statements as well as the patient's answers in that it leads to verbal economy on his own part and steers him away from unnecessary questions and interruptions—a fault all too common in beginners.

At the end of the initial examination when all that can be said has been said, the examiner should prepare a short précis of the case including all that seems to be relevant (*formulation*) together with a statement of what action is recommended (*prescription*). The formulation should be reasonably complete and about as detailed as a letter which might be sent to a referring doctor giving an opinion on the patient's case, a copy of which may often actually be used for this purpose. In simpler and more straightforward cases, this may be the end of the matter. In other instances, only an interim statement can be made pending subsequent interviews in which further information about the patient may be obtained.

Special investigations

There are three kinds of special investigation: physical, psychological and social.

Physical procedures

Any of the usual physical procedures may be required according to circumstances. A variety of biochemical tests, tests of thyroid or other endocrine and liver functions, haematological examination for anaemia, tests for folic-acid deficiency, may all be useful. The estimation of serum drug levels now seems likely to have the potential of making prescribing practices more efficient, while the employment of certain other procedures such as the dexamethasone suppression test seems currently to offer the prospects of greater diagnostic accuracy in at least some cases (see p. 106).

Many investigations, of course, may relate more or less directly to the function of the central nervous system, particularly so in those patients in whom the presence of organic brain disease or damage is suspected. In these a full and detailed neurological examination including perimetry of the visual fields may be required. An electroencephalogram (EEG) examination may throw valuable light on the nature of a patient's disorder, particularly where epilepsy or a focal brain lesion is suspected. It may also help to clarify diagnosis in cases of encephalitis and of various encephalopathies. Disturbed children and adolescents and some emotionally immature adults may show EEG tracings not compatible with their age or stage of physical development. Neuroradiological investigation may help to identify a variety of organic brain disorders. Cortical lesions may be demonstrated by carotid angiography or brain scan. Enlargement of the ventricles in dementia or in normal pressure hydrocephalus may be shown up by air-encephalography, either, if the CSF pressure is normal, by the lumbar route, or, if it is thought to be raised, by direct ventriculography via burr holes. In many centres these investigations have been replaced by computerized tomography (CT scan), a great advance on previous methods of investigation in that it is non-invasive. Biochemical examination of the cerebrospinal fluid (CSF) may also be needed. This is not only the best possible way to diagnose early neurosyphilis, especially general paralysis (GPI), but may occasionally throw light on the nature of some other organically produced mental disorders. Finally and in a few cases of obscure cerebral disease, brain biopsy may very rarely be justified.

Psychological tests

A number of psychological tests are available. Those that measure intelligence or defects due to brain damage or are an aid to the assessment of personality are likely to be of the greatest interest to psychiatrists. The tests which are of particular value are those designed to evaluate some or other aspect of a subject's behaviour and measure it in a standardized and objective way.

The term *standardization* has two important meanings. Firstly, it implies that any test should only be employed in a predetermined manner. All questions asked must be put in a particular way and in a particular order if for no other reason than that such tests may only properly be used in order to compare one individual's performance with that of others. Each individual must, therefore, be exposed to comparable questions. The second meaning of standardization involves establishment of the confines of normality. Any new test must first be tried out on a large number of people from different backgrounds, differing age groups and so on, the population sampled depending on the nature of the test. The results from all these groups are then used to set a standard against which the individual being tested is compared. Thus a 25-year-old man's intelligence test results are compared with the results of all the 25-year-old men in the standardization sample. Such tests do not give an absolute measure of a psychological function, but a relative one. A truly objective psychological test result is difficult to achieve, particularly when dealing with indefinite concepts such as those which surround personality or intelligence.

Intelligence tests

Intelligence tests, which were first devised in 1905 by Alfred Binet and developed in 1908 in collaboration with Simon, were primarily used for testing schoolchildren. Since then a number of other tests have been devised, most being designed to measure a variety of intellectual functions ranging from verbal through numerical to spatial abilities. One of the more widely used tests of adult intelligence is the Wechsler Adult Intelligence Scale (WAIS). This is made up of a number of subtests, some measuring verbal activities, such as general knowledge, comprehension and vocabulary; some measuring psychomotor and perceptual abilities, such as block design and object assembly. Such tests provide a measure both of verbal and performance skills as well as overall ability. Because other tests measure different aspects of intellectual function, the results obtained may not be comparable. The intelligence quotient (IQ) is an often-quoted (and equally often abused) measure of intelligence, the validity and reliability of which must always be clearly understood when trying to apply a figure to a particular individual. It is often very much more important to look at the scatter of subtest scores and the actual behaviour of the subject in the test situation rather than place too much reliance on a single figure.

Personality tests
Personality tests are usually derived from a particular theory of personality. The two prime examples currently in use are Eysenck's Personality Inventory (EPI) and Cattell's 16 PF questionnaire. As both tend to concentrate on particular aspects of behaviour in a variety of situations, it is possible to classify the subjects' behaviour on the basis of their responses. Because the validity of the data obtained must necessarily depend largely on the validity of the theoretical model underlying the test employed, it is by no means clear that the full range of a person's behaviour can be adequately described by a series of numbers. Despite this there would appear to be fairly strong experimental evidence to suggest that responses to particular situations and some behavioural predictions can be made on the basis of an individual's score on these tests.

While the two examples quoted are standardized tests, there is another group of personality tests which do not fulfil the criteria of standardization in the same way. These include *projection tests*, such as the Rorschach or the Thematic Apperception Test (TAT). Both use ambiguous stimuli (ink blots or pictures) to provide the subject with a stimulus about which he is allowed to talk, fantasize or freely associate. Alternatively the subject may be asked to find some meaning in the stimulus, his replies then being assessed by a skilled interpreter who is usually a psychotherapist. Because these tests are unstandardized their value tends to be limited. Not only is lengthy training required before they can be used possibly to good effect, but the amount of information which they may reveal about a patient's problems is limited, depending as it does heavily on interpretation, much of which is likely to be subjective. However, some useful information may be gained.

Brain damage tests
These were developed specifically as an aid to diagnosis. For example, it is often necessary to differentiate between depression and dementia in elderly patients. While it is likely that no fully accurate diagnosis can be made using psychological testing alone, tests such as the Halstead-Reitan Battery may be useful diagnostic aids. Likewise, when devising rehabilitation programmes, such tests may give important information

about the level at which an individual is functioning, thus allowing suitable rehabilitative measures and assessment of employability.

Because all psychological tests require skilled interpretation, the decision to undertake testing should never be made lightly. No psychological test should ever be given routinely and without a good clinical reason for requesting it.

Social investigations

Because social and environmental factors play a large part in the cause and outcome of psychiatric illnesses they can rarely be ignored. Except for domiciliary visits, the psychiatrist as a general rule sees his patients either in the outpatient clinic, in his private consulting room or, if they are admitted, as inpatients or day patients in hospital, or in some other setting such as a prison or remand home. Because, under these circumstances, the patient has, as it were, been artificially extracted from his usual surroundings, the psychiatrist must glean what he can of the patient's physical and social environments and the influence of these upon his problems from what he is told, either by the patient or his relatives. Often even this is not enough. To compensate for this deficiency the psychiatrist may need to lean very heavily on the services of a skilled social worker, preferably psychiatrically trained. One of the social worker's most important functions may be to carry out a home visit, thus allowing a view of the patient and family in their usual surroundings. Alternatively, it may at times be of considerable value to visit the patient's place of work and, if part of the problem is here, to discuss it with his employers—having, of course, obtained his permission to do so. As the social worker is often able to spend more time with a patient's relatives than a psychiatrist can usually do, he or she may also be in a better position to offer them such assistance as is required to help them to cope with the patient's problems, and any of their own, which may arise secondarily; relieving at the same time any pressures which relatives might otherwise put upon the psychiatrist and which might lead to some interference in his treatment of the patient.

Having obtained further information about the patient's problems, from his family and other relevant sources, a social worker customarily produces a written report for inclusion in the case history, and may be present to speak about this at a case conference in which the diagnosis and management of the patient's case will be discussed by all those who have a contribution to make.

In addition to investigating environmental and social problems, social workers have important contributions to make to treatment and rehabilitation. These and other aspects of their work are covered in Chapter 23.

Further reading

Institute of Psychiatry. Department of Psychiatry Teaching Committee (1973) *Notes on Eliciting and Recording Clinical Information*. Oxford: Oxford University Press for Institute of Psychiatry.

5

Aetiology and Classification

Mental disorder is seldom if ever due to any single aetiological factor but to many. Broadly, these factors fall into two groups: *endogenous* having a genetic or some other basis, and *environmental* (or *exogenous*) having a physical, psychological or social basis or a combination of these. It should be noted that these categories are not entirely distinct, there being considerable overlap. In assessing any individual patient, the fullest consideration must, therefore, be given to both, otherwise the formulation will inevitably be incomplete. Overemphasis of one set of factors to the exclusion of the other is a hallmark of poor psychiatric practice.

Heredity

Man inherits certain mental dispositions, just as he inherits a particular physical configuration, both being modified by environmental influences. However, in considering the likely basis of his emotional qualities, it may be difficult and often impossible to distinguish between what is innate and what is the product of conditioning or due to parental example. This is particularly true of abnormal emotional reactions and personality disorders. In the two major types of functional psychosis—manic–depressive illness and schizophrenia—it is clear that heredity plays an important predisposing role. Even then, the exact mode of transmission remains in doubt. While in manic–depressive disorder there is some evidence that a major autosomal gene is involved, statistical investigation of the relative frequency of the disorder in first- and second-degree relatives suggests that polygenic inheritance is more likely, but this is still undecided. Similarly, in schizophrenia two genetic models are available: one being polygenic, the other monogenic involving a single autosomal gene. Certainty must await further understanding of the biochemical bases of both these disorders. There is also growing evidence that hereditary factors are operative in a number of organic mental disorders such as Alzheimer's and Pick's diseases, although in only one—Huntington's chorea—is the mode of transmission known to be dominant. Many forms of mental handicap are also genetically determined (see Chapter 21).

Hereditary factors in mental illness are also reflected in the high proportion of instances—up to 50 per cent or more—in which both of a pair of monozygotic twins tend to develop the same type of mental disorder, often at about the same age. As a general rule, the closer the relationship between a relative and a mentally disturbed proband, the higher are the chances that the former will also develop a mental disturbance of a similar or related kind.

Inability to detect the *carrying* of recessive characters by persons who are apparently healthy often makes it difficult to give precise advice about hereditary risks when one or other proponent for marriage has a relative with an apparently inheritable mental disorder. It must be borne in mind that an adverse family history is not necessarily a 'sword of Damocles' and that while a *statistical* estimate of the likelihood or otherwise of the appearance of a mental disorder can often be made with fair reliability, an individual forecast carries nothing like the same degree of certainty. Furthermore, many important aspects of psychiatric genetics remain controversial, quite apart from the currently seemingly endless dispute as to the respective significance of genetic versus environmental factors.

Chromosome abnormalities

When present, chromosome abnormalities usually give rise to mental handicap. The best known example is Down's syndrome (*mongolism*) in which trisomy-21 and some other chromosomal aberrations are found to occur (see Chapter 21). Mental handicap also occurs in association with abnormality of the sex chromosomes. Thus, in males with Klinefelter's syndrome, two or more X chromosomes are present in addition to one Y chromosome. Mental retardation is a common though not invariable feature. In Turner's syndrome there is no Y chromosome (XO constitution) and although retardation and other psychological abnormalities may be evident, these tend to be less prominent than in Klinefelter's syndrome. Males with an extra Y chromosome may be taller than average, intellectually dull, impulsive and sometimes given to antisocial behaviour, although it is by no means fully established what proportion of those with an XYY constitution fall into this category.

Physical constitution and temperament

While almost throughout medical history a connection between physique and temperament has been recognized, interest in the relationship between body build and personality type has undoubtedly waned in recent years, having been seen as a matter having greater implications for prognosis than diagnosis.

Kretschmer defined several broad classes of body build which he associated with certain temperamental or personality characteristics.

1. A *pyknic* type (characterized by a rounded thick-set bodily configuration) having an affinity to manic–depressive illness with a tendency to mood swings (*cycloid personality*).

2. An *asthenic* or *leptosomatic* type in which the body tends to be long and lean with prominent bony joints. This is thought to be associated with the so-called schizoid personality and in neurotics with a high anxiety level.

3. An *athletic* type with strong skeletal and muscular development, showing some relationship with a 'sticky slow-to-move' (*colledothymic*) temperament.

4. A *dysplastic* type which may consist of a mixture of one or more of the types listed above, or include others difficult to classify both physically and temperamentally.

In England and the United States, Kretschmer's typology has been largely superseded by the work of Sheldon, who, using a photographic method against a grid, assessed his subjects on a seven-point scale according to the prominence of three types of bodily configuration: *endomorphy*, *ectomorphy* and *mesomorphy*. These, together with their associated personality types, *viscerotonic*, *cerebrotonic* and *somatotonic*, correspond more or less to Kretschmer's pyknic, asthenic and athletic types respectively, although in each instance where one form of bodily configuration is the more prominent the extent to which characteristics relating to the other two are present is also measured. However, even this more elaborate approach to the discovery of a relationship between physique and personality does not look like lasting the test of time.

Age, sex and marriage

Age

The majority of those seeking psychiatric treatment are middle aged. Even if younger people are included, and the numbers of first-time hospital admissions are calculated in relation to the proportion of the general population in each group, it will be seen that admission rates rise steadily with increasing age, especially after the sixth decade. The greater expectation of life through reduction in infant mortality, improved living conditions, and the effectiveness of modern medical and surgical treatment, particularly of acute formerly fatal illnesses, appears to have created what amounts to a population explosion among the elderly, this being reflected in the number of those now resident in mental hospitals. Thus, the number of persons liable to degenerative conditions, amongst whom, from the psychiatric standpoint, various forms of cerebral degeneration are especially important, is increasing. These (ESMI, *elderly severely mentally ill*) constitute a serious social and administrative problem. However, by no means all mental illness among the elderly is due to organic or degenerative brain disease. Changes in social structure leading to social isolation, lack of occupation and of a sense of purpose; having to exist on insufficient means; poor nutrition together with chronic physical invalidism caused by pain, discomfort, chronic respiratory and locomotor disorders, are all factors which not only tend to induce a state of depression in those growing older, but in the later stages probably contribute to the advancement of senility (see Chapter 19).

Apart from the aged, personality development may be seen as a succession of differentiated phases each punctuated by a change during which the subject may be more vulnerable than at other times. Erikson called these periods *developmental crises* and suggested that if *accidental crises* (e.g. bereavement) occurred during vulnerable periods, those exposed might experience special difficulties in adaptation. Such vulnerable periods or developmental crises may take place during the transition from infancy, from toddler to schoolchild, at *puberty*, during *pregnancy* or following *childbirth*, at the *menopause* and on *retirement*. All these may be stressful periods calling for a fresh level of emotional adjustment. Each, according to the particular disposition of the individual, tends to be associated with one or other form of mental disorder.

Sex

Since the overall prevalence of mental illness in the community is not known with any certainty, it is impossible to say how far, if at all, one sex is more vulnerable than another. Whereas in the past psychoses due to alcoholism, neurosyphilis and cerebral arteriopathy seem to have been mainly responsible for the higher proportion of male admissions to mental hospitals, the decline in frequency of the first two conditions has altered the ratio between the sexes. It may well be that the incidence of mental disorder in both sexes is more or less equal and that hospital admissions are no true guide. While women are in some respects more at risk in relation to the menarche, menstruation, childbirth and the menopause, it is easy to make too much of these. In contrast, crime is very much more commonly committed by men than women, and crimes associated with mental disorder are also much commoner in males.

Marriage

Some mental disorder is commoner in the divorced and those who are separated, with a lessening in turn among single people who have never married, the widowed and married. Mental instability is a common cause for failing to make the adjustments necessary for a satisfactory marital relationship. In the case of those who are single, psychological problems may render them disinclined for marriage. Widowhood also may be an important cause of mental disturbance, especially in those who suffer severe bereavement reactions as a result of which prolonged depression may occur.

Environmental factors

Although some have already been mentioned, a large number of environmental or exogenous factors remain to be considered. The evaluation of their aetiological significance can be difficult, it being sometimes hard to determine whether they should be regarded as a matter of cause or effect. For example, in the last century *masturbation* was thought to be an important cause of mental illness, particularly among young people. No doubt this idea arose not only out of Victorian morality but from the observation that young schizophrenics often masturbated unashamedly in public. Today, even if excessive, masturbation is now known to be only a symptom rather than a disease *sui generis*.

Much the same kind of problem arises in respect of alcoholism which, primary cases apart, may be seen as a symptom rather than a cause of mental disorder; the matter is further complicated by the fact that alcoholism may bring fresh symptoms in its wake, so that it becomes, as it were, a disease caused by a disease.

Physical factors

Apart from acute infections which may produce transient delirious reactions (see Chapter 9) and chronic infections, such as *neurosyphilis*, which is rare, drugs number among the more important physical agents responsible for mental illness. In drug abuse, such as *barbiturate dependency*, the same problem of cause and effect are operative as in alcoholism. Drugs, not taken primarily for therapeutic reasons, and which may be abused, particularly by adolescents, include *amphetamine, cannabis, heroin* and *cocaine* (see Chapter 11). Other kinds of drugs, even those having no sedative or stimulant properties and prescribed for some quite different therapeutic purpose, can cause mental symptoms. These include *reserpine* and *methyldopa* which, given to treat hypertension, may sometimes produce a severe state of depression. Some forms of oral contraceptives can also give rise to depression, while *steroid* hormones can produce a wide variety of adverse mental effects, some of which appear to depend on the disorder for which the patient is being treated (for instance *disseminated lupus erythematosus*) and others on any associated personality disorder which may be present.

Apart from drugs, industrial poisons such as *lead*, *arsenic*, and various '*dopes*' may produce mental symptoms. In small children *lead encephalopathy* leading to mental retardation may result from sucking lead paint from toys, cot sides, etc. In adults, *carbon monoxide*, inhaled accidentally or with suicidal intent (occurring much less often nowadays due to the detoxification of domestic gas), is a rare cause of permanent mental impairment. Complete recovery or death is more usual.

Currently, a very important cause of mental disorder is *cerebral trauma*, usually from road accidents. Apart from mental symptoms due to actual brain damage, almost any type of mental illness to which a patient may be predisposed can be precipitated by head injury. In addition, abnormal emotional reactions which may be the outcome of worry about financial loss from disability as well as concern about the possibility of compensation may arise. A surgical operation is yet another example of physical trauma which can precipitate a reaction prolonged as a result of psychogenic factors. Certain types of operation are thought to be more prone to produce such reactions than others, in particular *amputations*. It is often thought that *hysterectomy*, which is in effect amputation of the uterus, may also commonly give rise to adverse mental effects, although more recent studies have indicated that this may be less important than was once thought. *Mastectomy* may also give rise to depression and despair as a consequence of disfigurement.

Psychosocial factors

While blame for an apparent if not real increase in the prevalence of mental illness is often laid on physical environment, the operative factors are as much if not more likely to be psychosocial in nature. A finger is often pointed at the growing consumption in the Western world not only of alcohol and tobacco but also of stimulants, sedatives and tranquillizers. This, it is often said, is part of the increased pace of modern living, together with noise and other forms of physical and psychological pollution and an apparently constant need to 'try to keep up with the Joneses'. Such reasons, together with *overwork*, are frequently advanced by patients to account for their symptoms. While not all such reasons can be entirely discounted, it may be observed that there is a constant tendency for patients and their relatives to displace on to some common and more or less obvious environmental event, blame for a mental illness, the cause of which really lies elsewhere, such as abnormal heredity or a family disturbance which those concerned may find difficult to acknowledge. Furthermore, where the cause of mental illness is hard to find there is a natural tendency to try to allay anxiety by resorting to some kind of rationalization.

Although overwork is often invoked, this is much more likely to be a symptom than a cause. Thus a patient entering a depressive illness, who is caught up by an overwhelming feeling of inadequacy, may struggle hopelessly to overcome his disability by working harder and longer, although with ever-decreasing efficiency. If not checked, the outcome of this can be disastrous. Overwork may, however, be relative. Too much can be expected of one who, intellectually or emotionally, cannot measure up to required standards or to the pressures of his immediate environment. This is a frequently recurring problem for those concerned with student mental health.

Perhaps the most important message derived from psychoanalysis is that adverse environmental happenings in infancy and childhood may produce emotional maladjustment later in life. However, the assessment of the aetiological importance of these early life events can be very difficult. It is all too easy to ascribe adult emotional symptoms or personality problems to events which occurred in childhood, several decades before. However, viewed retrospectively, no one can say that any such chain of cause and effect is irrelevant or of no importance; it is also impossible to predict when such events do occur whether they will cause trouble later on. Despite this, there seem to be certain constellations of early environmental happenings which may lead to permanent malfunctioning. Generally, exposure to continuing parental disharmony, the loss or fairly prolonged separation from one or other parent, the creation by undue dominance or overprotection of a state of dependence, continuing inconsistency of parental attitudes and undue pressure towards conformity as a reward for approval grudgingly given, are some of the matters which may interfere with the steady emotional development of the growing child and may later augur badly for his mental health. Nonetheless, it is remarkable how often those who have been exposed in childhood to a seemingly most unhealthy emotional environment still appear to escape unscathed. It must be assumed, in such cases, either that powerful compensating factors are at work or that it is necessary to evoke the concept of differing predispositions.

The once-popular notion that a single traumatic event during childhood might be responsible for personality problems in later life has largely been discarded. Most children are in fact sufficiently resilient not to suffer permanently adverse effects following some isolated incident of psychic trauma, unless of course this is completely overwhelming. In contrast, continuing exposure over a sufficient length of time to a series of minor traumata is likely to be much more damaging. The principal exception is where an isolated traumatic incident which sensitizes the sufferer is reinforced by exposure at not too great an interval to a second sufficiently similar traumatic event. This development is particularly evident in the formation of *monophobias*, where the patient develops anxiety symptoms which relate directly to a specific object or situation to which he has become adversely conditioned. These, however, may often be easily cured by desensitization.

Apart from psychologically traumatic incidents long past, present adversities can prove to be important precipitants of mental illness, though once again they tend to be of greater significance in those previously sensitized. This explains the difficulty in assessing what is stressful and what is not. What is stressful to some may leave others relatively unmoved. In later life, situations involving loss may be important precipitants, particularly of depressive illnesses. These may take the form of bereavement, material loss, loss of status or job, retirement, redundancy, loss of 'face', failure to achieve expected promotion, and many other similar losses or demotions. In essence, psychological or emotional stress can be said to occur when an individual finds himself faced with a situation with which he cannot deal. This causes him to become anxious, frustrated or depressed or, alternatively, to develop a grudge or believe himself persecuted or victimized, according to his particular temperamental predisposition. Most mental illnesses and especially abnormal emotional reactions are precipitated by interpersonal problems with which the sufferer cannot deal in a normal or satisfactory manner.

Prevalence

Estimates vary according to the extent of facilities for inpatient and outpatient care and treatment. About 0.5 to 1.0 per thousand of the general population may currently be inpatients in psychiatric hospitals on account of a major mental disorder; however, it should be noted that approximately half of those resident are aged over 65 and another 1.0 per thousand are there because of mental impairment. At some time in their lives about 5 per cent of the general population will be admitted to a hospital for treatment of mental illness. About 8.5 per thousand are mentally handicapped and another 3.0 per thousand are dull enough to need to seek help from clinics and welfare organizations on account of emotional and economic difficulties. Some 10 per cent of children of school age need special educational provision because of backwardness.

It has been estimated that up to 30 per cent of patients attending general hospital out-patient departments may have symptoms having an emotional basis which may call for psychological attention in the way of advice, suggestion or psychotherapy. The same is true of those seeking primary care, although the number varies widely from one practice to another. As might be expected, those family practitioners who have an understanding of and are sympathetic to psychiatric problems tend to attract larger numbers of patients falling within this category.

Classification of mental disorders

As there are as many different psychiatric classifications as there are psychiatrists, there can be no logical basis for diagnosis so long as the underlying causes of some of the commonest and most important mental disorders remain largely unknown. Psychiatric diagnosis rests upon empirical, descriptive or psychological criteria about which opinion is often likely to differ, particularly among those working in different centres far removed from one another. Sometimes these differences are differences in approach, sometimes only in nomenclature.

The two systems of classification most widely used at present are the *International Classification of Diseases*, of which the ninth revision was published by the World Health Organization in 1977 (ICD 9), and the *Diagnostic & Statistical Manual of Mental Disorders*, third edition published by the American Psychiatric Association in 1980 (DSM III). The ICD 9 is used internationally, whilst DSM III is in general use in the United States. The manuals of both classifications contain descriptions of the different syndromes so that the clinician may match the symptoms of his patient with a standard. The ICD 9 is more flexible and more nearly conforms to diagnosis as most psychiatrists use it; DSM III is more structured and attempts to form a rational basis for research. The DSM III recommends a multi-axial system for evaluation. Axis I includes clinical syndromes and conditions that are not attributable to mental disorder but are a focus of treatment evaluation; Axis II covers personality and specific developmental disorders; Axis III various physical disorders and conditions; Axis IV psychosocial stressors; and Axis V the highest level of adaptive functioning in the past year.

The following classification of adult mental disorders should be regarded as provisional. The four major categories for diagnosis are: (1) organic psychotic conditions; (2) other or 'functional' psychoses; (3) a category that includes neurotic disorders, personality disorders and other non-psychotic mental disorders; and (4) mental retardation. The ICD 9 terms are used for the different conditions within the four categories listed. Terms used in DSM III are inserted in brackets [   ].

Organic psychotic conditions [organic mental disorders]

In these conditions there is impairment of memory, orientation, comprehension, calculation, learning capacity and judgement. There may also be alteration of mood, disturbance of behaviour and personality and impairment of volition. *Dementia* describes such disorders if they are chronic and progressive; *delirium* describes such disorders with a short course and the features above often over-shadowed by altered consciousness.

Senile and presenile organic psychotic condition [dementias arising in the senium and presenium]

Senile dementia, simple type [primary degenerative, senile onset, uncomplicated].

Presenile dementia [primary degenerative dementia, presenile onset].

Senile dementia, depressed or paranoid type [primary degenerative dementia, with delusions or depression].

Senile dementia with acute confusional state [primary degenerative dementia, with delirium].

Arteriosclerotic dementia [multi-infarct dementia].

Alcoholic psychoses [substance induced—alcohol]

Delirium tremens [withdrawal delirium]

Korsakov's psychosis, alcoholic [amnestic disorder].

Other alcoholic dementia and/or hallucinations [hallucinosis].

Pathological drunkenness [idiosyncratic intoxication].

Alcoholic jealousy.

Drug psychoses [substance-induced, type of drug, e.g. barbiturate, opioid, etc.]

Drug withdrawal syndrome [withdrawal].

Paranoid and/or hallucinatory states induced by drugs [delusional disorder].

Pathological drug intoxication.

Transient organic psychotic conditions

Acute confusional state [delirium].

Subacute confusional state.

Other organic psychotic conditions [chronic]

Korsakov's psychosis or syndrome (non-alcoholic) [amnestic syndrome].

Dementia associated with other illnesses [dementia].

Other Psychoses

Schizophrenic psychoses [schizophrenic disorders]

Simple type.

Hebephrenic type [disorganized].

Catatonic type [catatonic].

Paranoid type [paranoid].

Acute schizophrenic episode [schizophreniform disorder].

Latent schizophrenia.

Residual schizophrenia [residual].

Schizoaffective type [schizoaffective disorder].

Affective psychoses [affective disorders—major affective disorders]

Manic–depressive psychosis, manic type.

Manic–depressive psychosis, depressed type [major depression, single episode].

Manic–depressive psychosis, circular type but currently manic [bipolar disorder, manic].

Manic–depressive psychosis, circular type but currently depressed [bipolar disorder, depressed].

Manic–depressive psychosis, circular type, mixed [bipolar disorder, mixed].

Paranoid states [paranoid disorders]

Paranoid state, simple.

Paranoia [paranoia].

Paraphrenia.

Induced psychosis [shared paranoid disorder].

Other non-organic psychoses

Depressive type.

Excitable type.

Reactive confusion.

Acute paranoid reactions [acute paranoid disorder].

Psychogenic paranoid psychosis.

Neurotic disorders, personality disorders and other non-psychotic mental disorders

Neurotic and related disorders are not retained as a category in DSM III. The component conditions are listed under Affective, Anxiety, Somatoform, Dissociative and Psychosexual Disorders. Comparison of terminology becomes very difficult in this area.

Neurotic disorders

Anxiety states [anxiety disorders—anxiety states].

Hysteria [dissociative disorders, factitious disorder with psychological symptoms].

Phobic state [anxiety disorders—phobic disorders].

Obsessive-compulsive disorders [anxiety states—obsessive-compulsive disorder].

Neurotic depression [dysthymic disorder].

Neurasthenia.

Depersonalization syndrome [depersonalization disorder].

Hypochondriasis [hypochondriasis].

Personality disorders [Axis II]

Paranoid personality disorder [paranoid].

Affective personality disorder.

Schizoid personality disorder [schizoid].

Explosive personality disorder.

Anankastic personality disorder [compulsive].

Hysterical personality disorder [histrionic, chronic factitious disorder with physical symptoms].

Asthenic personality disorder [dependent].

Personality disorder with predominantly sociopathic or asocial manifestation [antisocial].

Sexual deviations and disorders

Homosexuality [ego-dystonic homosexuality].

Bestiality [zoophilia].

Paedophilia [pedophilia].

Transvestism [transvestism].

Exhibitionism [exhibitionism].
Trans-sexualism [trans-sexualism].
Disorders of psychosexual identity [gender identity disorder].
Frigidity and impotence [psychosexual dysfunctions].
Other (fetishism, sadism, masochism) [fetishism, voyeurism, sexual masochism and sadism].

Alcohol-dependence syndrome [alcohol intoxication]

Drug dependence
Morphine type [opioid]
Barbiturate type [barbiturate or similarly acting hypnotic or sedative].
Cocaine [cocaine].
Cannabis [cannabis].
Amphetamine type and other psychostimulants [amphetamine or similar-acting sympathomimetic].
Hallucinogens [hallucinogen].
Other [other].
Combination.

Non-dependent abuse of drugs
Alcohol [intoxication].
Tobacco [tobacco].
Cannabis [cannabis].
Hallucinogens [hallucinogen].
Barbiturates and tranquillizers [barbiturates etc.].
Morphine type [opioid].
Cocaine type [cocaine].
Amphetamine type [amphetamine etc.].
Antidepressants.
Other [caffeine, other].

Physiological malfunction arising from mental factors
Musculoskeletal.
Respiratory.
Cardiovascular.
Skin.
Gastrointestinal.
Genitourinary.
Endocrine.
Organs of special sense.

Special symptoms or syndromes not elsewhere classified
Stammering and stuttering [stuttering].
Anorexia nervosa [anorexia nervosa].
Tics
Stereotyped repetitive movements } [stereotyped movement disorder].
Specific disorders of sleep [sleep disorders].
Other and unspecified disorders of eating [bulimia, pica].
Enuresis [functional enuresis].

Encopresis [functional encopresis].
Psychalgia.

Adjustment reaction [adjustment disorder]
Brief depressive reaction [with depressed mood].
Prolonged depressive reaction.
With predominant disturbance of other emotions [with anxious or mixed emotional features].
With predominant disturbance of conduct [with disturbance of conduct].
With mixed disturbance of emotion and conduct [with mixed disturbance of emotions and conduct].

Specific non-psychotic mental disorders following organic brain damage
Frontal lobe syndrome.
Cognitive or personality change of other type [organic personality syndrome].
Post-concussional syndrome.

Disturbances of conduct not elsewhere classified [disorders of impulse control not elsewhere classified]
Unsocialized disturbance of conduct.
Socialized disturbance of conduct.
Compulsive conduct disorder [kleptomania].
Mixed disturbance of conduct and emotions [pathological gambling, pyromania].

Mental retardation [mental retardation]

Mild mental retardation [mild].
Moderate mental retardation [moderate].
Severe mental retardation [severe].
Profound mental retardation [profound].

The above is not intended as a comprehensive conversion table. The terminology of ICD 9 is generally used in this book and relevant DSM III terms are used above to make the former diagnoses comprehensible. 'Unspecified' and 'other' categories are usually omitted; there are other DSM III terms which are not exactly analogous to ICD 9 and have not therefore been included.

Further reading

American Psychiatric Association (1980) *Diagnostic and Statistical Manual of Mental Disorders*, 3rd edn. Washington: American Psychiatric Association.
Lewis, A. (1967) *Inquiries in Psychiatry*, Chapters 10–16. London: Routledge & Kegan Paul.
Slater, E. T. L. and Cowie, A. V. (1971) *The Genetics of Mental Disorder*. London: Oxford University Press.

6

Affective Disorders

The term *affect* means *feeling tone*, an ongoing, relatively constant emotional state governing activity. But while bearing some relation to one another, *affectivity* and *mood* are not, however, synonymous for although endogenous mood swings can occur, mood tends to be more immediately variable and responsive to environmental influences whereas affect has a greater degree of persistence and appears to be more dependent on inner factors. Affect also embraces the concept of *warmth* (in the psychological sense), together with an ability to make contact with others or, conversely, *coldness* or *flattening* of affect, as seen in the case of some, notably schizophrenic, patients with whom it may be very difficult to make affective contact.

Despite this, *affective disorders* are customarily taken to include those in which the primary or prominent feature is a persistent disturbance of mood ranging in all shades of quality and intensity, from depression to elation. All other associated symptoms are usually considered to be secondary to this mood disturbance, thus distinguishing primary affective disorders from those in which depression, elation or other mood changes occur as a symptom of schizophrenia, an organic mental illness or some other abnormal emotional reaction. Although a persistent alteration of mood is, as a general rule, the most striking manifestation of an affective disorder, closer scrutiny often reveals that this is part of a much more profound disturbance which influences function so that, in depressed patients, there is a marked *lowering of vitality* affecting all bodily and mental activity. In *mania* the opposite occurs.

Contrary to what is generally thought, lowering of mood is not by any means always the most striking symptom of a *primary depressive illness* and in some cases may be altogether absent. The same is true of *manic states*. Although *elation* is often to the forefront, this is not invariable, and in some cases anger, irritability and even frank hostility are much more evident. What stands out sharply, is that just as the patient with a primary depressive illness may be regarded as pathologically under-active, so is the manic patient pathologically overactive; both states being seen as morbid when the intensity, persistence and duration of activity are disproportionate to the circumstances which govern them.

Depressive and manic states are amongst the most important encountered in psychiatric practice; depressive illness the more so on account of its frequency, its liability if undiagnosed or improperly handled to lead to suicide, its ready treatability and, if successfully managed, its relatively good immediate prognosis. Depressive illness also presents a challenge to medical diagnosis owing to its tendency to present in a number of disguised forms often resembling various physical conditions as well as other mental illnesses.

Classification

There is as yet no universally agreed classification of affective disorders. The unresolved controversy, in which most psychiatrists are currently embroiled, is whether so-called *endogenous depression* (that form which is probably largely genetically determined and dependent on some type of biochemical disturbance) and *reactive* or *exogenous* depression (that form which is dependent on external misfortunes such as bereavement or some other type of loss) are distinct entities or two ends of a continuum. None of the attempts which have been made to solve this dilemma has so far been convincingly successful.

The classification used in this book does not completely subscribe to either of these views. In essence, *endogenous* and *reactive* depression are not seen as separate entities, nor as ends of a continuum, it being considered that it is those who are genetically or in other ways predisposed, in whom a depressive or even a manic illness can occur as a reaction to a wide variety of circumstances both of an internal and external kind. Based, however, on the phenomenological features of the illness and the presence or absence of so-called biological symptoms (loss of appetite, weight, sleep and libido; failure of concentration and other intellectual functions), affective disorders are divided into *primary* and *secondary*. In this chapter the main consideration is with primary affective disorders, whether or not these appear to have been precipitated by some untoward physical, mental or otherwise adverse environmental life event or whether they are of seemingly spontaneous occurrence.

Primary affective disorders

1. Manic–depressive psychosis (bipolar with both manic and depressive episodes).
   a. Depressive.
   b. Manic.
   c. Cyclothymic.
   d. Mixed states.
2. Depressed psychosis (unipolar without manic episodes).
3. Involutional depression ('melancholia').
4. Depression in old age.

Secondary affective disorders

1. Accompanying an abnormal emotional reaction (neurosis) (see Chapter 12).
2. Schizoaffective disorders (see Chapter 7).
3. As part of a chronic brain syndrome (see Chapters 9 and 19).

Combinations occur, particularly in old age where secondary brain failure may render chronic a depressive illness or manic state, which may or may not have been present previously.

Psychopathology of depression

In respect of mood, it must first of all be emphasized that there is a definite difference between the kind of depression which characterizes a primary affective disorder and that which may be a secondary reaction to some type of stressful occurrence in a normal or neurotic subject. While depression is an experience which is universally familiar and is a state of mind for which many synonyms exist in the English language, such as sad, gloomy, miserable, blue, fed-up, wretched and so on, *depression* in terms of a depressive illness has a very different meaning and, as already suggested, refers to an all-pervading *lowering of vitality*. Put colloquially, the subject operates like a machine which has partially 'seized up'. Many of his symptoms can, indeed, be understood on this basis. One patient, a sufferer from manic–depressive psychosis, stated:

At Whitsun, as an antidote to strain, we went fishing. However, I went high and spent a month in hospital. I came out feeling fairly miserable. By October I was depressed in the medical sense. I felt that my career was in a mess and I felt totally and utterly miserable. I felt utterly desolate and the drugs from the doctor didn't seem to help. Life seemed a totally hopeless proposition. I didn't realize that depression can be cured and my despair was almost infinite. I took an overdose of drugs and I cannot, at this point, honestly say whether or not I intended to commit suicide or draw attention to my plight or seek relief. The doctor thought it was a *cri de coeur*. I have never since that time felt so utterly lost and unable to cope. Looking back it seems idiotic that I allowed this comparatively trivial situation to assume such alarming proportions. Medical depression, in my experience anyway, has irrationality within it. It is as if the balanced logical mind fails to solve a problem and the emotions take control. Everything is viewed through black-tinted spectacles.

I think the main difference between ordinary depression and medical depression (meaning manic–depressive depression) is qualitative rather than quantitative. It becomes impossible to concentrate on anything as the depression digs deeper and deeper. Sleep is affected badly and one may become either lethargic or restless. Sometimes one thinks there is a rational cause for the depression but often there is not. At its worst it is entirely irrational since perception is utterly distorted.

Another patient, a young doctor, who gave a vivid retrospective account of the progress of his depressive illness wrote:

In April the whole of life slowed down and time seemed to stand still. I had begun to worry and I was aware that I was grinding my teeth constantly so that my lower incisors became loose. I did not mind as eating had become a chore. I could not remember anything about my patients . . . I had no power to help them . . . I was waking early in the morning, listening to the hours pass through the chimes of my neighbour's grandfather clock. I would lie worrying, feeling physically ill, unable to get up and make use of the time, but dreading every moment of it. When it came to getting up I did not mind what I wore. If I looked like a tramp than that did not seem inappropriate. I remember trying to shave one morning. It took about 10 minutes—I could not keep my mind on it. The morning walk with the dog gradually became shorter and shorter although it seemed to take as long as ever. It gradually dawned on me that I might be dementing. Somehow this seemed to fit. My memory and thinking capacity had gone. I was a changed person. Of this I was aware, but I could not say how, it was altogether too vague. I knew that the only reason people had faith in me was that I had managed to fool them all these years. Any good things I had done had been a matter of luck and any bad things overlooked or unmentioned. The latter seemed more likely. I knew that while my boss was pleasant, he despised me for my incompetence. Every comment he made was a guarded remark related to my uselessness.

One of the many interesting features which emerges from this second account is the patient's changed experience of the passage of time. Many patients when depressed appear to feel as if time were endless in its passing; on recovery, however, and looking back on their experience they often feel as if time had passed in a flash.

Apart from this and from any changes in mood it is quite clear from these and other accounts that *intellectual impairment* is a prominent feature in depressive illnesses. Thus *concentration* is affected so that the patient cannot bring his mind to bear on any subject which may be a cause of immediate concern. Decisions become well-nigh impossible. His *memory* tends also to be impaired, subjectively in most cases but sometimes to the point where in elderly patients, this taken together with other symptoms may give rise to an appearance at first sight of true dementia. Although slow and impoverished, speech together with indecisiveness and lessened concentration may reflect a parallel retardation of thought processes. This is by no means invariable, for there is often a considerable sense of inner restlessness which has been described as a constant press or surge of thinking, leading to agitation rather than retardation. These disturbances of intellectual function occur early on and are often insufficiently emphasized. They are important in that they frequently lead a patient into believing that his mental faculties are failing, and in turn tend to exacerbate his ever-increasing sense of inadequacy, causing him to fear impending insanity.

Psychomotor retardation may extend to include every form of motor activity. Mobility of facial expression may be greatly reduced, so that except in agitated cases, the patient may sit virtually motionless and almost parkinsonian-like with eyes downcast, wearing a tonic expression of grief and uttering but a few words in a monotonous and dreary fashion which in their content may reflect his misery and constant preoccupation with his obtrusively morbid and painful thoughts. On the other hand, in *agitated* cases there may be continuous restlessness, so that the patient wrings his hands and may bemoan his fate aloud in a reiterative fashion, uttering some stereotyped phrase such as 'Why did I do it? Why did I do it?' and so on.

The activity of the vegetative nervous system may be grossly impaired. Both skin and mucous membranes tend to be dry, the rate of salivary secretion reduced and tears impossible to shed. Reduced food intake, dry mucosae and slowing of peristalsis may give rise to constipation and disagreeable abdominal symptoms, which are readily susceptible to delusional misinterpretation and lead to hypochondriasis. Blood pressure is often raised, possibly due to sustained emotional tension. Apart from *lessened libido* which is almost invariable, other genitourinary symptoms may be present. Pain can occur almost anywhere, particularly in the face, chest and lower back. Indeed the multiplicity of somatic symptoms is such that it can be said that depressive illness enters into the differential diagnosis of any condition of which the origin is not otherwise immediately obvious particularly if *early morning insomnia* is present, with *diurnal variation* so that all symptoms tend to be worse on waking and to improve as the day goes on, a feature of high diagnostic importance.

Although a state of lowered vitality is not invariably associated with depression of mood this is usually the case. Those affected in most of the ways which have been mentioned do not, however, always express depressive thoughts, nor will they always admit to a depressed mood, particularly during the earlier stages of the illness (*depressio sine depressione*). There are also some who exhibit apathy or indifference rather than depression, answering such questions as are put to them in a remarkably laconic manner, almost coldly (*masked depression*). Others complain of a feeling of having lost all feeling. Some can even be moved to laughter—albeit hollow laughter and without real mirth—sometimes referred to as 'gallows humour'.

Some of these seeming incongruities can be accounted for by the state of *depersonalization* which accompanies many a depressive illness of any severity, but which may not be proffered as a primary complaint. Depersonalization also accounts for some of the more bizarre hypochondriacal delusions which depressed patients express, particularly those of a nihilistic kind (*délire de négation*). Such patients sometimes speak of themselves in the third person as if they had no real existence. Thus one, referring to herself, said: 'It's no good, take it away, wrap it up and throw it in the dustbin.'

Most of the kinds of delusion that characterize severe depressive states are mood determined, rather than due to some particular complex or constellation of ideas. However, both varieties can occur. The content of most depressive delusions is concerned with feelings of guilt, wickedness, worthlessness and hopelessness, all of which may be congruent with the patient's state of depression, although far in excess of the circumstances which occasion them. In lesser degrees, where the subject has not completely lost touch with reality, such ideas may not amount to full-blown delusions but, as it were, hover on the brink, so that he may proclaim his own inadequacy or feelings of failure in such a way as to indicate that his future holds nothing in store. Although it is seldom possible to persuade him of this at the time, a depressed patient will on recovery usually agree that such self-denigratory statements were 'due to his depression talking'.

Apart from frank delusions, sensitive ideas of reference which lead the sufferer to believe that others discuss his affairs in a derogatory fashion to look upon him askance may occur. Although they too are clearly evoked by an overall state of depression, they may, nevertheless, be said to rest on certain hidden complexes such as may surround problematic sexuality and about which a patient may have been sensitive long before he became depressed or, alternatively, may be derived from guilt over rather trivial acts of years gone by, of which he may accuse himself, or otherwise believe that others accuse him. Guilt complexes such as these may remain hidden until a patient becomes depressed, when he begins to believe that his sins have been bared for all the world to see.

While it has often been stated that true hallucinations can occur as a feature of depressive illnesses, it is now more generally believed that almost all who experience genuine hallucinations usually do so in a state of altered consciousness due possibly to drugs or other factors. Pseudo- or psychogenic hallucinations do, however, occur and are common in bereavement reactions, particularly in those whose personalities are characterized by a mixture of obsessional and attention-seeking traits. Pseudohallucinations may also occur in primary depressive disorders in which, however, they may be difficult to distinguish from vivid and strongly emotionally toned illusions, the content of which often clearly reveals the melancholic trend of the patient's thoughts.

It is clearly important to look more closely at the mood disturbance which characterizes a primary depressive illness with a view particularly to determining whether this has a different quality to that which occurs in depressive reactions secondary to disorders of other kinds. This brings into question the nature of the essential difference between the experience of the psychotic and the neurotic patient. Clearly, the criteria of severity or persistence will not serve, for whereas a primary depressive illness largely endogenously determined may often be relatively short lived, and readily responsive to treatment; a neurotic disorder with secondary depressive symptoms may, in contrast, be virtually life long, poorly responsive to treatment, and severe enough to inhibit productive life more or less completely. On closer examination the nearest that can be got to understanding the quality of psychotic depression is to discover that it contains something which is alien to normal experience. Thus it is completely unlike a normal depressive reaction brought on by some adverse circumstance or the depression from which a patient with an abnormal emotional (neurotic) reaction may suffer. One reason why this may at first be difficult to perceive is because, inasmuch as the patient is able to describe his depressed feelings at all, he has, like other people, to resort to everyday language in order to be understood. Everyday language may not, however, be an adequate vehicle for the expression of a psychotic experience. It is clear then that only a very careful and detailed phenomenological analysis will reveal that the depressed patient is not really describing a 'normal' state of depression, however mild this may be, but something which, while it may bear some resemblance to it, is nonetheless very much more profoundly disturbing, having a morbid quality which may be quite beyond the ken of one who has never experienced such a thing himself and is in this respect un-understandable. A good example is contained in the expression of nihilistic delusions (Cotard's syndrome) in which the patient may maintain that his bowels have turned to stone or even, perhaps, that he is dead.

Mania

The psychopathology and symptoms of mania are in most respects the polar opposite of depression. This can be clearly seen in the list of clinical features given on pages 100 and 101, where they are contrasted with those depressive symptoms against which they appear in parallel.

Psychodynamic aspects of depression

While endogenous and reactive depressive illnesses are not seen here as distinct entities, it is clearly necessary to give further consideration to those factors thought to precipitate depressive illnesses, regardless of the form in which they may present themselves.

Such factors may be either psychological, resulting perhaps from adverse environmental circumstances, or a physical event, such as an illness, accident, surgical operation or childbirth. In the latter case it must be assumed, whatever the precipitating event, that the sufferer is in some way predisposed. Prominent among psychological precipitating factors is some kind of loss which may be of almost any variety—bereavement, loss of status, occupation, worldly goods, loss of part of the body, failure to achieve some much cherished ambition together with a wide range of similar events.

While it is perfectly clear that a primary or endogenous depressive illness can come out of a clear blue sky—as happens not uncommonly in quite a proportion of cases of manic–depressive disorder—nonetheless it is not uncommon to find that the illness may also be triggered by some depressing circumstance such as has been mentioned. The same is true of mania, but seemingly much less frequently; it being thought by some that the precipitation of a manic attack by a depressing circumstance constitutes a denial of reality and with it a denial of depression (see p. 100). It should also be noted that in between full-blown attacks of manic–depressive depression it is common to find that mood swings occur, which may not be of such proportions as to incapacitate the sufferer severely or other than to lead to a slight or temporary slowing up or reduction of his everyday activities. Given this and the fact that any kind of loss will depress a normal person, albeit temporarily, it may be hypothesized that if a loss situation overtakes a manic–depressive subject or one prone to any form of primary depression, during a phase when he is, as it were, down, and therefore vulnerable, this may well push him into a continually deepening state of depression so that the expected 'getting over it' which occurs in a normal subject who is depressed by some depressing event, does not occur as expected.

It probably applies to depressive states of all kinds that loss is more severely felt when the subject has previously been sensitized. It has, for example, been shown that there is an increased incidence of depression and suicide in those who have lost one or both parents by bereavement before the age of 16. Applying the notion of a sensitizing experience to this, then it is perhaps easier to understand why a premature bereavement in later life may become a potent factor in precipitating a depressive state. This, however, does not detract from more fundamental theories of causation which rest upon genetic, biochemical and other as yet unidentified factors. How people react to loss may therefore depend both on whether they are sensitized by some previous unfortunate experience of a similar kind and on whether their particular constitution, genetically determined or otherwise, renders them liable to a prolonged and deepening depressive state to which those more fortunately endowed may be less liable.

Manic–depressive psychosis

Although both mania and melancholia have been well known and well described for centuries, it was only a little over 100 years ago that it began to be fully realized that the two were in some way connected. Finally, in 1896, Kraepelin formulated a group of morbid affective states under the general heading of manic–depressive insanity, having the characteristics of a good prognosis for the attack but with a liability towards recurrence.

Attacks of mania or depression may be intermittent or periodic, with many variations in the course of the illness. Some patients suffer recurrent attacks of depression only; others recurrent attacks of mania. Some have both manic and depressive attacks. These may either be discrete or the patient may swing from mania to depression and back to mania and so on without any intervening periods of normality (*cyclothymia*). More rarely, features of both may be present at one and the same time (*mixed states*). Any combination is possible. Recurrence is not inevitable though may occur even after many intervening years of normality. Although attacks are usually self-limiting there appears to be a tendency for their duration to increase as the patient grows older and for remissions to become shorter. In old age a chronic state of depression or mania may occur.

First attacks usually occur between 20 and 35 years, although these may be mild and pass unrecognized. With a patient in middle age apparently with a first and florid attack, careful history taking may uncover an account of a vague period of 'nervous' ill-health during late adolescence or early adulthood when the patient was unable to work or pursue his studies for a time and without good reason. This may be regarded as a 'larval' attack. Occasionally the disorder is evident in childhood but this is rare and may be difficult to diagnose.

Aetiology

Heredity is the most important known cause. The mode of inheritance is not known exactly; while there is good evidence for a single dominant gene of variable penetrance, the possibility of multifactorial inheritance remains. In at least 10 per cent of cases one or other parent has had an attack of mania or depression and a higher proportion of near relatives display cylothymic tendencies. Up to 25 per cent of the children of one manic–depressive parent may be affected. Women tend to be affected more than men, probably on account of stresses associated with childbearing. However, in men milder forms of the illness may be hidden behind some associated type of disturbance such as alcoholism.

In recent years considerable research has been undertaken into a possible biochemical basis for manic–depressive disorder. Although it cannot yet be said that this is firmly established, there have been interesting developments along several separate lines. The first—*the catecholamine hypothesis*—suggests that an abnormality of mood, particularly depression, may be the outcome of altered mid-brain concentrations of 5-hydroxytryptamine (5-HT) and noradrenaline (NA). Most of what is known about this has been derived from animal experiments. However, efforts have been made to tie this up with the clinical use of monoamine oxidase inhibitors (MAOI) which may relieve some cases of depressive illness and are known to produce an increase in the concentration of 5-HT and NA in lower human brain centres. There is some recent experimental evidence which suggests that electroconvulsive therapy may do likewise.

The other principal field of biochemical investigation concerns electrolytes in which alterations of water and mineral balance have been observed to occur in association with disturbances of mood, the most significant abnormality so far uncovered being intracellular retention of sodium. However, it is not yet certain whether this and other possible abnormalities such as changes in plasma cortisol levels are a cause or an effect.

Clinical features

A consideration of the principal symptoms of the manic–depressive complex seems to show that, from a phenomenological viewpoint, mania and depression are polar opposites, although it has also been postulated that mania is an extension of depression in terms of its severity. This latter idea is difficult to sustain, as very severe depressive states may be seen in patients who never exhibit manic symptoms while, conversely, manic illnesses are in themselves not necessarily always particularly severe (*hypomania*). Some patients oscillate remarkably quickly between the two: indeed it is not uncommon to observe what seems at times to be a manic façade, suddenly crumble so that the patient momentarily becomes tearful and depressed. This observation has led to the concept of *manic denial* which suggests that the patient in some way protects himself from being depressed by developing a manic pattern of behaviour. Interesting though this notion may be, in that it may contribute something towards a psychological understanding of the relationship between mania and depression, it is insufficient in itself as an explanation.

Expressed in terms of contrast, the principal symptoms and signs of manic–depressive illness may be laid out as shown in Table 1.

Table 1. Principal symptoms of manic–depressive illness

	Manic phase	Depressed phase
Mood	Elated, excited, jovial, euphoric, sardonic	Depressed, sad, miserable, wretched
Activity	Accelerated, restless	Retarded, reduced (sometimes agitated)
Behaviour	Erratic, eccentric, antisocial, aggressive	Indecisive, lacking in initiative
Thought	Pressure of thoughts, flights of ideas	Slow, laboured, restricted, repetitive
Concentration	Marked distractability	Impaired. Attention may be hard to gain

	Manic phase	Depressed phase
Memory	Hypermnesia	Subjective (and sometimes objective) impairment
Ideation	Grandiose, omnipotent, self-exalted ideas or delusions	Hypochondriacal ideas or delusions, also guilt, unworthiness, self-reproach, hopelessness, etc.
Speech	Rapid, garrulous, may be disjointed to the point of incoherence	Laconic, monotonous, slowed up almost to the point of mutism
Sleep	Overactivity may prevent sleep	Insomnia (usually of early waking type)
Appetite	Overactivity may interfere with eating	Reduced (a few patients overeat)
Weight	Variable (may be subject to sudden fluctuations due to alterations in fluid balance)	Steady loss (may be profound)
Libido	Hypereroticism may occur	Reduced. Impotence, frigidity, and amenorrhoea may occur
Variability	No special pattern	Usually worse in the morning with improvement as day goes on
Insight	Almost invariably lacking	Usually lacking but in recurrent attacks some degree of insight may be preserved

Not all the symptoms listed are present in every case and there are many individual variations. Whereas the mood of manic patients is often elated, some are more inclined to be harsh, irritable, sardonic and sarcastic, if not overtly paranoid. Depressed patients although functionally depressed do not invariably appear to be depressed in mood. Whereas the behaviour of manic patients is usually difficult and may be degraded, even violent, those who are depressed usually conform to social pressures as far as they are able. They may, however, be uncooperative and exhibit a degree of passive resistance. Occasionally depressives commit crimes or other antisocial acts.

Depressive stupor

Where retardation is extreme, thinking, speech and all activity may be brought virtually to a standstill. This is the condition known as *depressive* or *benign stupor*. Although marked it is seldom as profound as catatonic stupor, and rapport is not entirely lost. Usually and with great effort the patient seeks to reply to questions, although his attempts to do so may amount to little more than a faint but anguished murmur. What monosyllabic replies do emerge bear witness to his utter misery and self-abasement. In cases of doubt it is sometimes possible to clarify the diagnosis by the intravenous injection of some soluble barbiturate preparation combined perhaps, with methylamphetamine. This, as a rule, loosens the tongue of the depressed stuporous patient; in catatonic stupor it may do likewise but, in this event, thought disorder and delusional ideas characteristic of schizophrenia but not of depression usually become apparent.

Varieties of mania

Most varieties of mania are a matter of degree. Very acute forms are nowadays seldom if ever seen.

Hypomania

Hypomania, which literally means 'little mania', is now the form most commonly encountered. It is relatively mild, characterized usually by a moderate degree of elation or exaltation with excessive ego-valuation together with overestimation of personal ability and an undue feeling of self-importance. Other common features are garrulity, restlessness and instability of purpose and emotion. Ideas of grandeur are common. Actual grandiose delusions occur only in severer forms of the disorder.

Chronic mania

Chronic mania is rare, more so today than yesterday and presumably because more effective drug treatments are now to hand. Patients with this condition show long-standing manic features in an attenuated form; there is evidence of flight of ideas, mild restlessness and meddlesomeness. They are often somewhat paranoid in their general attitude both to those near to them and to the world at large. They may be given to voluminous letter writing to all and sundry, mostly of trivial content. They tend to espouse bad causes and often show an astonishing memory (*hypermnesia*) both for important and unimportant events extending years back. If they can be persuaded to cooperate in treatment, their condition can, in most cases, be controlled. Lithium carbonate appears to be effective.

Mixed states

Mixed states are those in which both manic and depressive symptoms occur in one patient at one and the same time. While Kraepelin thought all possible combinations of the components of mania and depression could occur, in practice the most commonly found is *agitated melancholia*. Much more rarely, *manic stupor* occurs. Agitated melancholia may not, however, be a true mixed state but merely severe depression accompanied by intense anxiety and restlessness as opposed to retardation. Manic stupor, which is a very uncommon condition, is characterized by elation of mood paradoxically linked with marked psychomotor retardation. A patient with this disorder may sit motionless and unresponsive to questions but with a broad grin on his face. Yet other mixed states occur in which feelings of depression are accompanied by racing of thoughts although movement is retarded so that an overtly depressed patient may exhibit typical *flight of ideas* although in a retarded fashion.

Mixed states such as have been described are not infrequently transitional and tend to occur in *cyclothymia* during a phase of fairly rapid transition from a depressed to a manic condition.

Unipolar depression

For some considerable time it has been thought that another form of endogenous depression, which possibly consists of a heterogeneous group of disorders made up of three or more separate illnesses, each with a distinctive mode of inheritance, may exist in addition to that of manic–depressive type, while bearing a close and possibly largely indistinguishable clinical resemblance to it. As this type of depression appears not to occur in those patients who are subject to bouts of mania, it seems now to have become customary to designate this as *unipolar* depression as against *bipolar* in the case of full-blown manic–depressive disorder. One difficulty is that a patient with manic–depressive disorder may well have one or more bouts of depression before developing any manic symptoms, so that until this occurs certainty of categorization may be impossible. One other difference between the two conditions may lie in their hereditary backgrounds: in the case of unipolar depression this is often negative or of a different kind as compared to many cases of manic–depressive psychosis, in which there is often a much more strongly positive family history. It would also appear—although this needs confirmation—that the response to lithium is less satisfactory in the case of unipolar than in bipolar manic–depressive depression. However, even if this does turn out to be correct, it must be considered bad practice to draw conclusions about diagnosis derived from the effects of treatment.

Involutional depression

The relationship of involutional depression (*involutional melancholia*) to other forms of depressive illness is still controversial. The issue is whether involutional depression is a distinct entity—some would not regard it as such—or whether it is a late primary manifestation of manic–depressive or possibly of unipolar depression having atypical components determined by ageing and all that goes with it, together perhaps with the very first signs of encroaching organic deterioration. By definition, a patient who may be said to be suffering from involutional melancholia is one who has undergone no previous depressive illness. Yet on examination of the life histories of these patients it is often apparent that up to the time of their becoming overtly mentally ill they have maintained an all too precarious level of adjustment. In becoming depressed, it would seem that they have undergone a type of decompensation, analogous perhaps to the patient who, owing to valvular disease, has some degree of cardiac insufficiency but gets by often for many years until superadded strains drive him into heart failure.

Patients who are prone to develop involutional melancholia are those who seem unable to 'grow old gracefully'. This is bound up with the very nature of involution, in that it is the period in which it has to be accepted that life is more than half over. During this time it becomes necessary to come to terms with increasing physical and psychological limitations. Many of these while taken by themselves are insignificant in the early stages. Taken together they may, however, possibly forewarn those in late middle age just what growing old means. A diminution in exercise tolerance, presbyopia, impaired hearing, loss of elasticity of the skin, hair and teeth and waning sexual powers may be only too obvious signs. In women the occurrence of the menopause, quite apart from any inconvenient symptoms this may induce, marks the end of the childbearing period. Also, on the psychological side, it may become necessary to come to terms with the fact that memory is failing, that understanding and the ability to grasp new ideas and concepts are lessening, that preferred ways of life, manners and established customs do not arouse the enthusiasm and respect of younger oncoming generations and, even more seriously, that old long-cherished ambitions, as yet unrealized, may have to be abandoned for all time.

Patients with involutional depressive states commonly present several of the following features.

1. A history of a tense, worrying, overanxious disposition with obsessional personality traits.
2. Absence of retardation of thought, speech and action, but in its place, morbid anxiety, apprehensiveness and agitation, often accompanied by stereotyped depressive utterances and gestures of despair.
3. Extreme depersonalization from which hypochondriacal ideas or delusions may arise, such as of cancer or that the body no longer exists or the bowels have rotted away (*nihilistic delusions*).

The onset of involutional depression is usually fairly gradual. Until recently the course of the illness tended to be prolonged although today it often responds remarkably rapidly to ECT. Particularly dangerous as potential suicides are those depressed patients in later life, of high intelligence, education, integrity and drive, all qualities which have brought them to responsible positions and calling for adherence to the highest standards, which in the face of an oncoming depressive illness are difficult if not impossible to maintain. Even after treatment when acute symptoms have subsided, such patients although remaining depressed are still inclined to struggle on. It is at this point that an overall sense of failure may lead to suicide.

Some patients with involutional melancholia show, in addition to the symptoms already listed, marked paranoid features. In these, schizophrenia may be suspected and the diagnosis of depression may need to be revised. For this reason, some authorities, begging the question, prefer to use the term *involutional psychosis* rather than involutional depression.

Diagnosis

Although often easy, diagnosis can at times be very difficult. Manic states, particularly those which have become chronic, are often misdiagnosed as schizophrenic though it has to be said that if chronic and unduly prolonged, symptoms which are highly suggestible or virtually indistinguishable from those seen in some patients with schizophrenia may be evident. Mixed states, other than transient ones, can also present an unfamiliar picture and, once again, being of bizarre appearance may be mistakenly thought to be of schizophrenic origin.

While an acute overt depressive illness can usually be recognized at a glance, it is necessary to watch closely for atypical examples. In adolescents, depression can be a prime manifestation of schizophrenia. Only after antidepressive treatment has been given may the true nature of the illness be revealed. However, the prevailing mood is often one of apathy rather than depression. In older patients depressive illnesses may present themselves in many guises. These are often seemingly physical so that the patient complains primarily not of depression but of pain or some other physical discomfort. Headache, various abdominal discomforts, facial or low back pain are common examples, although depression may be suspected in the case of almost any somatic symptom which is present without any good physical cause being apparent.

Another pitfall for the unwary is the not too infrequent expression of a depressive illness in the guise of an abnormal emotional or neurotic reaction. Many so-called anxiety states are really mild depressions, for anxiety is an integral part of depressive illnesses. In other patients obsessional or even hysterical symptoms may manifest themselves as part, and sometimes the most prominent part, of what is really an affective disorder. The key to recognition lies in the study of the manner of occurrence of the symptoms. Emotional disorders usually tend to be long standing and can often be traced back to childhood. In affective states, however, premorbid abnormal personality traits may not necessarily be prominent and are often largely lacking. Their sudden onset, particularly in an adult of mature years, should therefore arouse suspicion that they may be due to depression, as also should a pattern of remission and relapse. If this proves to be so, they will almost certainly disappear following treatment of the depressive state.

One new and possibly promising development in diagnosis is the finding that about 50 per cent of depressed patients may have a raised plasma cortisol which is not lowered by a low dose of dexamethasone (*dexamethasone suppression test*). This is most frequently found in bipolar depressives, those who are deluded and those with a positive family history. With clinical recovery, dexamethasone resistance usually disappears. In contrast, those with reactive and other forms of secondary depression including schizophrenia rarely show this abnormality.

Management and treatment

Because of lack of judgement leading to eccentric, antisocial and occasionally violent acts—profligacy, spendthrift, and (in women particularly) risky sexual behaviour—it is imperative that patients with manic illnesses should be brought speedily under control. In milder hypomanic states this can often be done without resource to compulsion, although handling such patients can demand the utmost skill and tact. In severer more excited cases of mania there may be no alternative to some form of compulsory admission order. Once in hospital the condition is usually readily controlled, in the first instance by the parenteral or oral administration of chlorpromazine or haloperidol and later possibly by lithium carbonate (see Chapter 24). In a few cases ECT may be indicated but, if used, may need to be given intensively, probably daily or more than once daily during the first few days.

In depressive states management is also an important consideration. While management includes treatment, such as ECT and antidepressive drugs, it is a more embracing term. Although psychiatric care is today much more permissive than it used to be and in this respect is appropriate to the treatment of many mentally ill patients, who need to be urged to take responsibility for themselves, this precept is much less applicable to those with depressive illnesses. Indeed, in treating depressed patients it is often imperative for the physician to take a large measure of direct responsibility. Because a depressed patient is unable to make his own decisions these must be made for him. Often the overconscientious, depressed patient must be ordered, when he is clearly unfit for work, to give this up, despite his protests: 'I can't let them down at the office', etc. He may need to be told firmly that he is ill, not idle as he may insist himself to be. He must be instructed about his need for treatment and told that if he cooperates he will certainly recover, for this is what almost invariably happens. This is what management means.

Management of the patient and his illness also rotates around the suicidal risk which is an ever-present danger. The assessment of this risk both in the initial and later stages of the illness must never be neglected (see Chapter 18). Most depressed patients can be induced to talk about their suicidal ideas fairly freely, although as they are unlikely to do so spontaneously they may need to be asked. A few dissimulate but this is rare. The doctor must also beware of the patient whose state of depression is coloured by delusions: those of guilt, worthlessness and, in particular, *hypochondriacal delusions*, such as a conviction of having cancer or venereal disease. The suicidal risk in these patients is high and almost invariably they should be admitted to hospital for observation.

Agitated patients are probably more at risk than those who are retarded. But it is unsafe to rely on this, as a retarded patient can quite suddenly become agitated. Also, apparent improvement does not necessarily mean that the risk of suicide has passed. Indeed, where suicide is considered a possibility, periodic assessment of a patient's attitude to himself should always be carried out. The only safe rule is to consider every depressed patient a suicidal risk unless proved otherwise. That such proof can never be forthcoming does not of course mean that every depressed patient should be in hospital. What it does mean is that continuing awareness of the possibility is probably the best way of forestalling disaster.

A large number of mild to moderately depressed patients can be adequately cared for at home. Specialist advice should, however, probably always be sought where there seems to be a real suicidal risk as in severe depression characterized by obvious retardation or agitation, where the patient is obviously deluded in some way, where he is socially isolated, perhaps living alone with inadequate social contacts, or where his condition fails to respond to treatment after a seemingly adequate period of time.

Some patients with milder forms of depression may need to be admitted to hospital to remove them from a disturbing environment. Although instructed not to go to work, a depressed patient at home may still feel he ought to be working and even if he does not actually go to the office, may try to have work sent home. He may also be unduly disturbed by well-meaning friends and colleagues who may call to see how he is getting on. Although they do not overtly do so they may, by their very presence, seem to him to be trying to urge him to get up and get going. Many mild or moderately depressed patients are indeed conscious of the fact that they do not look particularly physically ill, which may lead them to wonder whether they really are ill at all or just not pulling their weight. This, of course, stems from the idea many healthy people have, and depressed patients often share, that being ill means being sick in bed or obviously physically disabled in some way.

Two important aspects of treatment are attention to nutrition and to sleep. Many depressed patients lose a great deal of weight and in most cases appetite does not start to return until recovery begins. This, and a gain in weight in patients who have lost weight, is probably the best objective sign of progress. *All depressed patients should be weighed regularly* and under the same conditions. It is almost axiomatic that the depressed patient who apparently recovers with treatment but does not gain at least some of the weight he has lost during the course of his illness almost invariably relapses. In the case of one who has gained or is rapidly gaining weight, recovery is nearly always secure.

In treating insomnia, barbiturates, although still widely used, should be avoided and non-barbiturate sedatives and hypnotics such as dichloralphenazone, nitrazepam or temazepam used instead. If the effects of these are not powerful enough, they may often be potentiated by 50–100 mg of chlorpromazine. This is often better than increasing the dose of the hypnotic drug. With any hypnotics the usual precautions should be taken against the patient using them as a means of suicide. Many patients becoming depressed for the first time, to whom insomnia has hitherto been a stranger, either tend to feel that it is wrong for them to take sleeping tablets or fear that if they do so they will become dependent. They should be told that it is better to sleep having taken sleeping tablets than not to sleep at all; that insomnia is an enemy to recovery and that when they do recover they will no longer have need for them. A doctor may sometimes have to be quite forceful in persuading his patient of this. Indeed, depressives differ from those with abnormal emotional reactions who often take too readily to hypnotics and have an over-ready tendency to habituation.

The use of ECT and antidepressive drugs is discussed in some detail in

Chapter 24 and will not be gone into here, except to say that in patients with severe depressive illnesses, particularly those who are deluded, ECT is still the treatment of choice. Indeed, as antidepressive drugs are less certain in their effects, it may be neither charitable nor good treatment to allow a patient to linger on in mental pain while awaiting a response to drug treatment which could better and more quickly be achieved by ECT.

During recovery there are other matters to which attention should be given. It has been said of patients who are admitted to hospital for treatment that: 'Depressives tend to be discharged too early, schizophrenics too late.' This is often true. It also applies to those depressives, whether treated in hospital or not, who are considering the question of return to work. Premature attempts to return to work by patients who have been depressed are very common and should be strongly resisted. Cooperation from the family may have to be enlisted to ensure this. What depressed patients often do not realize is that when away from work and from having to take responsibilities and make decisions, they may seem to themselves to be better than they really are. Exposed too soon again to stress with which they are not yet ready to cope, they may well relapse. In many cases, return to work should therefore be accomplished gradually and by stages, if this is at all possible.

Depressed patients in the phase of recovery should also be warned that they are quite likely to suffer *bad days* which arise out of sudden unexpected swings of mood. If not forewarned of this and finding themselves plunged once again into a slough of despondency, they may rapidly come to believe that all indeed is lost. Such sudden despair can lead to suicide.

Finally, there are problems to be solved if recurrence is to be prevented. As stated earlier, there is a reactive element in very many depressive illnesses, even those seemingly the most endogenous. Indeed, it often seems that the occurrence of a depressive illness is in some way biologically purposive, in that it seems to draw attention to the fact that the patient has a problem in living, which he cannot solve. Depression, therefore, may sometimes represent a 'derailment' of the life pattern. This is often precipitated by some kind of loss such as bereavement. However, a loss which is significant may not only be one as profound as the death of a spouse, but apply equally to those who have lost face, status, job or a sense of self-purpose. Retirement from work with a lack of compensatory self-resourcefulness may be an important factor. In treatment, therefore, a depressed patient may need to be helped to come to terms with such events if his recovery is to be sound and secure. This part of treatment should, however, be left until his illness has been brought under symptomatic control, if only because during the actual period of depression, probing into such matters can be an intolerable experience. It should therefore be put on one side until the sufferer from depression feels better able to face up to the facts.

Further reading

Kendell, R. E. (1968) *The Classification of Depressive Illness*. Institute of Psychiatry Maudsley Monographs. London: Oxford University Press.
Lewis, A. (1967) *Inquiries in Psychiatry: Clinical and Social Investigations*, Chapters 3–5. London: Routledge & Kegan Paul.

7

Schizophrenia

The concept of *dementia praecox*, now known as *schizophrenia*, dates back to the second half of the nineteenth century, prior to which the disorder does not seem to have been distinguished from the amorphous mass of mental disorder. However, the use of the term *dementia* was misleading, since the type of deterioration which occurs is very different from that due to organic brain disease. In schizophrenia, the *formal* intelligence of the patient remains intact. What suffers is his capacity to use his intellectual powers in a realistic and purposeful way.

The term *schizophrenia* was first introduced in 1911 by Eugen Bleuler. Although this term means 'split mind', Bleuler did not intend this to be regarded as being split into two parts, as indeed is commonly misunderstood, but as fragmentation, leading to a basic disconnected-ness in the association of ideas and to the inappropriate expression of emotions in relation to thought and behaviour together with detachment from reality. Bleuler's original definition runs:

By the term schizophrenia is meant a group of psychoses the course of which is at times chronic, at times marked by intermittent attacks, which can remit at any stage, but probably never without leaving behind some defect of personality. The disease is characterized by a specific type of alteration of thinking, feeling and relation to the external world which appears nowhere else in this particular fashion.

Two aspects of this definition should be noted. The first is doubt as to whether it covers one disorder or several, an uncertainty which still persists. The second is that the three primary characteristics which Bleuler defined—thought disorder, flattening of affect and withdrawal from reality—are not always present. Currently, therefore, it is common practice to regard schizophrenia as a mental illness (or group of mental illnesses) characterized by a number of psychological symptoms not all of which are necessarily present in every case, some of which carry greater diagnostic weight than others.

It is variability of course and outcome which has led to the suspicion that the term schizophrenia may include several conditions having certain features in common. For example, acute short-lived episodes following some fairly well-defined precipitating event are not rare. These are sometimes designated as schizophrenic *reactions* for, despite a tendency towards recurrence, complete recovery is not unusual. In contrast is that form of the disease which begins so insidiously that its certain identification may be impossible for many years and which, once begun, runs an unremitting downhill course towards an apparently irreversible state of hebetude. This is the form designated as *nuclear* or *process* schizophrenia, the term *process* indicating an ongoing change in the patient's psychic life. Although these two conditions may seem to be distinct, it is because there are other schizophrenic disorders having a course and outcome lying somewhere in between, that it may well turn out that a schizophrenic reaction on the one hand and a schizophrenic process on the other are no more than two end-points of a continuum.

A more recent formulation (Mackay & Crow 1980) which does not necessarily do damage to the continuum theory is the division of schizophrenia into two different types. Type I is characterized by positive symptoms—delusions, hallucinations and thought disorder—but unrelated to intellectual deterioration; while Type II is associated with negative symptoms which constitute a defect state which is much less responsive to treatment and has a very much poorer prognosis.

Aetiology

Heredity

While heredity is an important aetiological factor in schizophrenia, the nature of the genetic disposition and mode of transmission remain unknown. Various theories have been advanced. Originally Rüdin favoured a two-gene theory; others have suggested a monogenic form of inheritance of recessive type; also, that some types of schizophrenia are not genetically determined. What is more certain, however, is that twin studies have usually shown a remarkably high concordance rate, up to 60 per cent, for monozygotic twins. Similarly, the risk of other relatives of schizophrenics developing the disorder—up to 11 per cent for parents (according to Slater), 8–17 per cent for siblings and from 14 to 46 per cent of children depending on whether one or both parents are schizophrenic—is considerably higher than the risk in the general population, usually taken to be somewhere in the region of 0.8–1.0 per cent.

Somatic factors

Once the disease concept of schizophrenia was formulated an extensive search for brain and other pathology began. Much research has been stultified by unsound methodology and uncontrolled observations. It is difficult, moreover, to know whether the biochemical changes reported have a causal significance, are due to the effects of a chronic illness or, in some cases, of treatment. At one time or another a dysfunction of almost every bodily organ has been considered. The knowledge that schizophrenia may be precipitated by puberty or may follow childbirth, and that severe mental disorders sometimes bearing a resemblance to schizophrenia can occur in association with diseases such as Cushing's syndrome, has led to many investigations of endocrine function. Once again nothing conclusive has emerged other than the somewhat paradoxical finding that schizophrenics on the whole tend to be rather less responsive to hormonal substances than are normal persons.

In 1939, Gjessing demonstrated that certain periodically recurrent catatonic states were associated with abnormal retention of nitrogen and could be successfully treated by thyroxine. Much of Gjessing's work has been confirmed by Jenner although it now seems likely that *periodic catatonia*, a remarkably rare condition, is not so closely related to schizophrenia as was once thought.

Biochemistry

The discovery that drugs such as mescaline and lysergic acid diethylamide (LSD-25) could produce states resembling though not identical to schizophrenia in otherwise normal persons (*model psychoses*) led to research into the possibility in schizophrenics of some naturally occurring substances of a similar kind. Such research was stimulated by the discovery that mescaline bears some structural resemblance to *dopamine* and that excess dopamine activity may possibly contribute to schizophrenia. Further support for this hypothesis comes from the knowledge that certain powerful tranquillizing drugs having an antipsychotic effect, notably phenothiazines and butyrophenones, block dopamine receptors and thereby inhibit its effects. Amphetamine does the opposite. Some support has been lent to this theory by the discovery that a number of schizophrenic patients excrete dimethoxyphenylethylamine (DMPE) in their urine as compared to controls, this giving the 'pink spot' reaction on the chromatogram. This also occurs in patients suffering from Parkinson's disease (*paralysis agitans*).

More recently, interest has been shown in dimethyltryptamine (DMT) which has been shown to be a potent hallucinogen with tryptamine, which is present in the brain, as its immediate precursor. For further information the reader is referred to more specialized works on the subject. (It may be noted also that some plants with a hallucinogenic action, such as *Acanthaceae* and *Rubiaceae*, contain tryptamines.)

Lately there has also been interest in the discovery of virus-like agents in the cerebrospinal fluid of a proportion of patients with nuclear schizophrenia, the same having been found in some cases of Huntington's chorea and multiple sclerosis. While it is postulated that there may be a causal relationship between the presence of such agents and these diseases, it is thought that genetic predisposition must also be invoked.

Pursuing the theme of a possible neurological basis for schizophrenia, it has also been recently discovered by CT scanning that ventricular enlargement is present in about 40 per cent of patients with chronic schizophrenia in whom a defect state characterized by affective flattening, loss of drive and poverty of speech and ideation is prominent (Crow et al., Type II). The significance of this finding and whether it is a cause of the disease process or an effect is unknown. Some have even suggested that it may be irrelevant.

Family and social relationships

Much attention has been paid, particularly in the United States, but also in the United Kingdom and elsewhere, to the role of environmental factors in the aetiology of schizophrenia. However, while the prevalence of schizophrenia varies, the degree of variation appears to be so slight that it is world-wide constancy of the prevalence of the disorder which is the more noteworthy, as such variation as does occur may be accounted for by differing diagnostic criteria employed in different countries.

Schizophrenia is known to be commoner among those who are single or divorced than those who are married. Indeed, schizophrenics taken as a whole tend to remain single, their social contacts outside the family circle tending to be very limited. Thus some who believe that schizophrenia is largely environmentally or psychologically determined, lay the blame for its occurrence on family disharmony. A peculiar disorder of communication between schizophrenics and their parents has also been postulated leading to a relationship in which the keynote is uncertainty of action (the 'double-bind'). Such parents have been said to be *schizophrenogenic*. However, precisely the same kinds of difficulty have been observed in the background of those who, while having other kinds of emotional difficulty, show no evidence of schizophrenia.

Furthermore, it must be said in defence of the so-called schizophrenogenic parent that living with a schizophrenic can in itself be severely disruptive of family life; a condition hardly likely to be ameliorated as a result of guilt-ridden parents being made to feel as if it is they who are in some way at fault on account of their offspring's wretched condition. In any event, and as in the case of biochemical theories of origin, the evidence for psychogenesis is every bit as inconclusive and controversial, although this is not to say that psychologically as well as physically traumatic events cannot at times act as triggering factors.

Socio-economic factors

Although the prevalence of the disorder is as great in rural areas as in the cities, most large-scale epidemiological studies have shown that schizophrenics tend to cluster in slum areas. In both the United States and the United Kingdom, schizophrenia is much commoner in the lower socio-economic groups of the community, so that poor living conditions have been blamed. The evidence is, however, that the illness itself tends to cause its victims to drift downwards in the social scale. That schizophrenia is commoner in urban areas may also be an outcome of the fact that the isolation which the schizophrenic patient so often seeks, may be easier to find when he is lost in the middle of a crowd. Thus chronic schizophrenia has long been known to be common among tramps and vagrants and the inmates of common lodging houses.

Psychopathology

As the causes of schizophrenia are unknown and cannot as yet be explained, either in terms of some organic lesion or as being psychogenically or environmentally determined, detailed study of its psychopathology is essential. It is vital, as in the case of other mental disorders, to distinguish *form* from *content*. Fundamental to this is the assumption of the existence of a pathological brain disturbance and a psychic process as already defined, analogous though not identical to that which underlies an organically determined psychosis. This expresses itself in symptoms which may be considered as primary in the sense that they are not susceptible to psychological analysis, and cannot be further broken down. Thus it is held that the occurrence of a *primary delusion* as such cannot be *explained* in psychological terms: Why, for instance, a delusion and not some other kind of symptom? The fact that the content of a delusion can sometimes be *understood* in terms of a patient's life situation and personality structure is seen as a secondary issue and one not directly relevant to the emergence of the delusion as a symptom of schizophrenia in the first instance.

Conversely, those who adhere more strongly to a psychodynamic viewpoint tend to minimize the significance of any underlying somatic factor, regarding schizophrenia essentially as psychogenically determined and a result of early experiences together with regression to an infantile or narcissistic level of development. Bleuler, who endeavoured to combine both viewpoints, saw the schizophrenic process as manifesting itself in a loosening of the associative bonds of thinking, regarding this as the fundamental disturbance which allows normally repressed infantile material to emerge and assume a characteristically distorted and bizarre form.

A great many other views on the nature of schizophrenia have been expressed. Some see it as an expression of a disturbance of interpersonal relationships resulting in isolation, withdrawal and a failure to establish enduring patterns of response, while to the existentialist schools schizophrenia represents a special way of 'being-in-the-world'.

Premorbid personality

Much attention has been paid to the 'prepsychotic' personality in schizophrenia, it having often been said that this is characterized by reticence, seclusiveness and failure to make environmental contact. Other features are lack of adaptability and stubbornness, in a passive rather than in any active sense. These are persons who show little interest in their surroundings; who do not share the pleasures and pursuits of those around them; are sensitive, shy and who tend to live in a fantasy world (Hoch).

Because of these tendencies, those predisposed may fail to meet everyday responsibilities and tend to shrink back into themselves. The frequency with which these anomalies precede the emergence of the overt illness has been widely commented upon. Indeed, such personalities are often referred to as *schizoid*.

The suggestion has also been made that schizoid individuals are heterozygotes expressing partial abortive manifestations of schizophrenia. In others the condition may represent a mild defect state, the result of an earlier and possibly undiagnosed schizophrenic attack. Some probably bear no relationship to schizophrenia at all. However, premorbid traits of the kind described occur substantially more often in schizophrenics than in their relatives and up to 50 times more frequently than in the population at large.

Clinical features

Precipitating factors

A wide variety of physical and emotional stresses may act as precipitating factors in predisposed individuals. These include febrile illnesses, surgical operations and trauma of various kinds, especially head injury. Sometimes a schizophrenic illness may be triggered by the abuse of alcohol and drugs such as amphetamine and lysergic acid. Childbirth is a not uncommon precipitating event.

The influence of psychic trauma is often more difficult to evaluate. Confronted by a disorder which to them is both alarming and inexplicable, relatives are prone to put forward as causes all kinds of minor environmental happenings, some of which may be no more than the last link in a chain of cause and effect or due to the early symptoms of the illness itself. Immediate external stress probably cannot be regarded as an aetiological factor. The incidence of schizophrenia is said not to rise in wartime or in relation to other major catastrophes, although there is still some argument about this. Nevertheless, environmental factors obviously do play some part although how and in what way are still ill-understood.

Onset

The differentiation of the earliest symptoms of schizophrenia from original peculiarities of character which may have existed almost from the beginning may make for considerable difficulties. Relatives accustomed to living with one always thought of as 'odd man out' may, for a long time, fail to notice an alteration or deterioration in the patient's aloofness.

But it is during adolescence, when schizophrenia so often has its onset, that recognition of the true nature of the illness presents the greatest problem. Even normal adolescence is a time of vacillation and unpredictability and is frequently accompanied by a period during which the subject becomes seclusive, suspicious and antagonistic towards the feelings and attitudes of older persons. Such a phase, while bearing some resemblance to an early schizophrenic development, is in most cases transient and benign. It has also been suggested because the schizophrenic is incompletely equipped to cross the bridge between childhood and maturity, that this is why adolescence is so often the time when the disorder first manifests itself. In fact some 75 per cent of schizophrenic illnesses first appear between 15 and 30 years of age and, as a rule, earlier within these limits than later.

In only a very small proportion of patients is the onset acute and in these there is often some clear precipitating event such as childbirth. In a substantial number it may be so insidious as to make it impossible to determine exactly when the illness actually did begin. In young persons still at school an at first inexplicable deterioration in academic performance may occur, accompanied by a loss of interest in family, friends and in pursuits hitherto followed with some enthusiasm. Increasing anergia and solitary behaviour may be accompanied by a tendency to remain in bed by day and to wander restlessly by night. This kind of depressive state, often having a marked element of apathy and occurring in an adolescent, should always arouse suspicion. Apart from depressive symptoms other types of presentation are not uncommon, particularly those characterized by obsessional symptoms and behaviour.

Rather more florid cases with a subacute onset may be marked by the occurrence of erratic, capricious or inexplicable behaviour; groundless suspicions, odd paranoid ideas, interest in strange cults, a sudden and excessive preoccupation with religious and metaphysical problems and perhaps above all hypochondriacal symptoms, sometimes of a sexual kind. All these are familiar precursors.

First-rank symptoms

Reference has already been made to primary symptoms deriving from a hypothetical *process*. In contrast, secondary symptoms are those regarded as the response of the patient to those fundamental changes which he feels have occurred in himself. Whether primary or secondary, certain symptoms are widely accepted as having greater diagnostic importance than others. Thus Kurt Schneider classified schizophrenic symptoms into those of *first* and *second rank*. First-rank symptoms consist of hearing thoughts spoken aloud, that is, 'thought resonance' (*écho de la pensée*); hallucinatory voices which comment in the third person on the patient's actions; bodily feelings of influence (*passivity feelings*); thought withdrawal and other experiences of thought being influenced; broadcasting of thoughts; certain types of delusion (see Chapter 2) together with other passivity experiences in the spheres of feeling, instinct and will. All other symptoms—other forms of hallucinations, emotional changes, catatonic symptoms and so on—were considered by Schneider to be second-rank symptoms, i.e. not specific to schizophrenia. However, this concept is considered by some to be too narrow and restrictive.

Ego disorder

Most of Schneider's first-rank symptoms can be explained in terms of the disorder of ego function which is central to schizophrenic symptomatology (see p. 29). This disturbance shows itself in all functions but notably in thinking. Apart from this the patient may feel compelled to do something such as mutilate himself or to perform some outwardly inexplicable action, sometimes one endangering life. It is not surprising that in seeking to explain this uncanny experience so alien to normal living he soon develops a delusion of a *secondary* character and comes to believe he is 'hypnotized' or 'bewitched'. Similarly, his bizarre bodily hallucinations may delude him into believing he is under the influence of radio waves, television and so on. Such delusions have a tendency to reflect the current developments of science, as popularly conceived.

One female patient, a middle-aged paraphrenic, complained that she was disturbed by two young male lodgers knocking nails into the walls of a room in her house, not because of the noise or the damage, but because each time a nail was knocked in she felt it in her own body. One of Bleuler's patients complained of feeling the pain of an injection given to the patient in the next bed. The sense of unity of the ego may be disturbed leading to the experience of a double personality (not to be confused with *alternating personality*). One patient told his doctor: 'Every time I talk to you I feel I am you.' Similarly, the identity of the ego may be disturbed so that the patient's memories of his past are attributed to another person. Another described his sensations as:

I feel a thumping of my head as though someone was swinging it, something inside as though someone else is shivering inside me and playing havoc with my nerves . . . as though they came from another body inside mine, as though someone else was living inside me and making me shiver.

    . . . when I stand up my ankle may be pushed because I feel I am possessed

. . . It is like someone else fitting inside me, like a glove, fighting to take over my body.

Thought disorder

A frequent, important and characteristic symptom of schizophrenia is a peculiar disturbance of the process of thinking. It is difficult to formulate the character of this thought disorder briefly. In essence it lies in an inability to *focus* on the main point of a statement or an argument. In general the patient retains a given concept, but seems unable to suppress irrelevant associations, with the result that the concept becomes blurred and hazy. Consequently productive conversation is impossible, the patient may lose himself in a cul-de-sac, or in elaborate irrelevances, often by dwelling merely on formal aspects of a word, or even on its sound or visual appearance. He himself is often aware of an inability to direct his thinking. One patient said: 'It is like a motor car stuck in the snow, the engine keeps running, but the wheels turn round and round in the same spot.' Another patient found particular significance in numbers, for example '5 equals "The Holy Trinity", like a Roman V, like a snooker triangle', the interpolation of which in an attempt at mental arithmetic was disturbing.

Sometimes the disorder is not immediately evident in conversation and to elicit it certain tests are commonly used. The patient may be asked to recite a story or fable and to give the moral, to interpret proverbs, or to state differences such as between a child and a dwarf. While these may have a ready appeal to those eager for a sign, they are often hard to interpret for, in the absence of standardized norms, it is often difficult to assess the degree of abnormality of a given response, thus two interpretations may be equally valid although one may be unexpected.

While eccentricity is not necessarily evidence of schizophrenia the following, however, provides a good example of a schizophrenic response. A young paranoid schizophrenic, a refugee from a totalitarian state who believed himself spied upon, when asked the difference between a wall and a fence replied: 'A fence you can see through; a wall has ears!' This shows the formal disturbance as well, the patient not only seeing aspects of each which are certainly unusual, but also peripheral aspects of the total concept which are irrelevant and inadequate to the task set. In the second part of his reply, the ordinary relevant concrete significance becomes transformed in a flash into the metaphorical. Further, the response often reveals a self-referent tendency which is largely determined by the prevailing paranoid trends as in the example just cited. The relationship of this kind of incongruity to certain types of wit has often been remarked upon.

Patients often report a sudden stoppage of their thinking—*blocking*—which occurs for brief periods, reminiscent of 'petit mal', which under the influence of the ego disorder is often interpreted delusionally as *thought withdrawal*. An unpleasant *crowding of thoughts* is sometimes reported. Later on, when the disorder becomes chronic, the patient's mind becomes relatively empty of thoughts and those that he has are ill-elaborated. He may seek to overcompensate for this by an appearance of exaggerated profundity and gravity.

Despite all this, basic psychic functions such as memory, grasp and orientation remain intact and, except occasionally in the very acute stages of schizophrenic illness and sometimes later during brief episodes, consciousness remains clear. (Schizophrenic thought disorder is dealt with in greater detail in Chapter 2.)

Speech

The speech in chronic cases of schizophrenia reflects the degree of thought disorder. This in association with *eccentricity*, and with withdrawal into a private personal world (*autism*), leads to a loss of the social use of language. In consequence, speech becomes stilted, pedantic and mannered, words are given an individual meaning, syntax suffers and strange new words may be coined (*neologisms*) so that in time speech may become a meaningless hotchpotch (*word salad*). Writing and drawing may be similarly mannered and odd, although schizophrenic art may at times be startlingly original and meaningful.

Delusions

The term delusion (also discussed in Chapter 2) refers to a *primary* delusion, that is a delusion which does not derive from any antecedent emotional state, which appears without reason or occasion and which is incomprehensible to the normal individual. It is a highly characteristic symptom of schizophrenia although found transiently in other conditions such as temporal lobe epilepsy.

A primary delusion is the expression of a fundamental disturbance of function in which percepts acquire in addition to their everyday meaning another which is symbolic and which usually has direct and specific reference to the patient. For example, a patient seeing a railway engine stopped on a bridge, interpreted this as meaning that all stations, even those in foreign countries, were blocked to prevent his escape from a 'syndicate' of persecutors. Another patient whilst with his wife in a café had his order taken by one waitress, but was served by another. He said: 'That was funny, I thought it was a way of telling my wife I had taken one of the waitresses out.' Sometimes this kind of experience is preceded by an emotional state which is hard to describe in which the patient feels that his environment has become endowed with a threatening, sinister, uncanny quality. He feels something strange is going on; those around him seem odd, like machines, the shops look different, there is some vague meaning to it all, but what? Thus a young naval officer returning to his ship suddenly became convinced that other naval personnel in the train were spies, that the food in the dining car tasted queer so that he suspected it was poisoned. This type of experience has been called the *delusional mood*. Suddenly a *secondary* delusional explanation emerges and with it a sense of relief from tension and anxiety.

Hallucinations

Hallucinations, which are frequent in schizophrenia, often have their own peculiar quality which differentiates them from those which may accompany organic reactions and certain other conditions. Auditory hallucinations are the commonest, but hallucinations of bodily experiences, notably sexual, occur especially in women in middle age. Vestibular, gustatory or olfactory hallucinations, such as of 'odourless' gases pumped into the room, again are common in later life. Hallucinations are much less frequently visual, except sometimes in the early stages of acute paranoid illnesses. If at all prominent, an organic cause should be suspected and the diagnosis reviewed accordingly.

Because schizophrenic hallucinations are so often inextricably linked with the ego and thought disorder, it is sometimes difficult to be sure whether they have a true perceptual quality or not. In auditory hallucinations the voices which the patient hears may range in distinctness from a vague mumbling to apparently clear speech. Their content is almost invariably unpleasant and of a mocking or accusatory nature, often having a sexual content. Most characteristically, they seem to address him in the third person, thus he expresses no surprise when told that others do not hear the voices he hears, seeming to recognize them as being particularly personal to him. They are often located in some part of his body and blending with hallucinations of other sense modalities is not infrequent. Thus he feels a pain in his genitals and hears a voice coming from his penis.

Affective changes

Although not generally considered a primary symptom, affective changes of any kind can occur in schizophrenia and may be the first indication that all is not well. Firstly, there may be a loss of finer feelings in response to social situations; later, the degree of affective response is inadequate or inappropriate. Thus a schizophrenic laughed when a wreath fell off the hearse carrying her mother's body to the cemetery. A loss of contact develops and a sense of isolation from others is painfully experienced. Inexplicable emotional outbursts may occur. In young schizophrenics the onset of the illness is often masked by a depressive state.

Catatonic symptoms

Under the heading catatonic symptoms are included a number of quasi-neurological, 'psychomotor' symptoms which are by no means specific, since many catatonic states may be due not to schizophrenia but to a variety of medical and neurological states such as encephalitis and various types of encephalopathy, metabolic disorders, toxic agents, etc. Indeed, there is some evidence that catatonic forms of schizophrenia are diminishing in incidence. However, where catatonic symptoms are of schizophrenic origin they may be seen as representing the overt expression of thought and ego disorder and the splitting of the personality in the form of an alteration in motor behaviour. They can also be psychologically construed as disturbances of volition, e.g. the stuperous patient refuses to move because he *will* not bring himself to do so, an extreme form of *negativism*. Some of the symptoms are polar opposites, such as those of catatonic excitement as against those of stupor.

Forms of schizophrenia

Schizophrenia is traditionally divided into four main types: *simple*; *hebephrenic*; *catatonic*; and *paranoid*. None of these is mutually exclusive. Some patients show mixed pictures, in others the clinical state may alter with the progress of the disease. Other less well-defined varieties are described as *undifferentiated* (mixed) *pseudoneurotic*, *paraphrenic* and some cases of *paranoia* and *schizoaffective states*.

Simple schizophrenia

Simple schizophrenia consists of progressive mental deterioration beginning about the time of puberty or in early adult life, sometimes in those who already have some degree of intellectual defect. Emotional dullness is notable. Hallucinations and delusions are usually absent. Mannerisms and negativism may be present. Probably many simple schizophrenics pass unrecognized, at least for long periods of time. They tend to be shiftless, unable to hold a job and gradually sink lower in the social scale, having a tendency to vagrancy.

Hebephrenia

Hebephrenia, which some do not differentiate from simple schizophrenia, is commoner in late adolescence or early adult life. The sufferer may make various physical complaints and appear to be in indifferent health. He may be depressed, dull, irritable and apathetic, tending to avoid the company of others. While realizing that some change has come over him, he usually tends to ascribe it to some external influence. Suicidal attempts are not uncommon. As his condition progresses he becomes childish and inconsequent in behaviour so that his apparent state of depression may be interspersed with outbursts of giggling and laughing, thus offering a marked contrast to the consistency of a primary depressive state. Bizarre hypochondriacal delusions affecting any part of the body and often having a sexual content are common. Hallucinations occur, usually auditory in type. Mannerisms, peculiar antics and other oddities of behaviour may be observed. Deterioration is usually fairly rapid, remissions are rare and the prognosis is poor.

Catatonia

Catatonia is rather more common in females and occurs generally round about the age of 25, although occasionally in those much younger. The disorder appears in two main forms, catatonic *stupor* and *excitement*. These may alternate.

Stupor

After a prodromal period of indefinite ill-health characterized by insomnia, depression, limitation of activity, and a gradual withdrawal from contact with the environment, the patient may start to express delusions of a persecutory or self-accusatory nature. Hallucinations are commonly present. A peculiar rigidity develops which is uniform in distribution and different from that seen in melancholia with its distinctive downcast attitude. Moreover, catatonic patients do not show the characteristic facial expression of the melancholic, but grimace and display curious tremors and spasms of the facial muscles, especially a pursing or protrusion of the lips (*schnauzkrampf*). *Negativism* is often present in the form of resistance to any attention, *mutism*, and refusal of food. *Echolalia* and *echopraxia* may occur. Some also show *automatic obedience* carrying out any command put to them, however seemingly distasteful. Sometimes a single phrase may be repeated over and over again (*verbigeration*).

If severe, actual stupor may develop, although this also can be of relatively sudden onset. The stuporous patient stands, sits or lies in various and often uncomfortable attitudes. He may adopt the 'fetal position' or lie on his back with his head uncomfortably raised from his pillow (*psychic pillow*). If untreated, he may remain completely motionless for many hours or days, is mute and unresponsive to painful stimuli showing both retention of urine and faeces or occasionally incontinence. Muscle tone may be increased and he may be as rigid as a board or exhibit a curious waxy flexibility in which his limbs can be placed in some awkward position which when achieved he will maintain sometimes almost indefinitely (*flexibilitas cerea*). Although at the time he may appear to be unable to do so, he may be well able to take in quite clearly what is going on around him and give an accurate account of this on recovery.

Excitement

Excitement may occur at the outset, may follow suddenly upon catatonic stupor or may complicate other varieties of schizophrenia. The condition may be mistaken for, and be difficult to distinguish from, acute mania. The main points of difference however are that the behaviour of the manic patient while showing a press of activity is mostly purposive, while that of the catatonic is absurd, stereotyped, purposeless and often violent and impulsive. Manic speech is characterized by flight of ideas, while that of the catatonic is usually incoherent, a hotchpotch of words resembling some forms of aphasia (*word salad*). Manics, though not by any means cooperative, are not truly negativistic; catatonics usually are. The mood of the manic patient is infectious and expansive whereas in the catatonic the striking feature is absence of rapport. In mania, hallucinations are uncommon but in catatonia are almost invariably present.

States in between catatonic stupor and excitement may be observed wherein the subject may take up an almost statuesque position in some corner of the room, occupying himself with ceaseless repetitive stereotyped movements of various kinds. The range of variation of these is wide if not endless. Other such patients will cover countless sheets of paper with meaningless writing of words, symbols and other hieroglyphs which tend for the most part to be indecipherable.

Paranoid schizophrenia

Paranoid schizophrenia represents the extreme end of a spectrum of which *paranoia* is at the other end with *paraphrenic* forms in between. All these tend to begin somewhat later in life than the other types, those occurring over 35 and onwards being the most attenuated. While all are characterized by relative preservation of the personality, this appears to depend on the severity or character of the process. At one end of the scale signs of deterioration are manifest fairly early on and the prognosis is bad, while in not a few who suffer from paraphrenia, behaviour may be compatible with quite a useful existence outside hospital. Primary delusions are often evident and under the influence of hallucinations and secondary delusional formation, quite elaborate systematization takes place. These secondary delusions may be grandiose or persecutory. Passivity is prominent, but thought disorder may not be so readily apparent, especially in those in whom the personality is better preserved. Erotic hallucinations and delusions are common, especially in women.

Undifferentiated and other forms of schizophrenia

There are varieties of schizophrenia in which the picture is so mixed that it is impossible to designate the clinical form or type. Undifferentiated forms appear to be becoming commoner, possibly because of earlier application of more effective means of treatment. It is also likely that some of the more classic manifestations of schizophrenia may have been in part the outcome of institutionalism. More intensive care under better conditions, together with energetic rehabilitation, has done something to overcome this.

Pseudoneurotic schizophrenia

The presenting symptoms of pseudoneurotic schizophrenia are similar to, and may be mistaken for, those of an obsessional illness which, as already shown, is a not uncommon mode of onset. This diagnosis is less favoured in the United Kingdom than in the United States where the diagnosis of schizophrenia appears to be made on the basis of criteria which many British psychiatrists would not regard as being sufficiently strict.

Schizoaffective states

This diagnosis should only be used as a last resort and then probably only provisionally. Too ready resort to the term *schizoaffective disorder* often indicates a failure to assess properly the significance of psychopathological criteria. It is also wise to consider that although almost any kind of affective symptom may be present to a lesser or greater extent in schizophrenia, *true* schizophrenic symptoms are not part of primary affective disorders. Where, therefore, these are indubitably present the diagnosis of schizophrenia should be favoured. A schizophrenic illness with a marked affective component often carries a favourable prognosis and may remit completely. Then, at some later date, the patient may be seen again, apparently on this occasion suffering from a pure affective disorder. This observation has led some to postulate the occurrence of a *unitary psychosis* sometimes manifesting itself in schizophrenic form and at other times as an affective or schizoaffective state. Another possibility is that a mixture of genetic factors may affect a single patient, the type of illness occurring being due to whichever genes are, at the time, exerting the greatest effect.

Diagnosis

Diagnosis can be extremely easy in advanced cases or extremely difficult, if not at times actually impossible, in early cases, at least on the basis of a single interview. It must be made with the greatest care and, owing to its serious implications, not until certainty is achieved—especially before being communicated to the patient's relatives.

Feighner et al. (1972) have advanced the following criteria for diagnosing schizophrenia.

1. A chronic illness with at least six months of symptoms prior to evaluation without return to the previous level of social adjustment.

2. Absence of a period of depressive or manic symptoms of a quality sufficient to justify a diagnosis of affective disorder.

3. The presence of delusions or hallucinations without associated perplexity or disorientation.

4. Verbal production lacking logical or understandable organization.

5. At least three of the following.

    a. Single status.

    b. Poor premorbid work history or social adjustment.

    c. Family history of schizophrenia.

    d. Absence of alcoholism or drug abuse for at least one year before onset of psychosis.

    e. Onset of illness before 40 years of age.

Apart from these, the most decisive symptoms may be *passivity feelings, thought disorder*, if this can be elicited, and *primary delusion*, if clearly established.

The greatest difficulties arise when schizophrenic symptoms occur in the course of other psychoses, particularly when arising in the puerperium in which a mixture of affective and schizophrenic symptoms occur in a setting of mild clouding of consciousness—a common clinical picture after childbirth. It is often impossible to predict whether this will turn out to be a benign psychosis with recovery in a shorter or longer time, or a more malignant form which will quickly lead to a severe deterioration.

The problem of mixed affective and schizophrenic psychoses has already been mentioned. No doubt most of these will be seen later to be either schizophrenic *or* affective, but a small group of mixed atypical psychoses, some of them possibly specific, remain. The most important practical point is identifying those which are likely to remit and those which are not; here, only experience can guide. It is the difference in outcome and remission rate which has furthermore led to attempts to separate out *schizophreniform psychoses* with a benign course from more malignant forms of schizophrenia with marked disorder of ego function.

Where *obsessional symptoms* are prominent the true diagnosis, being masked, may be difficult. Much will depend upon the presence or absence of passivity symptoms. The general impression the patient makes is important. The obvious emotional tension of the obsessional, his usually good rapport, his strong desire for help and his reassurability, however transient, together with his history, usually enables a correct diagnosis to be made. There remain, however, a number of cases where doubt persists for a long time or indefinitely.

A *hysterical* type of presentation may also sometimes make for difficulties. It is not too uncommon to find an individual who has presented evidence of a gross, apparently hysterical personality disturbance for years who later develops an undoubted schizophrenic illness. A curious interweaving of hysterical ungenuineness in the schizophrenic—coolness, oddity and unexpectedness—a natural blend which may remind the observer how closely the two conditions can sometimes resemble each other may also occur. Confusion may also arise with certain types of personality disorder so that for some time the true diagnosis may remain in doubt.

Paranoid states require careful assessment. About 50 per cent or possibly even more patients with ideas of reference later turn out to be schizophrenic. Care must be taken to separate out those forms (see Chapter 8) which can be regarded as developing out of the premorbid personality of the patient, such as transient paranoid reactions to stress, paranoid symptoms occurring in the course of other psychoses, especially in affective disorders, the paranoid ideas of the deaf and of the 'infected' partner in *folie à deux*, in immigrants and in the mentally subnormal in whom the diagnosis of schizophrenia may often be difficult.

Stupor occurs in other psychoses such as toxic-confusional states, severe depressive disorders in which retardation is extreme, also in association with epileptic psychoses and sometimes in hysteria.

Treatment

Since the causes of schizophrenia are unknown, there is no rational therapy. Insulin treatment which led the field for over 20 years has now fallen into disuse. Acute cases may be brought under control by ECT which may be particularly valuable in catatonic stupor and in states of schizophrenic excitement.

Neuroleptics, particularly phenothiazine derivatives, of which chlor-promazine is the oldest and best known, have replaced insulin. Others such as trifluoperazine may be particularly effective in controlling hallucinations, although they may produce troublesome side-effects, notably parkinsonism and other extrapyramidal symptoms such as *tardive dyskinesia*.

Butyrophenones, such as haloperidol, also appear to be of con-siderable value. Their effect is very similar to that of phenothiazines (see Chapter 24). They are also more safely administered together with ECT than is chlorpromazine which may cause a fall in blood pressure and sometimes confusional states. When drugs are effective they often need long-term administration even after the patient has left hospital.

Difficulty in ensuring that non-compliant patients needing such long-term treatment actually receive it has recently been lessened by the introduction of certain long-acting phenothiazines such as fluphenazine decanoate, which given in a single injection, either when the subject attends as an outpatient or at home by a community psychiatric nurse, may exert an effect lasting two to four weeks.

Rehabilitation

One advantage of modern drug therapy in the treatment of schizophrenia is that it exerts a measure of control which allows the application of social, occupational and rehabilitative measures where these might not previously have been possible. Indeed, the importance of the therapeutic milieu in the treatment of schizophrenia cannot be sufficiently stressed. The value of work for psychiatric patients has been recognized from the beginning, but only in recent years has it been developed more fully. This consists not only of occupational therapy, which is useful in many cases, but the setting of the patients to gainful employment. Out of this has arisen the concept of the hospital factory and, even more recently, that of community industrial therapy units where patients can earn the fruit of their labours and are thus provided with a sense of belonging, even if at first only tangentially, to the community. This is a useful preparation for work outside on discharge from hospital. Vigorous efforts must be made to place the schizophrenic patient on discharge in suitable employment and to keep him out of hospital as long as possible, for good, if this can be achieved.

Whether to return him to home or not may be a vexed question. Thus for some, a suitable hostel may be a more satisfactory environment, this depending on the patient's social background and his relationship with his family. Treatment of the schizophrenic in hospital is only the beginning; the next and all-important step is his rehabilitation for which there is still all too little provision in the United Kingdom. Industrial rehabilitation units under the Department of Employment and Remploy factories are often helpful though with certain limitations, and the Disabled Persons Act may help in placing such patients in jobs outside hospital. An appreciable number of schizophrenics will, however, always require permanent hospital or long-term hostel care.

Prognosis and outcome

A schizophrenic illness must never be regarded lightly. Nevertheless, as has long been recognized, the outcome is not always unfavourable. The risk is that even if the first attack ends in apparently complete remission, subsequent attacks are likely to be followed by an increasing degree of personality defect, mostly after the third attack.

The difficulties of determining the outcome in general of schizophrenic illness are considerable. These depend on lack of agreement among psychiatrists on what should be included under the rubric of schizophrenia, on securing an adequate follow-up, on the predominant type of population from which a clinic or hospital draws its patients, on changes of view, or on insufficient examination. Too narrow an operational concept of schizophrenia such as that defined by Schneider (see p. 118) may have a poor predictive value as regards outcome, carrying with it a worse prognosis than the more broadly based diagnostic criteria since advanced by Feighner and others.

Apart from this generalization, it appears that catatonics have a better outlook, at least in the short term, than simple or hebephrenic patients, whilst the paranoid patient, even if not symptom free, may yet be capable of leading a tolerably useful life in society. Illnesses with a delirium-like character and those associated with clouding of consciousness tend also to have a favourable prognosis. Acute onset—thought by some to be the most reliable pointer of all—good prepsychotic personality, good intelligence, affective features especially if associated with *pyknic* physique, a lively affectivity and good rapport are also all favourable features. *Asthenic* or *leptosomatic* body build, a strongly positive family history, insidious onset, marked ego and thought disorder, affective flattening and lack of resistance to symptoms are generally unfavourable prognostic indicators.

Further reading

Clare, A. (1976) *Psychiatry in Dissent*, chapters 4 & 5. London: Tavistock.

Feighner, J. P., Robins, E., Guze, S. B., Woodruff, R. A., Winokur, G. and Munoz, R. (1972) Diagnostic criteria for use in psychiatric research. *Archives of General Psychiatry* 26: 57–63.

Fish, F. J. (1976) *Schizophrenia*, Hamilton, M. (ed.) 2nd edn. Bristol: John Wright.

Forrest, A. and Affleck, J. (eds.) (1975) *New Perspectives in Schizophrenia*. Edinburgh: Churchill Livingstone.

Mackay, A. V. P. and Crow, T. J. (1980) Positive and negative schizophrenic symptoms and the role of dopamine. *British Journal of Psychiatry* 137: 379–386.

8

Paranoid States

The term *paranoid* defines a tendency towards self-reference either of external events, which include the behaviour and attitude of others, and which may seem to the paranoid person to contain some special meaning for him; or of certain bodily happenings, the nature of which may be subject to delusional misinterpretation. Paranoid disorders, therefore, are those conditions in which the central clinical feature is the presence of delusional attitudes, or delusion-like ideas—such as are derived from the subject's affective state, or closely bound up with his personality structure—or primary delusions in the sense already defined. Although the content of such delusions is commonly persecutory, this is by no means invariable. Grandiose, religiose and hypochondriacal delusions are common. Certain special forms also occur such as delusional misidentification, and those which centre on the notion of loving and of being or not being loved, including delusions of jealousy.

Aetiology

In many instances, although paranoid symptoms are the most prominent feature, the disorder may be seen to be secondary to, or part of, a schizophrenic illness. In others the primary disorder is clearly of affective origin, the delusions which occur being potentiated by a depressive or manic condition. Paranoid delusions are also a common accompaniment of organic brain disease and may herald an oncoming state of dementia. There remains however, a group of disorders in which paranoid symptoms appear to be virtually the only mental abnormality to be discovered, at least for a substantial period of time. Some of these may possibly be largely of psychogenic origin.

Paranoid disorders may also occur transiently or lastingly in seemingly normal people either under the influence of adverse circumstances, such as isolation through physical causes or such as may be due to deafness or some other form of sensory deprivation, or where communication with others is grossly impaired as in the case of those in a foreign land who may perhaps be refugees among people whose language and customs they do not understand, or in prison or even for no discernible or seemingly adequate external reason at all.

When things go wrong human beings tend to split into two groups: those who blame themselves and those who blame others. Likewise, under the influence of strong emotion, balanced judgement may be impossible to achieve. In all paranoid states a sense of personal isolation and inner insecurity is prominent. In severer and overtly psychotic paranoid states this sense of isolation may be associated either with feelings of oppression or persecution or alternatively with an overwhelming sense of personal superiority. In both, however, and in varying degrees, awareness of the opposite tendency is also present. Thus he who feels himself exalted is also uneasily aware of his fundamental weakness and inferiority—his 'Achilles heel'—while he who feels persecuted is sensible at the same time of his own worth and individual value. To these feelings, together with a tendency towards the *projection* of blame for one's own shortcomings on to those of others, the term paranoid is given.

In view of the universality and hence the understandability of such conditions, it is not surprising that psychiatrists have often sought to explain paranoid states largely in psychological or psychodynamic terms. It is indeed often possible to do so in the case of certain sensitive, querulous or aggressive individuals who, under the impact of adverse experiences, are likely to respond with paranoid symptoms. Psychological mechanisms do not, however, adequately explain those states which arise from a primary delusion which is considered not to be *understandable* in terms of ordinary human experience. Paranoid states may therefore be separated into two fairly distinct groups: the first, an outcome of deviant personality development; the second, psychotic, and the result of an as yet unidentified somatopsychic *process*. Because in practice it is often difficult and at times impossible to draw a clear line between the two, the problem of the exact nature of paranoid states has for long been a battleground of dissension among clinical psychiatrists.

Psychopathology

The term *paranoia* has a long history. Among the early Greeks it was often used as loosely, as in the present day, to define a variety of mental disorders. Kraepelin, whose views on the nosological status of the disorder tended to fluctuate, defined it as:

The insidious development of a permanent and unshakable delusional system arising from internal causes, which is accompanied by perfect preservation of clear and orderly thinking, willing and acting.

In its original definition, the essential feature of paranoia is that other psychopathological phenomena, notably hallucinations, are absent, thus differentiating it from paraphrenia and attenuated forms of schizophrenia in which hallucinations are present as well as delusions, but in which personality deterioration is either absent or only of very gradual occurrence. Paranoia, it was originally said, runs a chronic course and although deterioration does not occur, recovery is never observed. Cases which answer all these criteria are rare, this being one reason for doubting the existence of paranoia as a clinical entity. Kraepelin also separated from *true* paranoia those patients who, following a specific traumatic experience in which they believed themselves to have been wronged, made this the starting point and focus of a delusional development. The *paranoid litigant* is the classic example.

However, in 1931, a follow-up study by Kolle, one of Kraepelin's pupils, showed that, sooner or later, the majority of his cases proved unmistakably to be schizophrenic, having furthermore a close hereditary relationship to schizophrenia. Kolle also observed that schizophrenia occurred very much more frequently in the families of paranoiacs as compared with the population at large. In contrast no cases of manic–depressive illness were found. Kolle concluded, therefore, that Kraepelinian paranoia was an attenuated form of schizophrenia. Taken overall, the available evidence is strongly in support of the essential unity of a range of variation extending from paranoia via paraphrenia to more overt forms of paranoid schizophrenia.

The opposing view has, however, had many eminent and influential supporters, all of whom have sought to explain paranoia essentially as a psychogenic illness; thus some have described mild abortive forms of paranoid illness which tend not only towards social recovery but in which the previous personality of the patient is of prime importance. Kretschmer, notably, described a group of conditions characterized by delusions of reference arising on the basis of a sensitive *character*. (*Note.* Those designated as *sensitive*—in the psychiatric sense—are those unduly impressionable persons who exhibit an undue tendency to ruminate about the possibly hidden meaning of some or other painful experience and who have a low capacity for release or the discharge of resulting emotional tension.)

Kretschmer postulated three cardinal factors in the genesis of these disorders—character, environment and experience—although he also assumed a hereditary or constitutional background. He saw these subjects as tender or vulnerable on the one hand; and, on the other, ambitious and self-affirmative, often with exaggerated ethical ideals almost impossible to attain. Any slight departure from these standards, possibly of a trivial kind such as a lapse from decorum in an ageing spinster (masturbation also figured prominently in Kretschmer's male cases), produces a sense of humiliating inadequacy which cannot be resolved and in the end, following some traumatic experience (*key experience*)—usually one in which the patient believes his particular weakness was revealed—an illness appears of which paranoid ideas of reference are the prime feature (*Sensitiver Beziehungswahn*). At this juncture the sufferer becomes convinced that others know of his moral lapse and that it has become a subject of widespread gossip. In a number of Kretschmer's cases, however, unmistakable *process* symptoms appeared, making it impossible to regard these reactions as other than schizophrenic episodes in which in view of their mildness psychological mechanisms seem to be unusually clear and consistent. In others, however, the basis of the condition may be primarily affectively determined rather than due to the insidious development of schizophrenic psychosis. Here and with adequate treatment the course and outcome of the disorder are likely to be benign.

Eugen Bleuler thought that paranoia arose from a disproportionate strength and stability of affect relative to the strength of the patient's power of logical association. This, he believed, gave rise to *katathymic delusions* based on a strong emotional or affective charge. A katathymic idea or delusion is that which is derived from a repressed or hidden complex, often having a sexual or some other content about which the sufferer is morbidly sensitive and secretly concerned. Nevertheless, Bleuler also thought, as some others do, that the illness might have taken root on the basis of a slight residual defect, the result of an earlier and possibly unrecognized schizophrenic episode.

Freud, taking the notion of the repressed complex somewhat further and on the basis of his celebrated Schreber case, ascribed paranoid illness to repressed homosexuality in patients whose psychosexual development had been fixated at the homosexual level. However, while many might still agree that, from a psychodynamic viewpoint, complex-determined thinking may play some part, the specificity of latent or buried homosexuality as an activating factor has in recent years been called into considerable doubt.

While, therefore, the majority of paranoid illnesses belong to schizophrenia, some may accompany affective psychoses, particularly manic states and depression in late middle age and among the elderly. In such cases a paranoid state may be *holothymically* rather than *katathymically* determined, that is, due to pervading mood rather than due to some concealed complex. Thus the depressive who feels himself shunned by his fellows does so because of his sense of utter worthlessness or guilt, feeling that others point to him as a 'leper' or outcast. Doubt has been expressed as to whether such delusional ideas should be regarded as paranoid in the strict sense. However, as projection and a sense of isolation are present, and sometimes, because of the patient's belief in the very uniqueness of his case, a note of grandiosity may not be entirely lacking, many would agree that the term paranoid is justified.

Clinical syndromes

Delusions of jealousy

The ideas and sometimes delusions of jealousy of the alcoholic are discussed elsewhere (see Chapter 11). Some of these can be understood psychologically as a reaction to sexual impotence and to a wife's growing aversion to her alcoholic husband. Probably, however, such ideas may either be of schizophrenic origin—for delusions of jealousy are by no means confined to the alcoholic or to those impotent due to some other cause—or possibly even more likely due to a fundamental personality defect which makes the formation and sustainment of a truly intimate personal relationship impossible.

From a psychodynamic viewpoint the notion of repressed homosexuality may again be evoked, for cases are certainly to be found which can at least be speculatively formulated in such terms. In these the jealousy of the spouse over his wife's supposed infidelity may best be understood by a consideration of his fantasy of himself indulging in a sexual relationship with the 'other man' whom he desires for his own. In view of this he therefore may be seen to be not so much jealous of his wife but of her lover (*Othello syndrome*).

Clinically delusional jealousy may give rise to a great deal of misery, sometimes to violent behaviour and occasionally to homicide. The jealous man tends constantly to spy on his spouse, observing her every movement, while subjecting her to perpetual cross-examination as to her daily doings. He may read her letters, go through her personal belongings and scrutinize her underwear for seminal stains. Curiously enough, however much he may torment her, it may be observed that he often stops short at any actual confrontation with her supposed lover, even if he really believes he knows who this is. Indeed it would appear almost as if he may actually realize that his suspicions of her infidelity are groundless but cannot, in the last resort, allow himself to be brought face to face with the truth.

Erotomania

Erotomania, which is not too far removed from delusional jealousy, is a state in which the subject, usually an unmarried woman, begins to believe that some exalted person is in love with her, but refuses to admit it. Once again the background of the condition ranges from an attenuated paranoid state with little in the way of personality deterioration and no other psychotic symptoms other than a monoideistic delusion (*'pure' erotomania; de Clèrambault's syndrome*) via a frankly paranoid psychosis to full-blown paranoid schizophrenia having as its central symptom a delusion of loving or of being loved. It is noteworthy that males are rarely affected and that the majority of the love objects are not only unmarried but possibly unmarriageable also, by virtue either of being already married or, if unmarried, homosexual, or in any event by being of higher economic or social status—sometimes even of royal birth—than the erotomanic subject. Thus stars of screen and stage, doctors, Roman Catholic priests and so on, are more than especially liable to become the subject of the erotomanic patient's fantasies.

Such patients can at times be a great nuisance to the target of their affections especially if they confront them. Until then they may have no knowledge whatsoever of the situation and, not infrequently, of the very existence of the lady concerned. Alternatively no confrontation may take place. Under this circumstance the delusion of being secretly loved may turn into one of persecution in that the patient may become publicly abusive or complain about the behaviour of her luckless and completely mystified victim to all and sundry, or even report him to the police ('Old Maid's Insanity'). As in the case of delusions of jealousy, erotomania can frequently be construed as a denial of repressed abnormal sexuality. Once having emerged, it tends also to be remarkably intractable.

Folie à deux

Folie à deux is essentially a variety of paranoid psychosis in which more than one person is involved. *Folie à trois, à quatre,* even *folie à famille* have all been described. There are several varieties of the condition which depend on the relationship between those affected, of which the commonest and most important is *folie imposée*, in which the more forceful individual imposes his delusions upon his partner. Although some maintain that strictly speaking those involved should not be blood relatives, a common heredity is evident in about 90 per cent of the reported cases.

The principal features which give birth to a *folie à deux* relationship are: firstly, the occurrence of a paranoid psychosis in the dominant partner—the *inducer*; secondly, a prolonged and intimate association between both partners; thirdly, the relative isolation of both partners from the community; and lastly, a personality disorder or latent psychotic tendency in the *recipient* which, after an initial period of resistance towards the acceptance of the inducer's delusions, leads him or her finally to accept them as fact. The content of the delusions can be of almost any kind but almost invariably has a persecutory quality. Separation of the affected partners or family members does not necessarily bring about a resolution of the condition of either, although this is said to be more likely in the case of the recipient or passive partner.

Hypochondriacal delusional states

There are several varieties of hypochondriacal delusional states, none of which is particularly uncommon. It is important to recognize that such ideas differ from the undue worries about health from which patients with abnormal emotional reactions may suffer and from obsessional preoccupations with disease. The essential difference between a hypochondriacal obsession and a hypochondriacal delusion is that the patient with the former, while able to accept temporary reassurance, can never quite convince himself that he has not got whatever disease it is that concerns him, whereas in the case of he who is deluded reassurance is completely without effect, so that never for one moment can he be convinced that his delusional belief is false. It is appropriate to include hypochondriacal delusional states under the heading of paranoid psychoses because in these conditions the patient may be regarded both as accuser and accused. Thus if he maintains he has cancer or venereal disease—both of which are diseases which carry some stigma—by virtue of his delusional belief he becomes in effect the person who is accusing himself by insisting in the face of all evidence to the contrary that he actually has the disease which he insists he has.

The most striking example of this is seen in the *nihilistic delusions* (*délire de négation*) which are the central feature of *Cotard's syndrome*. In this the patient may insist that his bowels are blocked or have turned to stone or even accuse himself of being dead. Although commonest perhaps as a manifestation of severe melancholia, nihilistic delusions may also occur in schizophrenia or with organic brain disease.

Sensitivity reactions

Sensitivity reactions are hypochondriacal states characterized by sensitive ideas or delusions of reference, as described by Kretschmer (see p. 132), which relate to some imagined or minor bodily deformity (*dysmorphophobia*) which, the patient is convinced, is a constant subject of discussion by acquaintances, workmates or even total strangers who, he believes, look meaningfully in his direction and at one another as he passes, making at the same time barely overheard but clearly derogatory remarks. The disorder most often effects sensitive and socially inadequate young men, although women are not altogether exempt. The sensitive focus is most frequently the patient's nose which he believes is too small, too large or in some way deformed. Usually no real deformity is evident or, if present, is so slight that those who learn of the patient's never-ending and intensive preoccupation with his supposedly offending organ may be left wondering just what all the fuss is about. Less frequently, the patient's concern is with his over-prominent ears and in the case of women with the size of the breasts. Such patients commonly importune plastic surgeons, some of whom may have learned by bitter experience the fallacy of trying to correct by surgery deformities which are more apparent than real.

Other varieties of sensitivity reactions include those who wrongly believe that they emit a foul anal or sexual smell and that others cough, sniff or avoid them on this account. Yet another group consists of those who react adversely to a variety of physical diseases or surgical operations (see Chapter 18).

Delusions of infestation

Delusions of infestation are clearly a form of hypochondriasis related also to sensitivity reactions, although tending to affect those in middle age. Here the content of the delusional belief is that the patient herself (the condition appears to be commoner in women) is infested, or the house in which she lives is overrun, most often by insects of various kinds. Sometimes the infestation is internal, such as the case of a middle-aged lady who believed she had a worm in her bladder. More often the delusion is of ants or other small insects running over the skin (*formication*) or a belief that such creatures have lodged themselves in one or other of the bodily orifices such as the auditory meatus. Such delusions tend to be extremely refractory to almost any form of treatment, leading in some cases, and as a last resort, to psychosurgery, which may sometimes be effective.

Where the delusions are of infestation of the house in which the patient lives, considerable trouble may be caused on account of repeated and importunate requests to the local health authority for disinfestation procedures. One difficulty is that many houses, especially older ones and those in which birds nest in the eaves, may actually be infested with fleas, mites, lice, thrips, etc., so that the patient's delusions may at first sight appear to have a basis of truth—a matter which may be nothing if not difficult to disentagle. However, the persistence of the complaints made usually and in due course reveals their delusional basis. Delusions of infestation are also a ready vehicle for the emergence of *folie à deux*, in which the spouse or some other person living with the patient comes to share her belief with seemingly equal conviction. Occasionally a whole family may be involved.

Paranoid personalities

Many active, self-righteous and dogmatic people who stand up for their rights, or protest on behalf of others and who react to real or supposed infringements, are often designated as *paranoid personalities*. They are often dominated by some overvalued idea and are given to founding or joining strange religious or political sects or odd movements of other kinds. The term, however, may not be justified unless the characteristic tendency to self-reference is present, which is by no means always the case. Where, however, such persons are subject to inevitable snubs and setbacks, as is sooner or later almost certain to happen, they may develop a growing feeling of certainty that some other person or group of persons is acting in concert to deprive them of their rights. Under this circumstance the term *paranoid* may be justified. Such a reaction is also not uncommon in those unsuccessfully seeking compensation for real or supposed injuries (*paranoid litigants*).

Diagnosis

Diagnosis may be difficult since the patient's ideas may in the first instance strike the observer as bearing the stamp of truth, so close to real and understandable experience do they seem to be. Furthermore, it must not be forgotten that the content of a delusion, such as that of marital infidelity, may be true in fact and yet still be a delusion. While paranoid features in depression or mania usually clear up with the disappearance of the basic illness, in a few cases the clearing away of depression uncovers an overt paranoid schizophrenic illness. Most difficult to assess are the *sensitivity reactions* for, despite the often clear psychogenesis of the subject's ideas and complete personality preservation over the years, together with normal working capacity and no other signs of illness, the probability is that many, possibly most of such cases, are very mild schizophrenics who will sooner or later show other symptoms of this disorder. Some, however, may respond to antidepressive treatment. Such conditions often so closely resemble obsessional states that differentiation may be difficult at times and require prolonged study and observation. In querulant patients, the sincerity of their aim must be questioned whatever the degree of justification of their complaints, however exaggerated, and however much supported by pettifogging detail, since it is often clear that the complaint is the thing and its removal merely a secondary matter.

Course and treatment

In general, the outlook for confirmed paranoid illnesses is poor as far as the delusions are concerned, with those exceptions already noted. Nevertheless many, even some paranoid schizophrenics, manage with ups and downs to exist in the community, alone or with psychiatric support or the support of an understanding general practitioner. Indeed, more paranoid individuals are to be found outside rather than inside psychiatric hospitals. Many such patients have enough insight to conceal their delusions, although they often strike others as odd, withdrawn and having a curious coldness and stiffness of manner. The condition of some who are seekers after compensation might clear up following a satisfactory settlement of their claim were it not that the injury which is sustained provides an occasion for the emergence of symptoms which commonly derive from a deep-seated dissatisfaction of the subjects with themselves and their life situations. Thus the injury serves to mobilize a latent paranoid personality development.

In more overtly psychotic patients with paranoid states, these may sometimes be partially or considerably relieved by ECT or by the long-term administration of phenothiazines or other tranquillizers.

However, for such treatment to be effective, the patient's cooperation must be sought, which in such cases is by no means easy to achieve. On the psychological side there is also some evidence that firm handling may sometimes be effective. Indeed, although patient and therapist may have to agree to differ (it is imperative that the therapist should never in any way subscribe to the patient's delusions), it is surprising how often a supportive relationship can be formed thereby preventing the patient's delusions from getting out of hand.

Further reading

Enoch, M. D. and Trethowan, W. H. (1979) *Uncommon Psychiatric Syndromes.* Bristol: John Wright.

9

Organic Disorders

The term *organic* is used in psychiatry to define those disorders due to some form of tangible brain pathology or a fairly well-defined metabolic or biochemical disturbance which disrupts brain function and produces mental symptoms. In early life, before, during or after birth and in the formative years, brain disease gives rise to mental impairment (*amentia*). In adults in whom brain and mind have matured normally, a disorder affecting the central nervous system may cause temporary disorganization (*delirium*) or, in the event of progressive neuronal damage, a persistent and continuing loss of mental faculties (*dementia*).

Leaving mental impairment aside (see Chapter 21), there are two main types of organic mental disorder to be considered, together with certain special varieties. The first, *delirium*, is an acute potentially reversible state often transient and due to a wide variety of causes. Providing that the underlying disorder which gives rise to delirium does not prove fatal, the sufferer will usually recover his mental equilibrium as his physical health is restored. There are exceptions, however. For example, a patient who has had several bouts of *delirium tremens* and has recovered more or less completely on previous occasions may subsequently not fully recover. Although his acute delirious state may pass, it may leave in its wake a chronic disabling amnesic-confabulatory state (*Korsakow's syndrome*). Acute brain infections giving rise to delirium, such as encephalitis, can also give rise to some degree of permanent impairment. The same is true of some cases of head injury.

The other primary type of organic mental disorder, *dementia*, is an outcome of destruction or degeneration of brain tissue. Once again, there is a large number of possible causes. Dementia tends to be of insidious onset. Most cases are irreversible and run a protracted course during which progressive emotional and intellectual impairment occurs. But while, on the whole, the outcome of delirium is favourable, the prognosis of dementia is not; although there are several conditions such as *myxoedema, vitamin B12 deficiency* and *normal pressure hydrocephalus* which produce a state closely resembling dementia, but which if diagnosed early and adequately treated may be reversible. Likewise, the progress of *general paralysis* (GPI) may be halted if treatment for neurosyphilis is begun soon enough.

The next point to be made is that the clinical picture of delirium is more or less the same whatever its basic cause, although it may vary considerably in severity and duration. Much the same applies to dementia where the kind of emotional and intellectual deterioration which occurs is manifestly the same whatever the basic pathology. All other variations are bound up with the premorbid personality of the patient. Thus life experience and premorbid personality may colour, although not fundamentally alter, the main manifestations of an organic mental illness.

What has been said so far applies to those mental conditions which are primarily the outcome of widespread or generalized brain dysfunction or disease. Where *focal* lesions predominate, certain more specific clinical pictures may emerge according to the particular area of the brain involved. A good example is the *frontal lobe syndrome*. Other focal lesions which may give rise to special defects of brain function include various forms of *aphasia, apraxia*, etc. which may occur either as isolated phenomena or in a setting of dementia. A full description of these is not, however, within the scope of this book.

Delirium

Delirious states are most often encountered in general hospitals, usually as a complication of some physical illness. In the past, infectious conditions accompanied by high fever were often accompanied by delirium; these, however, have become rarer since the introduction of antibiotics.

Aetiology
Whatever the cause it appears that some people are more prone to delirium than others. This susceptibility may be constitutional or of hereditary origin, or may stem from some previously acquired form of mental instability, such as may occur in alcoholics or drug takers. Age is also a factor, delirium being common at the two ends of life; when the nervous system is immature or, as it were, postmature. There are many causes of delirium.

1. *Infections.* Septicaemia, many febrile illnesses including malaria, typhoid, pneumonia, meningitis, encephalitis, and a variety of viral infections.
2. *Exogenous intoxications.* Alcohol, hypnotics, amphetamines, drug abuse, belladonna, acute poisoning with lead and other heavy metal poisons, industrial chemicals, etc.
3. *Metabolic disorders.* Hepatic and renal failure, acute porphyria, electrolyte disturbances, hyperglycaemia and hypoglycaemia, also malnutrition and avitaminoses.
4. *Cerebral catastrophes.* Head injury; subdural haematoma; cerebral

thrombosis, haemorrhage and embolism; raised intracranial pressure, neoplasm; demyelinating disorders, etc.

5. *Cardiovascular disorders.* Cardiac failure, severe anaemia, anoxia, blood dyscrasias, hypercapnia.

6. *Postanaesthetic and postoperative complications.*

7. *Epilepsy.*

8. *Profound physical exhaustion.*

Clinical manifestations

The cardinal feature of acute delirium is *clouding* or *partial impairment of consciousness* which waxes and wanes according to a variety of circumstances. Other manifestations, all of which are secondary to clouded consciousness, can be ascribed to lack of communication between the delirious patient and his immediate environment.

Delirium tremens

Delirium tremens may be regarded as the prototype. It occurs in chronic alcoholics and is usually brought about by sudden deprivation of alcohol—*abstinence delirium*. This may be precipitated by an accident such as fracture, a head injury, a surgical operation, a febrile infection such as pneumonia, or an excessive bout of drinking leading to arrest on account of drunkenness or any combination of these. However, despite the well-recognized circumstances which can precipitate an attack, the exact aetiology of delirium tremens is still obscure. It seems likely, however, that its immediate cause is some kind of metabolic disturbance.

Delirium tremens is usually of rapid onset, sometimes within a few hours of stopping drinking, at which point an attack of 'the shakes' may begin. Alternatively, there may be a short prodromal phase of 24 to 48 hours duration characterized by increasing uneasiness and perplexity, impaired and distorted comprehension, insomnia and terrifying nightmares. These are soon succeeded by illusions and hallucinations, commonly visual, but affecting other sensory modalities also, and all commonly horrific; disorientation in time and place; defective registration of current events; marked restlessness, agitation and apprehension. The subject's emotional state, which is extremely labile, is characteristically one of fear and terror. He may imagine that those around him are enemies against whom he may violently endeavour to defend himself. Between such excited episodes there may, by day, be intervals of relative clarity. By night when darkness looms his condition may worsen. Hence the basis of the old fallacy that the delirious patient should be treated in a quiet, darkened room, thus adding to his already existing state of sensory deprivation.

Apart from his abnormal mental state, the patient with delirium tremens is physically ill. He may suffer from fever and his pulse, though full in the early stages, tends later to become feeble. He may be severely dehydrated so that his urinary output is greatly diminished. Motor weakness, severe irregular tremors or continual movements of his hands and fingers and disordered articulation are usually evident. Epileptic fits may occur. Occasionally severe twitching of muscles due to *hypomagnesaemia* may be observed. However, with adequate drug treatment delirium tremens can now be brought readily under control; untreated it usually lasts five to seven days, following which remission occurs. A small number of patients may die of circulatory failure, but with modern methods of treatment this is now much less likely to happen.

Encephalitis

Because of the many ways in which it may initially manifest itself, encephalitis is considered separately. Epidemic *encephalitis lethargica*, the classic form of the disease, is now rare, although occasional examples are seen. However, encephalitis due to a variety of other viral infections is common enough. These include *mumps, measles, glandular fever* and encephalitis caused by *herpes simplex* virus and *acute inclusion body encephalitis* which may possibly be identical to that caused by herpes simplex, and some others the exact cause of which may be hard to find. As in epidemic encephalitis, the presenting clinical picture is highly variable and may at the onset mimic almost any form of functional mental illness, although the organic nature of the disease becomes apparent sooner or later when clouding of consciousness and other symptoms of delirium supervene. Other states resembling mania and catatonic schizophrenia sometimes accompanied by hyperpyrexia are also seen. A variety of fits, often midbrain seizures, may occur. Electroencephalography, CT scan and serological investigation may aid diagnosis. However, even following these and brain biopsy diagnosis may remain obscure.

The *prognosis* of encephalitis varies although it is always guarded. While death does not occur even in some severer cases, neurological and mental sequelae are common. Postencephalitic parkinsonian symptoms may follow; likewise, compulsive thoughts and actions and violently aggressive and sometimes self-destructive behaviour. Alternatively, complete recovery is possible.

Children may undergo a marked change in character as a result of encephalitis. From being well behaved they may become restless, irritable and unrestrained in behaviour. Attention suffers markedly; they may become so distractable as to be incapable of learning. There is some evidence to suggest that their deficit in attention span and concomitant difficult behaviour may be improved by amphetamine. It is possible, therefore, that in some cases encephalitis may have some lasting adverse effect on the alerting properties of the reticular-activating system.

Encephalopathy

As with encephalitis, there is a large number of basic causes of encephalopathy. Two are considered here.

Wernicke's syndrome (polioencephalitis haemorrhagica superior) is probably due largely to thiamine deficiency, although other types of avitaminosis may play a part. Alcoholics having a restricted diet over a prolonged period may be liable to develop this condition, although it can occur as a result of malnutrition or malabsorption from other causes, such as gastric carcinoma. Haemorrhages into the grey matter around the walls of the third ventricle and into the mamillary bodies occur. The onset is usually fairly acute with ataxia, somnolence progressing to torpor, delirium, ophthalmoplegia and diplopia, followed, if the patient recovers from these by the *amnesic (Korsakow) syndrome.*

Lead encephalopathy occurs primarily in children, although it may be seen in adults following massive exposure to lead fumes in industrial accidents. The presenting symptoms usually consist of a disturbance of behaviour in which the child is irritable and restless and may show symptoms suggesting schizophrenia. This tends to be followed by delirious or maniacal behaviour. Raised intracranial pressure giving rise to severe projectile vomiting may cause coma. Marked pallor may be present. The mortality rate is high and permanent neurological sequelae or mental impairment (see also Chapter 21) are common.

Confusional states

Milder delirious states are sometimes referred to as confusional states. This is not altogether desirable as *confusion* is a vague and ambiguous term. Once again, clouding of consciousness is the key symptom, unaccompanied, however, by the more florid symptoms of delirium. Thinking is scanty and loses its sequence so that *incoherence* is a prominent feature.

All true confusional states are of organic origin, although their causes are often difficult to determine. They occur most prominently and in an episodic fashion in old people in whom they may be superimposed upon *arteriopathic* or other forms of *dementia.*

Head injury

This is a common and important cause. When of any degree of severity, the immediate effect is loss of consciousness (*concussion*). This occurs primarily in closed head injuries, but not necessarily with penetrating wounds. The period of unconsciousness may last from a minute or so to several hours or days. On recovery there is usually a period of clouding of consciousness of some duration. In severe cases there may be noisy delirium with all its characteristic features or, in less severe cases, a confusional state. Some patients following head injury appear after a time to be almost normal, although subsequently it may be discovered that they are behaving automatically or are confabulating, later professing complete amnesia for this phase. The more chronic and long-term effects of head injury are described on p. 156.

Twilight states

In twilight states a type of alteration of consciousness occurs, described as 'narrowing of the field of consciousness'. It occurs in certain forms of epilepsy, when it is sometimes known as *automatism*. Under this circumstance the condition appears to be due to a prolonged psychomotor seizure, characterized by altered consciousness, automatic, unmotivated and sometimes aggressive behaviour, together with hallucinations which are often visual and vivid (see Chapter 10).

Twilight states are, however, not always of organic origin. They may also occur in depression and in hysterical disorders, in particular in the *Ganser syndrome*. Here, there is a disturbance of attention occurring under the influence of strong affect which singularly engages the patient's mind—that is, he dwells on one idea and one idea alone—to the virtual exclusion of everything in the periphery of his field of consciousness. During a twilight state complicated actions, sometimes occupying days or even longer periods of time, may be carried out. The patient may wander, often many miles from home (*fugue*) and, since his attention is engrossed almost exclusively by a dominating topic, little or nothing else is apprehended and nothing retained (*amnesia*). Where the basis of a twilight state is psychogenic and the subject, having something to hide, is amnesic, the formula for many can be summed up in Nietzsche's famous words: 'I have done that says my memory. I have not done that says my pride. Finally my memory yields.'

Other acute states

There are other acute psychiatric disorders which, at first sight, may resemble or be mistaken for delirious and confusional states.

Acute mania, now rare, may present as a state of wild overactivity together with incoherence. As a result of exhaustion, an element of true delirium may be superadded.

Catatonic excitement may present a very similar picture though the previous history, together with careful observation, will usually reveal the true diagnosis.

Acute paranoid panic may occur in some schizophrenic patients who are overcome by delusional threats which lead them to believe their lives are in danger. A similar acute paranoid psychosis, possibly of psychogenic origin, may occur postoperatively in those of a different cultural background who, in a strange land or surroundings, may misinterpret their environment and fear the intentions of those around them.

Treatment

A delirious or confused patient almost invariably requires admission to hospital. Once there, he should be nursed in a well-lit room as sensory deprivation through darkness enhances existing confusion and disorientation. Where possible, such appliances as bed rails are to be avoided, as the subject may understandably mistake these for prison bars. The secret of control is not physical restraint but good nursing and adequate sedation. Delirious patients should never be left on their own.

Symptomatic control is essential. Close attention should be paid to fluid intake and output and the correction of any electrolyte imbalance. Most confusional and delirious states can be quickly and adequately controlled by phenothiazine drugs, such as chlorpromazine in doses of 50–100 mg, 4–6 hourly as required, there being no case nowadays for the use of such anachronistic remedies as paraldehyde. Haloperidol appears to be better than phenothiazines and has the advantage of not causing hypotension when administered parenterally, as chlorpromazine sometimes does. Haloperidol is relatively non-toxic and may be given in variable doses of 10 mg or more. Although an antiparkinsonian drug such as procyclidine may be required, this does not appear to be as necessary when haloperidol is given parenterally as when it is given orally. Chlormethiazole is also useful in controlling confusional states in the elderly. Finally, delirium tremens and other delirious or confusional states due to avitaminosis will often respond strikingly to intravenous Parentrovite. Otherwise, their treatment must depend upon cause, which would be sought vigorously once acute symptoms have been overcome.

Chronic brain syndromes

Included under the heading *chronic brain syndromes* are various forms of diffuse and degenerative brain disorders which, as a general rule, give rise to progressive and irreversible dementia of which the primary features are loss of intellect and deterioration of personality. Also included are the mental effects of certain focal brain lesions such as the *frontal-lobe* and *Korsakow's syndrome* which may produce more circumscribed mental symptoms.

Dementia

As indicated at the beginning of this chapter, symptoms of dementia are of two kinds: *basic* or essential—these being present to some degree in every case—and *accessory* or idiosyncratic. The basic symptoms, which are intellectual and emotional, are due directly to whatever brain disease underlies them. In contrast, the accessory symptoms are derived largely from the personality of the patient. Because brain disease tends to cause disinhibition, personality traits previously kept under control may become exaggerated. Thus a thrifty man becomes a miser, while one always hard to please becomes increasingly crotchety and cantankerous. Many symptoms, notably a delusion of being robbed by relatives—notwithstanding this having an occasional basis of truth—are related both to the previous personality of the patient and to the intellectual impairment which interferes with his understanding of other people's actions and motives.

The intellectual deficit in dementia consists of a progressive loss of memory, initially for recent events but tending in due course to extend further backwards in time, although somewhat irregularly, so that even when profound, islets of memory may be preserved. Initially the difficulty may not be so much one of actual memory loss, but of slowness in remembering. This underlying psychological malfunction also comprises an inability to grasp, understand, retain and recall new impressions. Disorientation in time occurs, later in space or place and in very advanced cases approaching mindlessness, disorientation of person may be evident. Distractability, impairment of judgement and distortion of the critical faculties are soon apparent. This progressive loss of mental functions tends roughly to follow the phylogenetic pattern of their development, although in reverse order, so that it is the most recently acquired functions which are often the soonest affected. However, even in severer cases islets of memory tend, nevertheless, to be preserved.

These deficits are accompanied by emotional lability and loss of control (*emotional incontinence*), both of which may occur early, even before intellectual deficit is apparent. The dementing patient, therefore, is easily provoked to anger or tears. Alternatively, he may become foolish or flippant. In other cases more sustained changes of mood occur so that continuing depression, apathy or chronic excitability colours the clinical picture. Because of narrowing interests, the subject tends to become increasingly self-centred, hypochondriacal and indifferent to the feelings of others. He may thieve or commit sexual or other offences. As time passes his manner, habits and standards of personal hygiene inevitably deteriorate, so that he becomes dirty and dishevelled. Suspicious of others, he may become increasingly secretive, tending to hoard rubbish and even his own excreta.

Classification

It has long been customary to classify states of dementia according to age of onset. Thus the term *senile dementia* refers to cases occurring in old age; that is after 65 years when, in a chronological sense, an ageing person may, conventionally, be deemed to be senile. Because this distinction has become progressively blurred it would seem that the time has come to drop this somewhat pejorative term, it being generally realized that the clinical features of dementia in the aged differ in no very essential respect from those encountered in younger persons.

The term *presenile dementia* carries with it an even more dubious connotation, although one accepted by general usage. While at first sight the term may appear to refer to cases of dementia which occur in those under the age of 65, used more strictly it defines certain degenerative brain diseases of which two, *Alzheimer's* and *Pick's diseases*, are usually regarded as the most important. Because, however, there are a number of other pathological processes which may give rise to dementia in middle age, such as *cerebral arteriopathy, syphilis (GPI)*, and *Huntington's chorea*, there seems to be little point in retaining presenile dementia as a special category. In any event, the pathology of dementia in old age bears a close resemblance and may in its essential aspects be identical to that of Alzheimer's disease, although arteriosclerotic and other changes may be added (see Chapter 21).

A logical classification of the various causes of dementia is difficult to devise. The following should, however, prove fairly satisfactory in practice. Nonetheless, and as will be readily perceived, there is in the present state of knowledge an inevitable overlap between the various aetiological categories which have been suggested. In certain cases the placement of a cause in one category can, therefore, be considered as no better than including it in another.

1. *Infections.* Encephalitis, syphilis, trypanosomiasis, Jakob–Creutzfeld disease (slow virus).

2. *Exogenous intoxications.* Chronic alcoholism, lead and other heavy-metal poisoning.

3. *Metabolic disorders.* Myxoedema, vitamin B12 and folic acid deficiency, pellagra, hepatolenticular degeneration.

4. *Cerebral disasters.* Trauma, haemorrhage, stroke, multiple infarcts, thromboangiitis obliterans, tumour, disseminated lupus erythematosus, normal pressure hydrocephalus, anoxic damage, hypoglycaemia, etc.

5. *Demyelinating disorders.* Multiple sclerosis, Schilder's disease, Devic's disease.

6. *Heredofamilial and degenerative disorders.* Huntington's chorea, Pick's and Alzheimer's diseases.

7. *Epilepsy.*

Not all of the conditions listed above will be dealt with in detail;

only those which are the commonest and most important will be considered.

Cerebral arteriopathy

Although until recently it was considered that cerebral arteriopathy with or without accompanying hypertension was the commonest cause of dementia from middle age onwards, this idea probably arose out of the fact that some degree of arteriosclerosis is the commonest autopsy finding in the brain from the fifth or sixth decade onwards. However, it has proved impossible to correlate the extent of arteriosclerosis evident at autopsy with the sufferer's state of mind prior to his death. There is, however, no doubt that multiple small infarcts which may not necessarily give rise to gross physical signs during life, but which lead to areas of cerebral softening or, alternatively, a single massive lesion causing a stroke, can give rise to intellectual deficit varying in degree according to the amount of cerebral softening present.

The relationship between cerebral arteriopathy and loss of intellectual functioning is further complicated by the fact that arteriosclerotic and other pathological changes of different origin may coexist.

Physical signs

Peripheral arteriosclerosis, even that affecting the retinal vessels, is no guide to the extent to which the cerebral arteries are involved. Hypertension is present in roughly half of those with arteriopathy; in the other half the blood pressure may lie within, or even below, the normal range. Focal neurological signs when present are very variable; aphasia, apraxia and agnosia are common but not constantly demonstrable.

Symptoms

The earliest physical symptoms are those often associated with hypertension; the most frequent is headache of vague character, described as a feeling of fullness and associated with non-vertiginous dizziness. Insomnia—chiefly difficulty in getting to sleep together with flickering lights in front of the eyes—tinnitus and increased fatiguability are common complaints.

Among a wide variety of mental symptoms, difficulty in recalling names and other familiar matters is usually evident. On testing, *nominal aphasia* may be demonstrable (see p. 69). Lack of concentration is common, so that the sufferer feels he can no longer cope with the day's work. He is frequently depressed, is often irritable and commonly emotionally labile. A striking feature is a relatively good preservation of personality, together with a degree of awareness of mental disability which may lead him to become tearful and depressed over his failure to perform adequately during a psychometric test or indeed any other test procedure ('*catastrophic reaction*'). He may express paranoid, self-reproachful, self-pitying or hypochondriacal ideas. Episodic confusion lasting several hours or days is common; this is more prone to occur at night. All these symptoms are characterized by the irregularity and variability of their occurrence, together with a striking tendency to periodic and sometimes quite remarkable remissions, not usually apparent in dementia due to other causes.

In more advanced cases, possibly following a series of minor cerebrovascular accidents, conduct may become much more grossly disturbed especially when consciousness is impaired; although this, too, varies greatly in intensity. As the condition progresses, disorientation both in time and place, together with severe memory changes, aphasic disturbances, delusional ideas and some occasionally quite extraordinary visual hallucinations occur, all of which may lead to a serious problem of management at home. However, even despite continuing general disintegration, the *core* of the patient's personality may remain remarkably well preserved.

Diagnosis

The organic nature of the disorder is not infrequently overlooked in its earlier stages. This is especially true of those who present with seemingly hysterical symptoms. However, consideration of the history together with evidence of increasing emotional lability and of remarkable fluctuations in the patient's mental state should point to the diagnosis. While formal mental examination may offer confirmation, this does not usually reveal the underlying cause of dementia which, in the case of cerebral arteriopathy, can only be made with complete assurance in the presence of focal neurological signs. Even then it is still necessary to rule out other conditions such as a cerebral tumour or general paralysis. The latter is usually easily excluded by negative serological tests, while the former may be revealed by electroencephalography or by a CT scan where available.

Alzheimer's disease

Alzheimer's disease, although relatively rare in middle age, is considerably commoner than Pick's disease; both taken together have a morbidity risk of about 0.1 per cent. Over the age of 65, Alzheimer's disease is said to affect one person in six. Both disorders, which may first occur in those between 55 and 60 years of age, are often clinically indistinguishable. Thus, although pathologically distinct, it is convenient initially to consider them together. Both, during life, are characterized by progressive and relentless dementia accompanied in due course by focal signs. In Alzheimer's disease the sex incidence appears to be about equal, whereas in Pick's disease twice as many if not more women are affected. The genetic background of the two conditions is also distinct. In Pick's disease the influence of a dominant autosomal gene has been suggested, whereas in Alzheimer's disease multifactorial inheritance appears more likely.

Pathology

The characteristic pathological appearance of the brain in Alzheimer's disease consists of generalized atrophy chiefly involving the frontal, temporal and parietal lobes, together with the basal ganglia. The histopathological changes consist of loss of ganglion cells, together with the formation of *argentophil plaques, neurofibrillary tangles, granulovacuolar degeneration* and *congophilic angiopathy*.

Recent investigations have indicated that a selective destruction of the cortical cholinergic system is an important factor underlying these pathological changes. There is apparently a quantitative relationship between choline acetyl transferase activity, which may be considerably reduced, and the extent of the neurofibrillary changes and the formation of argentophil plaques, there being a correlation between the number of these and the degree of dementia.

Clinical features

After a prodromal period of vague symptoms—headaches, insomnia and irritability—*memory changes* begin to attract attention. A degree of forgetfulness inappropriate in the case of one still comparatively young, leading perhaps to important opportunities being forgotten, may soon become a cause for concern among a patient's relatives and friends. Severe *spatial disorientation* may occur quite early, leading to episodes of wandering and becoming lost even in familiar surroundings. Likewise, a disorder of body image may be apparent so that the patient cannot correctly identify parts of his own body and may have difficulty in dressing himself correctly (*dressing apraxia*). Despite such eccentricities, the subject's behaviour may still be socially acceptable, even appearing superficially normal for a considerable period (*presbyophrenia*).

With progress focal symptoms such as aphasia, apraxia and agnosia may appear, together with extrapyramidal signs leading to rigidity and alteration of gait. A curious speech disorder, *logoclonus*—an incomprehensible and staccato repetition of the last syllable uttered—may become evident. Fits may occur and finally progression towards the most profound stages of dementia, with all its tragic and inevitable consequences, not only for the patient but also for his friends and relatives who must, perforce, bear witness to the ultimate tragedy which increasing cerebral degeneration brings.

Pick's disease

Pathology

Whereas in Alzheimer's disease cerebral degeneration is more or less diffuse, in Pick's disease it is more circumscribed, and confined to the phylogenetically newest parts of the brain, the frontal or temporal lobes or both. This type of atrophy which may be asymmetrical can be recognized at autopsy immediately the skull is opened. In the frontal lobes the atrophic process spares the motor area; in the temporal, degeneration is mostly limited to the lower portion. Histopathologically there is an absence of plaques and neurofibrillary changes; the cortical cells show *ballooning* together with an associated reactive gliosis. Only rarely are the basal ganglia affected.

Clinical features

The onset is gradual. Initially a disorder of memory is prominent as in Alzheimer's disease. Involvement of the frontal lobes may give rise to gross disorders of conduct such as lying or thieving, and promiscuous and sometimes violent behaviour. As the disorder progresses the sufferer tends to become apathetic. Character change and poverty of judgement become more marked. Focal symptoms appear. Where the frontal lobes are most involved there is increasing anergia with perhaps mutism, with temporal lobe involvement. Sensory aphasia may occur. Extrapyramidal symptoms are occasionally seen. The final stage is similar to that seen in Alzheimer's disease. Diagnosis during life may sometimes be made by air-encephalography, by CT scan, or with greater certainty by brain biopsy although today it would seem rarely justifiable to submit a patient to this procedure.

Jakob–Creutzfeldt disease

Jakob–Creutzfeldt disease (*cortico-striato-spinal degeneration; spastic pseudosclerosis*) is due to a diffuse degeneration of the brain, having its onset during the fourth decade or later. It runs a fairly rapid course leading to death in the course of a year or two. The main features are spastic weakness of the limbs, extrapyramidal symptoms, cortical blindness, myoclonic jerking and progressive affective and intellectual deterioration. It is a rare condition and although some doubt has been cast on its existence as an independent entity it has relatively recently been shown to be possible, as in the case of Kuru, to transmit the disease to monkeys, though at present the aetiological significance of this finding is not clear. The causative agent is believed to be a 'slow' virus, the exact nature of which has yet to be determined.

Huntington's chorea

The two principal features of Huntington's chorea are jerky choreiform or choreoathetoid involuntary movements and dementia. As a general rule the movements precede the occurrence of dementia, often by many years, although, owing to frontal lobe involvement, behavioural changes sometimes occur before other manifestations of the disease become evident. Because the condition is due to a non-sex-linked dominant gene, approximately 50 per cent of the children of an affected parent are themselves liable to be affected. The pathological basis of the disorder comprises degenerative changes which involve the frontal lobes, the basal ganglia and ultimately the rest of the cerebral cortex. The tragedy of Huntington's chorea is that its manifestations do not usually appear before the fourth decade so that gene carriers have, by then, often given birth to children, a number of whom having inherited the gene will inevitably develop the disorder. So far no means of identifying the gene carriers is known although there are perhaps grounds for believing that this may soon be discovered; thus allowing the promotion of a positive eugenic programme which could—apart from occasional genetic mutations which are believed to occur—lead to complete prevention of the disorder.

Initially the choreoathetoid movements tend to involve the face and upper limbs, spreading in due course to involve the whole body, giving rise to explosive articulation, ataxia and continuous movement of body and limbs while awake. One half of the body and limbs may be affected in advance of the other. Mental symptoms comprise emotional instability, outbursts of irritability and slowly progressive intellectual deterioration. These symptoms, while differing in no essential way from those of dementia due to other causes, may remain relatively slight for many years. The duration of the disorder tends to be lengthy, extending over a period of 10 to 20 years.

There is no treatment which will halt the inevitable progress of Huntington's chorea, although some limited control over involuntary movements can be achieved by the use of phenothiazines such as chlorpropazate.

Neurosyphilis

In view of the decline of syphilis as a cause of mental illness and the now relative infrequency of neurosyphilis in the Western world, it would now appear necessary to deal only briefly with this subject.

General paralysis

This is a diffuse meningoencephalitis caused by *Treponema pallidum*, having its impact mainly on the frontal and temporal lobes. The manifestations of the disease are threefold: serological, neurological and psychiatric, in that order of diagnostic importance, the diagnosis resting on this triad. The incubation period is long, ranging from 8 to 20 years, the average age of onset being in the mid-fifties.

Clinical features

The first sign is frequently some gross error of judgement, tact or propriety, as, for example, when a male patient unconcernedly passed water in front of a large crowd at the first tee of a well-known golf club. The symptoms may, however, be much more indefinite and of a *neurasthenic* kind, the danger in this instance being that they may be dismissed as psychogenic. Alternatively, an epileptic fit may be the first sign. Whatever the form of onset, the progress of the disorder may well, if untreated, lead to dementia differing in no essential respect from that due to other causes. However, and in the initial stages, other pathoplastically determined symptoms, derived from the patient's premorbid personality, may be evident. It is these which determine the particular form the established picture will take: expansive, depressed, schizophrenic, paranoid, and so on. It is, however, the simple dementing form which is the most common. There is also a juvenile type which is congenitally determined. The principal neurological signs of general paralysis include Argyll Robertson pupils, slurred speech, tremor and spastic quadriplegia although a hemiplegic onset can occur. Sensory symptoms due to posterior column loss are present only if the spinal cord is involved (*taboparesis*).

In active neurosyphilis the CSF is serologically positive in 100 per cent of cases, and the blood in 90–100 per cent. The CSF protein is raised, being usually in the region of 0.05–0.10 g per cent. There is a lymphocytosis of up to 100 per mm^3.

Diagnosis

It is essential that diagnosis should be made so far as is possible before the appearance of physical signs and by examination of the cerebro-spinal fluid. In more advanced cases the clinical picture of digital, labial and lingual tremor ('trombone tongue'), together with dysarthria, sluggish pupils and absent knee and ankle jerks (if tabes is also present) may suggest chronic alcoholism (*alcoholic pseudoparesis*). This is a fairly uncommon condition which may be distinguished from general paralysis by an examination of the blood and cerebrospinal fluid. Cerebrovascular accidents, other forms of dementia and cerebral tumour also enter into the differential diagnosis. It should also be noted that while nowadays cerebral neurosyphilis is considerably rarer than it used to be, atypical forms have become relatively commoner.

Treatment

The introduction of penicillin marked a new era in the treatment of neurosyphilis. It should be given intensively beginning with 20 000 units every six hours intramuscularly for two or three days followed by 1 000 000 units of benzyl-penicillin daily up to a total of 20 million units. If the CSF remains serologically positive after six months, a further course of treatment is indicated. Electroconvulsive therapy (ECT) may be given to excited and delirious patients in preference to heavy sedation, and to depressed cases, concurrently with penicillin. By these means good remissions may be obtained in some 30 per cent of those patients treated whose degree of mental deterioration has not progressed very far, while in less favourable cases the extremes of physical enfeeblement with persistent incontinence and secondary infection may be postponed for many years.

Meningovascular syphilis is usually accompanied by severe headache. There may be episodes of delirium, and focal signs are common, also epileptiform seizures. A *gumma* may produce signs and symptoms of cerebral tumour, and the mental state may be dull and clouded. The blood is usually serologically positive although this is not invariably so in the case of CSF. The condition usually responds readily to antisyphilitic treatment.

Cerebral tumour

In the later stages, tumours of the cerebrum all produce dullness and dementia, ending in coma and death. Prior to this such symptoms as may occur are predominantly of focal origin or due to raised intracranial pressure.

Prefrontal tumours may give rise to mental changes in the early stages before physical signs have become well marked. Of these, *character changes* stand out: irresponsibility, facetiousness (*Witzelsucht*) or sometimes frankly antisocial behaviour. The same may occur in patients with atrophy of one or both frontal lobes following head injury—the so-called *frontal lobe syndrome*. However, it should be noted that a similar clinical picture can occur as a result of focal lesions elsewhere in the brain. In frontal lobe lesions, however, the presence of a grasp or sucking reflex may be an important localizing sign. Motor aphasia may also be present.

Temporal lobe tumours may give rise to *psychomotor attacks* (see Chapter 10). Sensory aphasia may be present, mostly of the nominal variety, followed by a syntactical disturbance with paraphasia which may lead very easily to the erroneous diagnosis of dementia. Visual field defects, quadrantic or complete homonymous hemianopia are common, resulting from involvement of the visual pathway.

Parietal lobe tumours may cause a considerable number of symptoms of great interest to the psychiatrist, the understanding of which is still very far from complete. Appreciation of spatial relationships is impaired, causing defects in the ability to construct designs (*constructive apraxia*). There may be unawareness of the opposite side of the body and other disturbances of the body image, also impaired comprehension and expression of speech. A combination of symptoms, finger agnosia, acalculia, agraphia, and right–left disorientation (*Gerstmann's syndrome*), may arise from lesions in the area of the angular gyrus.

Tumours of the corpus callosum lead the subject to become dull, apathetic and clouded. Disorientation and loss of memory for recent events are common and severe dementia may be present. At the same time, general or focal signs of a cerebral tumour may be slight or even absent. Pyramidal signs, at first more marked on one side, may occur, sometimes with other neurological signs and symptoms deriving from damage to adjacent structures.

Cerebral trauma

The more chronic sequelae of head injury are the outcome of its original extent, its site and, particularly, the premorbid personality of the sufferer. Open or penetrating head injuries are usually easier to assess than closed head injuries, in which diagnostic appraisal may initially be difficult. Apart from focal defects, which are usually readily identifiable, head injuries appear to bring about four main types of psychiatric disorder: intellectual deficits, affective disorders, behaviour problems and somatic complaints having no obvious basis. An association between intellectual deterioration and temporal or parietal lobe damage has been demonstrated, whereas disturbances of behaviour apparently occur more frequently when the frontal lobes are involved. It is difficult, however, to correlate with any exactitude the degree and site of brain damage following head injury with the occurrence and extent of post-traumatic affective disorders.

Apart from dementia and specific neuropsychiatric defects, aphasia, apraxia etc., which depend upon the site and overall extent of brain damage, any type of psychiatric illness, whether functional or organic, may be precipitated by cerebral trauma. The nature of this depends upon predisposition; being determined both by heredity and by environmental factors. While a single severe head injury may produce dementia, this is more likely to occur when head injury is recurrent, as in the case of professional boxers who after a series of reverses may develop symptoms of 'punch-drunkenness' (*traumatic encephalopathy*). The commonest manifestations of this condition are slowing and impaired coordination of muscular reactions, tremors, ataxia, extrapyramidal and cerebellar signs and symptoms together with intellectual deterioration. The 'scars of battle' usually indicate all too clearly the source of this disorder.

Post-traumatic epilepsy is a common complaint following head injury. It may be of any type and attended by any of the complications of epilepsy whether of traumatic origin or not, such as disturbed behaviour, amnesic attacks, fugues, and so on.

Other symptoms tend to be rather less well defined, so that it is often difficult to assess how much of what is residual is functional as opposed to what is the result of organic damage. However, how much does this really matter? Is it not, in large part, an artificial problem? The head-injured patient often presents with a number of seemingly emotional symptoms. While he may complain of memory loss and difficulty in concentrating, it is often, at the same time, difficult if not impossible to demonstrate this objectively. He tends to suffer from irritability and is easily provoked to outbursts of anger or bad temper, sometimes on the slightest provocation and especially when under the influence of drink or drugs, to the effects of which he appears unduly susceptible. He often complains of headaches, of blackouts or of attacks of dizziness. He lacks energy and seems unable to undertake any task demanding sustained effort. He may show frankly hysterical or obsessional symptoms.

Compensation

It is all too easy and probably largely unjust to dismiss too much of the head-injured patient's complaints as malingering in the hope of compensation. While this certainly applies to some who are head injured at work, cognizance should be taken of the fact that many patients are very considerably depressed and may believe themselves, by virtue of the nature of their injury, to have become, or be likely to become, more or less permanent invalids. Such beliefs tend to be fostered by the lengthy delays and multiple examinations by one side or the other, which the legal procedure requires. There is evidence to suggest, however, that if the depressive element is recognized and treated early enough, the outcome may be improved and much demoralization and disability prevented thereby.

Prognosis

Even following severe head injury, the ultimate prognosis may be better than might at first appear. The prognosis is less favourable in alcoholics, the elderly and young children. Nevertheless, a remarkable degree of recovery can occur with the passage of time. It may be wise, therefore, to defer final assessment until two or even three years have passed.

Normal pressure hydrocephalus

Normal pressure, or *occult*, hydrocephalus is an uncommon although important condition in which a block occurs between the ventricular system and the subarachnoid space which interferes with the circulation and reabsorption of cerebrospinal fluid. This may result in severe dementia, ataxia and urinary incontinence, the condition being mistakenly regarded as due to other causes. However, if correctly diagnosed, the condition may be greatly improved in certain cases by the insertion of an in-dwelling catheter into one of the lateral ventricles and connecting this with the jugular venous system.

Korsakow's syndrome

Korsakow's syndrome occurs most often following an attack of delirium tremens but may also develop gradually during the course of chronic alcoholism or from some other cause of thiamine deficiency. It may occur as a phase during the recovery from head injury (see p. 145) or be due to heavy-metal or carbon-monoxide poisoning.

Pathology

Various parts of the brain may show small haemorrhages, necrosis or a glial reaction. The *corpora mamillaria* or their connections are frequently involved, sometimes the *hippocampus* and occasionally other basal nuclei.

Physical signs

If caused by alcoholism, peripheral neuropathy is likely to be present giving rise to tender calves, muscular weakness, foot-drop and ataxia, wrist-drop, absent jerks, peripheral impairment of all forms of sensation and sometimes trophic changes. The condition may also follow upon Wernicke's encephalopathy.

Mental symptoms

Mental symptoms may occur in the absence of neurological signs. The essential feature is a defect of registration and of retentive memory. Patients with Korsakow's syndrome may be completely unable to remember an event which occurred only a few moments before. This leads to gross disorientation. Being unable to register or retain environmental events, they have no continuing signals whereby to orient themselves either in time or place.

Another characteristic feature of the disorder, often, though not invariably present, is *confabulation*. This is the outcome of the memory defect together with suggestion which may lead the patient to give the most circumstantial account of events which if not obvious soon turn out to be entirely a figment of the imagination. Memories in existence prior to the onset of the disorder, which may be sudden, may in contrast be perfectly preserved.

A patient with Korsakow's syndrome has no insight whatsoever into his intellectual deficit. This may lead him to claim acquaintance with total strangers. His emotional state tends to be exaggerated or of shallow indifference.

Prognosis

Prognosis depends upon cause but must always be guarded. Recovery may occur over 12 months or so but some degree of permanent impairment may persist.

Treatment

Parentrovite or some other combined vitamin B preparation should be given intensively and may do good. Polyneuropathy may call for rest, splints and other physiotherapeutic measures. Due to his mental state, the patient is likely to need the kind of care and protection that only an institution can provide. Efforts have been made to assist patients with Korsakow's syndrome to learn, but so far these remain at the level of experiment.

Frontal lobe syndrome

This may not by itself give rise to dementia but to a disturbance of behaviour characterized by euphoria, lack of judgement, tactlessness and fatuity (*witzelsucht*). Finer feelings are lost so that the subject appears to be largely unaware of those of others. Lack of drive and sustained effort may lead to a deterioration of working ability. Personal habits and hygiene may be neglected. At the same time there may be little in the way of actual intellectual impairment.

The condition may be due to a variety of causes: cerebral tumour, head injury, psychosurgery, or focal lesions elsewhere in the cerebral cortex.

Further reading
Lishman, W. A. (1978) *Organic Psychiatry: The Psychological Consequences of Cerebral Disorder.* Oxford: Blackwell Scientific.
Pearce, J. and Miller, E. (1973) *Clinical Aspects of Dementia.* London: Baillière Tindall.

10
Epilepsy

Epilepsy is a symptom rather than a disease, although often so closely associated with brain pathology as to be regarded as an illness *sui generis*. Even the normal brain sufficiently provoked may respond by generating a convulsion as, for example, when ECT is administered. Thus epilepsy should only be regarded as pathological when it occurs spontaneously or is evoked in response to stimuli to which most brains are inert. Each person can be regarded, therefore, as having a *convulsive threshold*—a level of response at which an epileptic seizure may be generated and which is probably largely genetically determined.

Prevalence

About 5 per cent of all persons have an epileptic fit at some time during their lives. The majority, however, are not epileptic in the sense of having a recurrent tendency to seizures, among whom the prevalence rate for epilepsy is about 0.5 per cent. About 4 per cent of young children have febrile convulsions, but only one in seven develops epilepsy on growing up. Ten per cent of those with cerebral atherosclerosis have fits; while those suffering from traumatic, toxic, metabolic or infective brain disease are also prone. Alcohol and certain drugs may cause epileptic attacks, either as a side-effect or when withdrawn.

Clinical features

Classification

Epilepsy can be divided into two main types: *centrencephalic epilepsy* which probably originates in the thalamic nuclei and the reticular activating system (RAS), and *cortical* or *focal epilepsy* which originates in the cerebral cortex or in subcortical structures. The latter includes *temporal lobe* or *psychomotor epilepsy* which, being commonly accompanied by mental symptoms or disturbed behaviour, is of most interest to psychiatry.

Centrencephalic epilepsy

Centrencephalic seizures are of two types—*grand mal* (*tonic–clonic*) fits and *petit mal* (absences). In grand mal or major epilepsy there is abrupt loss of consciousness, an immediate onset of tonic spasm and frequently a cry as air is squeezed out of the lungs through the closed glottis. This phase is followed by a series of clonic jerks of varying intensity and duration involving the whole body. Incontinence of urine and, much more rarely, of faeces, may occur. The sufferer may become deeply cyanosed and produce copious quantities of saliva, often blood-stained. Following cessation of the clonic phase a period of confusion and drowsiness is usual.

Petit mal

Other types of centrencephalic epilepsy are a variation on the theme of the *absence*—a brief loss of consciousness. The purest form of absence is *petit mal (generalized simple absence)*. This consists of temporary impairment of consciousness so that the victim is momentarily cut off from his surroundings. He is usually unaware of the spell. Occasionally eyelid flickering occurs; rarely he may fall or be incontinent. Petit mal occurs largely in children and adolescents and hardly ever over the age of 20 years. The EEG is pathognomic—bilateral and synchronous 3 per second spike and wave activity—although clinical attacks do not necessarily correlate with EEG activity. Patients with petit mal may also, but not invariably, have grand mal attacks.

Occasionally simple absence attacks are prolonged so that the patient lies flaccid and unrousable for many minutes. This is sometimes accompanied by urinary incontinence or automatisms (*generalized complex absence*). Such phenomena may still be compatible with a centrencephalic focus, although not all absence attacks are of centrencephalic origin. In particular, brief psychomotor (*temporal lobe*) attacks may mimic centrencephalic attacks so that close observation may be required to distinguish the two.

Other varieties of petit mal include *myclonic absences* in which a transient impairment of consciousness may be accompanied by jerking of the arms, head or whole body. Such attacks tend to occur in the early morning, are often associated with grand mal seizures and may indicate widespread brain damage.

In *akinetic epilepsy*, absence is accompanied by a sudden complete loss of postural control so that the patient falls to the floor (*drop attacks*). Recovery is usually instantaneous. Occasionally absences may be accompanied by an increase in muscle tone (*retropulsive absence*).

Cortical epilepsy

Partial seizures

Cortical epilepsy originates either in some part of the cortex or in subcortical structures. The focus is usually situated in the vicinity of an area of damaged or scarred cortex or near a new or abnormal growth. While such a focus may be found anywhere, the two commonest sites are the temporal lobes and the sensorimotor cortex of the frontal and parietal lobes.

Sensorimotor epilepsy

The most characteristic feature of sensorimotor epilepsy is the Jacksonian attack, which may lead either to motor or sensory symptoms, or a mixture of both. The attack usually starts in a small area of the body such as the thumb. It may remain localized (if for a long time, this is known as *epilepsia partialis continuans*) or may spread up the limb—the '*Jacksonian march*' until every cortically unilaterally represented muscle on one side of the body is twitching and jerking or alternatively in a state of tonic spasm. At this point the attack may die away or may spread to the centrencephalic area so that a *secondary generalized grand mal* seizure occurs. On recovery the limb or side of the body in which the attack began may be temporarily paralysed for a few hours or days (*Todd's paralysis*). In sensory epilepsy, symptoms of burning, tingling, heaviness or paraesthesiae replace muscle twitching. This too may remain localized or progress as in motor epilepsy, and may, in due course, be followed by temporary anaesthesia in a manner analogous to Todd's paralysis.

Temporal lobe epilepsy

The temporal lobes are by far the commonest site of cortical epileptic foci. This is because the temporal lobes, especially the hippocampal structures, are particularly sensitive to the effects of anoxia, especially in infancy. In addition, the temporal lobes are commonly the site of small benign tumours which frequently become epileptogenic. The evidence for this comes from post-mortem material and studies of temporal lobes resected at operation for temporal lobe epilepsy. However, in about 25 per cent of cases no lesion can be found. In these, therefore, it may be presumed that there is a biochemical or metabolic lesion affecting one or both temporal lobes. If in both, then the two foci may 'fire' in synchrony or independently (*mirror synchrony*).

The temporal lobes are complex structures serving a wide variety of functions including memory storage, thinking, the experience of emotion, the expression of emotion via the autonomic nervous system, and the cortical reception of the senses of hearing and smell. Epileptic disruption and disturbance in these lobes may, therefore, give rise to many symptoms.

Visceromotor and viscerosensory epilepsy

The autonomic nervous system is involved in visceromotor and viscerosensory epilepsy, the symptoms of which include skin changes such as flushing, blanching or sweating and activity in the gastrointestinal tract. Stereotyped chewing, swallowing and lip-smacking movements are common. Such signs are often accompanied by a peculiar churning or rising feeling in the epigastrium which is distressing but almost impossible to describe—the so-called epigastric aura. Occasionally physical sexual feelings may occur.

Alteration of conscious level (clouding)

An alteration of consciousness is common. However, during an attack the subject may still respond to some extent to environmental stimuli. Occasionally he responds quite normally, but is unable to remember this afterwards. If such automatic activity continues for a long time, this may be referred to as a *fugue*.

Likewise, illusions and misinterpretations are common. The shape of objects may alter and *micropsia* or *macropsia* may occur, making it seem to the patient that his surroundings are becoming smaller or larger, often in a somewhat threatening manner. More complex types of illusion also occur; such as complete misidentification so that the faces of friends are seen as devils or something of the kind. Frank hallucinatory experiences—visual, auditory and particularly olfactory—are common. More rarely, *autoscopy* (hallucinations of the self) are described.

Memory disturbances

Disturbances of memory may lead to an intense feeling that a particular situation or event is familiar to the sufferer when it is not—*déjà vu*, or its converse, *jamais vu*. Such experiences are not, however, confined to temporal lobe epilepsy. Alternatively, a patient may vividly relive a stereotyped auditory or visual memory experience as part of his ictal experience ('playback').

Affective changes

Affective changes consist of feelings of fear or panic which may or may not be accompanied by signs and symptoms of anxiety or intense feelings of elation, sadness or anger leading occasionally to outbursts of rage and aggression. Depersonalization and derealization also occur.

Automatism

Automatisms are stereotyped repetitive episodes of behaviour which occur as part of a seizure. They may be fragmentary, brief, complex or prolonged and sometimes bring the victim into conflict with the law. Automatism is still sometimes proffered as an excuse for criminal behaviour, but can only be accepted as a defence if there is a previous history of epilepsy and of similar stereotyped behaviour in the past. Crime committed during an epileptic attack is very rare.

About 80 per cent of patients with epilepsy emanating primarily from the temporal lobe have secondarily generalized tonic-clonic seizures. Thus an initial symptom such as an olfactory hallucination may commonly be followed by a grand mal attack. It is important to recognize that such a so-called *aura* is not a warning that a fit is about to happen, but part of the actual attack. Almost all patients who have an aura followed by a tonic–clonic fit have temporal lobe epilepsy. The converse, however, is untrue. Often the spread of epileptic activity from the temporal lobe to the centrencephalic area is so rapid that the patient either has no time to experience an aura or fails to remember it. The absence of an aura does not, therefore, mean that the patient does not have temporal lobe epilepsy.

In those who do not have tonic–clonic fits, the most typical form of temporal lobe seizure is the *psychomotor attack*. More rarely, such attacks result from epileptic activity occurring elsewhere. During a *psychomotor seizure* consciousness is clouded so that the subject becomes distant and unreachable. He may experience hallucinatory perceptions which later he may or may not remember. Blanching or flushing may occur. Chewing, swallowing, lip-smacking and automatism occur very frequently, during attacks which may last for a few seconds or for many minutes. Occasionally, prolonged states occur lasting several days or even weeks, during which the subject remains in a state of clouded consciousness with accompanying perceptual, affective or behavioural symptoms. This *twilight state* is, of course, the psychic equivalent of *epilepsia partialis continuans*.

Other varieties of epilepsy

Both *frontal* and *occipital lobe* epilepsy may express themselves clinically via pathways to the temporal lobes and in consequence give rise to psychomotor attacks. The true origin of a frontal lobe seizure may, however, be revealed by an *adversive attack* in which there is a sustained turning movement of the eyes, head or even of the whole body to one or other side. Likewise, an attack emanating from an occipital lobe may give rise to unorganized elementary visual hallucinations such as flashes of coloured lights followed by a tonic–clonic seizure.

Differential diagnosis

The diagnosis of epilepsy rests largely on the history of the attack given by the patient and on accounts given by witnesses. While the differential diagnosis is wide, epilepsy can often be distinguished by its conspicuous tendency to recur and its relatively stereotyped nature. In psychiatric practice, epilepsy may have to be differentiated from a simple faint, an anxiety attack, from hysterical seizures or from conscious simulation.

Fainting

Fainting usually occurs when erect and is of brief duration. Complete recovery is rapid. There is often a warning feeling of giddiness, light-headedness or faintness. During the faint itself there is gross pallor, marked hypotension and bradycardia. Injury seldom occurs, although occasionally there may be incontinence and minimal muscle twitching (*jactitation*).

Anxiety attacks

In anxiety attacks, the sufferer develops a rising feeling of fear and panic, together with tachycardia, palpitations, profuse sweating, nausea, etc. Hyperventilation may occur so that carbon dioxide is washed out of the bloodstream leading to paraesthesiae, which in turn may be followed by tetanic spasms of the hands and feet. If the patient continues to overbreathe, he may eventually lose consciousness and may indeed occasionally suffer an epileptic fit.

Simulated epilepsy

Very occasionally, epilepsy may be simulated either as part of an hysterical illness or consciously as part of the repertoire of a malingerer. Such 'fits' are, however, usually easy to distinguish from those which are genuine. Unless the patient is very knowledgeable, what he tends to simulate will be no more than a layman's idea of what an epileptic attack should be, not what it actually is. Thus he may fall to the ground with a dramatic cry and thrash about in a way entirely different from a true epileptic seizure. There is no real evidence of loss of consciousness; injury is uncommon and incontinence rare. However, when there is debate about the nature of a patient's attack it is usually safer to assume that it is in fact epileptic as most simulated seizures occur in those who actually do suffer from epilepsy. It must also be remembered that epileptics can faint and that this can precipitate a convulsion. Epileptics are also likely to have anxiety attacks which may trigger their seizures. In addition those who are brain damaged and socially deprived are prone to develop attention-seeking symptoms.

Electroencephalography

The EEG is subject to misleading artefacts, both positive and negative. However, it is an important investigatory tool in epilepsy and can help to localize the anatomical origin of epileptic attacks. It should, however, be emphasized that a normal EEG tracing does not exclude epilepsy.

Epilepsy, indeed, is a clinical diagnosis to which an abnormal EEG may add confirmation.

In centrencephalic epilepsy, symmetrical paroxysmal activity—spike, spike and wave or paroxysmal slow activity—is found over the entire hemisphere in all EEG channels; this is a reflection of the projection of midbrain activity in all areas of the cortex. In cortical epilepsy, paroxysmal activity may be confined to a particular area of the brain in which case a focus may often be accurately localized by means of phase reversal. Independent slow-wave activity accompanying epileptic activity suggests a pathological basis such as brain damage or an expanding lesion. Nevertheless, the localization of cortical epileptic activity is not necessarily always precise as the actual site of an epileptic discharge may be far removed from where the activity appears in the EEG tracing to be. Epileptic activity may even appear in the opposite cortex and not at all over the actual lesion or, appearing over one side of the brain, may excite a mirror focus on the other side so that a spurious interpretation of bilateral foci is made (*mirror synchrony*).

Many cortical foci lie deep and are not accessible to conventional scalp electrodes. Various methods are used, therefore, to enhance or provoke epileptic activity. There is value in taking serial recordings over a period of time and sometimes hyperventilation and photic stimulation are rewarding. Sleep recordings may also be valuable, as sleep enhances epileptic activity in the EEG. It may also occasionally be necessary to inject drugs, such as methohexitone (Brietal), which provoke epileptic activity. Special electrode placements can be useful, in particular sphenoidal leads, using needle electrodes pushed under the zygoma so as to lie under the greater wing of the sphenoid thus picking up an epileptic discharge occurring in the buried inferior and medial portions of the temporal lobes. These will very often demonstrate abnormal temporal lobe activity when conventional EEG tracings will not.

In addition to EEG studies, other investigations such as CT scanning may be extremely useful in screening patients who possibly have cerebral lesions.

Epileptic mental disorders

Emotional disturbance or frank psychiatric illness occurs in epileptics for several reasons.

Firstly, many epileptics are rejected by their families and by society. Because their employability is restricted—they cannot work in potentially risk situations: at a height, with machinery, where driving a vehicle is necessary, etc.—they may find it difficult to obtain work and often have to accept employment at a level far below their real or potential capacity. In addition, they may have difficulty in establishing and maintaining personal relationships. The attitude of others towards the epileptic and his attacks may cause him to struggle both with feelings of inadequacy and with a sense of being an outcast. The mentally ill or handicapped epileptic having a double handicap is especially vulnerable.

Secondly, many epileptics—particularly those with temporal lobe epilepsy—are brain damaged; this, even when minimal, can be critically disabling. Because memory, thinking and emotional control may all be impaired, tolerance of stress and the ability to surmount environmental, personal and emotional difficulties are hampered.

Thirdly, an epileptic attack may be no more than the tip of an iceberg. In between actual fits there is often much disruptive activity going on in affected brain areas. If such subictal activity occurs in the temporal lobes, it may have a marked effect on a patient's ability to concentrate and may obliterate newly laid down memory traces. Thus an epileptic child may find it difficult to pay attention and learn, leading to lifelong handicap in terms of intellectual deficit and personality difficulty. In adults in whom clinical attacks are completely suppressed, subictal activity may still continue. Under these circumstances a subject's mental state may paradoxically become worse so that he may be better off having an occasional grand mal seizure as this may temporarily suppress such subversive subictal activity.

Lastly, medication may occasionally affect a patient's mental state either by inducing a toxic psychosis or possibly by inducing a disturbance of folic acid and vitamin B12 metabolism.

Prevalence

The actual prevalence of mental illness in epileptics in the United Kingdom is unknown, although it is generally agreed to be commoner than expected by chance. One-sixth of epileptics treated in general practice—mostly patients with centrencephalic epilepsy—suffer from neurotic or stress disorders. Ten per cent of all epileptics require psychiatric hospital admissions at some time or other, usually for a short period. Those with temporal lobe epilepsy may have difficulty with schooling and employment because of personality and learning difficulties. A third of temporal lobe epileptic children have educational difficulties, mostly behaviour disorders. About 75 per cent of chronic epileptics also present serious social problems. However, lest it appears that too much emphasis is being placed on the psychiatric aspects of epilepsy, it should be remembered that about 85 per cent of epileptics have fits which are well or completely controlled and suffer no more mental symptoms than the average citizen.

In more serious mental disorder requiring hospital admission, epileptics are certainly over-represented. Remembering that the prevalence rate of epilepsy in the general population is 0.5 per cent, one study has shown that 5 per cent of chronic patients in mental hospitals are epileptic. The equivalent figure for those in hospitals for the mentally subnormal is much higher.

In considering the mental disorders associated with epilepsy certain important questions need answers. Firstly, what is the time relationship of the disorder to the patient's attacks: do they occur before, during or after an attack or is there no relationship whatsoever? Secondly, is consciousness clouded at the time mental disorder is present? Thirdly, is the occurrence of mental symptoms preceded by a marked increase or decrease in fit frequency? Lastly, what evidence is there of concomitant brain damage?

Mental disorder having a time relationship to fits

Before a fit.   There may be prodromal symptoms lasting several hours or days before a fit takes place. Some patients become depressed, others aggressive or paranoid. This is sometimes described as 'working up for a fit'. Occasionally more bizarre prodromata occur, for example the patient who regularly develops an urticarial rash several days before an attack.

Whereas an epileptic aura is not a true prodromal feature but the initial manifestation of an attack, an aura as a recurrent phenomenon, without a full-blown seizure following, may be experienced. If it is of an emotional, behaviour or perceptual kind, such as a hallucinatory voice, it may be difficult to distinguish from symptoms caused by other types of mental illness. It may not be until the patient has his first grand mal attack that the true nature of the disorder is recognized.

During a fit.   Epileptic automatisms and twilight states may be misdiagnosed as primary mental disorders. The patient who sits mute and appears to be hallucinated and who occasionally shows bouts of aggressive behaviour may be thought to be suffering from catatonic schizophrenia. Indeed, catatonic symptoms can occur as part of an epileptic attack. A child in *petit mal status* may also present a diagnostic puzzle and may be seen in terms of behavioural disorder or mental retardation.

After a fit.   Automatisms, twilight states, together with fugues, may occur as postictal phenomena following upon a major seizure. Another type of postictal disturbance is *furor*, a state in which the patient develops an outburst of rage even to the point of going berserk. Such rages can be very difficult to control. A patient who has had one attack of furor is likely to have another, though sometimes this can be prevented by the continuous administration of benzodiazepines. Furor is probably the result of a complex interaction between anoxia, producing a degree of delirium, a disturbance of personality and continuing abnormal brain activity. It is best treated by *not* restraining the patient but allowing the outburst to settle spontaneously.

Mental disorder having no time relationship to fits

Confusional states.   Confusional states are common and are often associated with a sudden increase in fit frequency, as in the case of the patient who usually has four to five grand mal attacks a year but who suddenly has seven or eight in the course of a day or so, possibly as a result of stopping medication. Such confusional states probably arise out of relative hypoxia induced by frequent attacks and continuing subictal activity and may be so pronounced that the subject becomes delirious. Often a paranoid element enters into the illness, and very occasionally depressive features. Providing the attacks can be rapidly controlled, the prognosis is good. Occasionally acute delirium leaves dementia in its wake, but epilepsy *per se* is only rarely a cause of dementia.

Affective disorders. Depression is not only the most important mental illness of epilepsy but severe depressive illnesses are commoner in temporal lobe epileptics than in the general population. *Suicide* also occurs more commonly in epileptics than can be expected by chance. The clinical features of severe depression occurring in temporal lobe epileptics are indistinguishable from those occurring in non-epileptics, although they often have a rather sudden onset. Such states are relatively resistant to medication with antidepressants and sometimes need treatment with ECT. Interestingly, depression seems particularly likely to occur in patients whose fit frequency is declining. It may therefore be a side-effect of successful anticonvulsant medication or surgical treatment. It is more likely to occur in patients with non-dominant temporal lobe discharges.

Paranoid states. Paranoid states are common in temporal lobe epilepsy. Indeed, a paranoid schizophrenic-like state tends to appear several years after the inception of temporal lobe epilepsy, often at a time when fit frequency is declining. This may be difficult to distinguish from paranoid schizophrenia occurring in the non-epileptic, although affective contact is said to be better preserved. The aetiology of this condition has excited considerable interest and is now thought to be related to temporal lobe dysfunction. Indeed, it has been shown that paranoid schizophrenia may be *followed* by epilepsy, suggesting that temporal lobe dysfunction is common to both conditions.

Abnormal emotional reactions. All types of abnormal emotional reactions occur commonly in epileptics as an over-ready reaction to stress. The principles of treatment are the same as in non-epileptics, but treatment may be more difficult in those who are also brain damaged or who face insoluble environmental difficulties.

Sexual disorders. Temporal lobe epilepsy may interfere with sexual function, giving rise to impotence in male patients. Occasionally better control of attacks restores potency. The notion that other sexual problems are commoner in patients with epilepsy than in the general population has not been convincingly substantiated.

Personality disorders.   Some varieties of personality disorder are said to be commoner in epileptics than might be expected by chance, but the evidence for this is slender. These include those who are unduly aggressive and liable to suffer from outbursts of rage, often with very little provocation. These outbursts are not dissimilar to attacks of epileptic furor but do not occur in direct association with a seizure. Because a patient can become destructive and at times violent during such an outburst, some are commited to mental hospitals. This kind of patient is the source of an undeservedly bad reputation for epileptics. There is good modern evidence to show, however, that aggression is not a personality trait of epileptics in general, but only of a few individual patients.

The aetiology of these aggressive states is not well understood. It is suggested that they are common in temporal lobe epileptics and that they may represent a kind of 'sham rage'. Aggression in the epileptic also appears to have something to do with age at the inception of attacks: the earlier this is, the more likely is the patient to be aggressive. Such aggressive traits may, therefore, be a result of the influence of others on the patient's personality development rather than due to brain pathology. Most people with epilepsy, it must be emphasized, are *not* aggressive. Indeed, epileptic children have been shown to be less aggressive than their peers. There is also no relationship between violent crime and epilepsy.

The so-called *epileptic personality*, although often denied as an entity, is a type of personality disorder seen in many epileptics with temporal lobe damage, who have become institutionalized and who display a constellation of personality symptoms which seem relatively consistent. Such patients show an irritable or hostile response to environmental change, are liable to sensitive paranoid thinking and readily develop overelaborated ideas of personal affront. Thinking is sticky and viscid together with *global perseveration* or difficulty in shifting from one topic to another. Marked hypochondriasis is often present and sometimes an undue tendency to religiosity. This personality profile, although common in epileptics, is probably not caused by epilepsy as such but is an outcome of temporal lobe damage.

Mental subnormality.   Mental subnormality occurs more commonly than by chance expectation in epileptics, but almost invariably because both mental handicap and epilepsy are secondary to some other disorder, such as severe brain damage at birth, tuberous sclerosis, etc. Occasionally continuous subictal activity or petit mal status may produce a gross but reversible limitation in intelligence. However, full-blown *status epilepticus* in children can give rise to complete and irreversible amentia probably due to anoxic damage to the temporal lobes and involving the hippocampus. If patients with brain damage from whatever cause are excluded, however, there is no real correlation between epilepsy and intelligence, although extensive subictal activity will interfere with learning and produce a spuriously low result on testing.

Treatment

It is sensible practice not to treat the first epileptic attack as it is possible that there will never be another. Its occurrence should, however, be thoroughly investigated. Of those who have repeated attacks, about 70 per cent respond well to anticonvulsants (although minor cortical attacks are particularly resistant to treatment), the aim being to achieve the maximum therapeutic effect with minimal side-effects. In recent years, the importance of monitoring the blood levels of anticonvulsant drugs has become established (so that the patient's dose is tailored to produce an effective but non-toxic level) as has the concept of *monotherapy* (using one drug at a time).

Monitoring serum drug level appears to be of the greatest value in the case of *phenytoin* and *carbamazepine*. Although monitoring *ethosuximide* is also of some value, because this drug is used largely in children frequent blood sampling may lead to non-compliance. It has also been shown that most anticonvulsants need only be given once or twice a day. All anticonvulsants, if given to excess, may actually provoke seizures. They also have complex interactions with each other. The most commonly used anticonvulsants are as follows.

Barbiturates. Phenobarbitone (30–300 mg daily) is the best known. Currently it is falling into disuse. It is contraindicated in petit mal and, in children, may cause hyperkinesis. Habituation and dependence may occur and sudden withdrawal can induce grand mal attacks. Chronic exposure may cause megaloblastic anaemia, also skin rashes. If used it need only be given once a day.

Hydantoins. Phenytoin (150–600 mg daily) is the main representative of this class (therapeutic serum level up to 80 μmol/l). It is one of the most effective anticonvulsants for all types of epilepsy except petit mal, particularly if blood levels are controlled. There are numerous side-effects of which cerebellar ataxia, lymphoma syndrome, megaloblastic anaemia, gum hyperplasia, hypertrichosis, skin rashes, and facial coarsening are the commonest. It is known to cause minor fetal malformation in about 6 per cent of pregnant women, as is phenobarbitone.

Succinimides. Ethosuximide (500–1500 mg daily) is the most widely used, especially in petit mal (serum level up to 700 μmol/l). A toxic psychosis is a well-recognized complication.

Primidone. Primidone (120–2000 mg daily) is an anticonvulsant chemically related to the barbiturates and therefore not of much use if combined with them. It should be introduced fairly slowly (in increments of 100 mg weekly) otherwise marked drowsiness and ataxia may occur. It is reasonably effective in temporal lobe epilepsy.

Sulthiame. Sulthiame (200–800 mg daily) is a carbonic anhydrase inhibitor, said to be effective in temporal lobe epilepsy, but there is some doubt as to whether it actually has any anticonvulsant effect. Paraesthesiae, visual blurring, vomiting, and hyperventilation from an induced metabolic acidosis and a toxic psychosis are the main side-effects.

Benzodiazepines. All the benzodiazepine group of drugs have anticon-vulsant activity. Diazepam (6–40 mg daily), nitrazepam (5–20 mg daily) and clonazepam (2–12 mg daily) are the most useful. They are sometimes highly effective in resistant generalized epilepsy. Side-effects include ataxia and drowsiness which can usually be avoided by introducing the drug slowly: benzodiazepines may provoke seizures.

Carbamazepine. This drug (400–1200 mg daily) is effective in cortical epilepsy and is probably the most effective drug for minor cortical seizures (serum level up to 50 μmol/l). Some authorities regard it as the drug of first choice for cortical epilepsy. Side-effects are ataxia, vomiting and water intoxication. Contrary to popular belief, blood dyscrasias appear to be rare.

Sodium valproate. Sodium valproate (600–1600 mg daily) is a new but highly effective drug, possibly the first choice for the generalized epilepsies. Side-effects are nausea and vomiting, drowsiness (if given with phenobarbitone) and abnormal hair growth or loss.

Surgical treatment

Surgery is occasionally indicated. In unilateral temporal lobe epilepsy uncontrolled by medication, temporal lobectomy may be successful. Careful selection of suitable cases is necessary together with certainty that the other temporal lobe is intact. Otherwise dementia may result. In some patients with bilateral temporal lobe epilepsy, stereotactic lesions can be made in those areas of both lobes from which epileptic activity originates without destroying the integrity of the rest of the lobes and interfering with their other functions.

Status epilepticus

In status epilepticus a succession of grand mal seizures occurs without return of consciousness. This is a medical emergency which must be treated vigorously. Otherwise the subject may die or his brain may be irrecoverably damaged by anoxia. The most usual cause is a sudden withdrawal of anticonvulsants or failure to take them regularly. Heroic efforts are sometimes needed to stop repetitive fits, including intravenous phenytoin, paraldehyde or sodium thiopentone. Probably the most useful control drug is diazepam (Valium) 10–50 mg given by slow intravenous infusion over 12 hours. One advantage of diazepam is that the patient will usually wake when his attacks have stopped; whereas if paraldehyde or phenytoin are used, he may well remain unconscious. Clonazepam may be even more effective than diazepam.

Psychiatric treatment

Treating epilepsy calls for much more than drugs or surgery. Management is highly important. Attention must be paid to social problems and to helping patients adjust to emotional and personal difficulties. Failing this, control of seizures may often be hampered. Those who are bored or lonely, anxious or under stress, are more likely to have attacks than those who are hard at work. Recently, experimental behavioural methods of treating epilepsy have been developed including intensive relaxation and EEG biofeedback training. While these seem to hold considerable promise, they need to be fully evaluated.

The treatment of mental disorders of epilepsy is in general no different from the treatment of similar disorders occurring in the non-epileptic. In psychotic states, haloperidol is probably superior to chlorpromazine because the sedative effects of the latter may possibly increase the number of the patient's attacks. Benzodiazepine drugs are particularly useful in combating explosive aggressive disorders, and may be useful in controlling twilight states. Tricyclic antidepressants need to be used with caution as they can be epileptogenic and may cause some epileptics to develop increased seizure frequency.

Apart from drugs, much other treatment is concerned with environmental adjustment—prevention of boredom, bolstering of relationships, support, the provision of work and suitable accommodation and, in general, helping the epileptic to find a meaningful place in the community.

Largely on account of its unpredictability, epilepsy is a frightening, anxiety-provoking illness, to those who suffer from it and their families, friends and workmates. Perhaps the greatest service a psychiatrist can offer any epileptic patient, whether or not he is mentally ill, is to help him to come to terms with his illness. There may, therefore, be no treatment so effective as the doctor himself.

Further reading

Rose, F. R. (ed.) (1982) *Progress in Epilepsy*. Edinburgh: Churchill Livingstone.

11

Alcoholism and Drug Dependence

Alcohol problems and drug abuse, although not identical, have enough in common to make it appropriate to consider both together. Both drugs and alcohol may relieve tension and, as Berton Roueché stated, have the power to satisfy man's need to obtain 'release from the intolerable clutch of reality'. He wrote:

All men throughout recorded history have known this tyranny of memory and mind, and all have sought and invariably found some reliable means of briefly loosening its grip. The most conspicuous result of their search, if not the most effective is . . . alcohol. It is also the oldest, the most widely esteemed and the most abysmally misunderstood. (*New Yorker*)

Whereas alcohol induces feelings of warmth, well-being and general exhilaration, it is not a stimulant but a cerebral depressant. Such relief as it may bring results from stifling self-criticism and the nagging voice of conscience. Put simply, alcohol, by dampening down cerebral activity tends to keep anxiety at bay, allowing certain otherwise inhibited impulses to gain at least momentary ascendance largely unencumbered by embarrassment, guilt or even fear of the consequences. As Samuel Johnson put it: 'In the bottle discontent seeks for comfort, cowardice for courage and bashfulness for confidence.'

When taken in large amounts, the psychological effects of alcohol become exaggerated and lead ultimately to mental as well as physical incoordination. More imbibing then leads to greater drunkenness and ultimately to coma. Death may result, particularly if a large amount of alcohol is rapidly consumed by a person unaccustomed to drink or where alcohol and certain drugs, notably barbiturates, are taken together.

How much alcohol the average adult can metabolize and how fast he can do so depend on several factors: dilution, whether he has recently eaten and, in particular, how used he is to taking alcohol. A normally abstemious person can metabolize 7–20 ml of absolute alcohol per hour; chronic drinkers as much as 25 ml. Some degree of intoxication is usually apparent when the blood alcohol level is in the region of 100 mg per 100 ml. At levels over 150 mg per 100 ml, drunkenness may be obvious. The effects of alcohol intake do not, however, appear to be entirely related to intake or to the rate at which it is metabolized, but to tolerance built up within the central nervous system. Tolerance in so-called hardened drinkers may, with the passage of time, be considerable. Nevertheless, this should not be taken to mean that the subject's reaction time or his other faculties are unimpaired. Although he may appear sober, he may be quite unfit to carry out complex tasks such as driving a car.

Alcoholism

There is no completely satisfactory definition of alcoholism. Perhaps the best so far is still that put forward in 1952 by the World Health Organization Expert Committee on Mental Health:

Alcoholics are those excessive drinkers whose dependence on alcohol has attained such a degree that they show a noticeable mental disturbance or an interference with their mental and bodily health, their interpersonal relations and their smooth economic and social functioning; or who show prodromal signs of such developments.

In lesser degrees it may be difficult to distinguish alcoholism from heavy social drinking which may merge with the passage of time into a state of more obvious dependence. There are also several patterns of excessive drinking. Those who progress from psychological to physical dependence with loss of control, increased tolerance at least initially, withdrawal symptoms and craving, constitute Jellinek's *gamma* type. Those in whom there is no loss of control but in whom several other features of alcoholism are present are referred to as the *delta* type, also called by some the *inability to abstain* type. This can be regarded as a form of *controlled* alcoholism; for although the problem does not, at least for a time, get out of hand, the drinker is nevertheless alcohol dependent. This, probably, is the pattern which comes nearest to heavy social drinking. Another less common form is periodic alcoholism, so-called *dipsomania*, in which after a period of total abstinence taking only a single drink may be sufficient to trigger a bout of alcoholism of such intensity as to cause the subject to reach with remarkable rapidity a state of considerable degradation. Such bouts may alternate with periods of relative or complete abstinence so that the pattern becomes one of remission and relapse. The condition is sometimes thought to be linked with manic–depressive disorder.

Prevalence

This is difficult to determine, estimates depending, among other things, upon definition. Much alcoholism is concealed so that even when the subject still has insight into the fact that he is drinking too heavily he may hide this from others, hesitating to seek help, because he fears ridicule or a hostile reaction. Where insight is lacking and before organic factors become operative, denial is an important mental mechanism.

Applying Jellinek's formula, which is based on the consideration of several variables, including reported deaths from cirrhosis, a proportion of which are due to alcoholism, the percentage of alcoholics with other complications who die of cirrhosis, and the ratio of all alcoholics to those with other complications, suggests that the prevalence of alcoholism in England and Wales is in the region of 11 per 1000, and considerably higher in Scotland. Currently over one-third of those killed in road accidents in the United Kingdom are found to have a blood alcohol level in excess of 80 mg per 100 ml (not only drivers but many of their passengers and pedestrians also). In Europe and elsewhere the prevalence of alcoholism varies greatly from one country to another; the manner in which alcohol is used and abused being governed by a variety of economic, social and cultural circumstances.

In Italy, for example, where a considerable amount of wine is drunk this, it is said, is largely confined to meal times. Insobriety is frowned upon which, if true, provides an example of how the pattern of alcoholic indulgence may be governed by social attitudes. Alcoholism tends to be prevalent in the Western world and in some though not all of those countries which are wine producing, for example France. Prevalence is low among Jews and in those Arab states with total prohibition. This, however, does not necessarily mean that alcoholism is unknown in Islam, it being said, for example, to be quite frequent among the Bedouin in Kuwait. In the Far East alcoholism is known to be commonest in Japan where its incidence has been estimated to be as high as 3 per cent, a figure similar to that in the United States, France and some Scandinavian countries which have the highest rates in the world.

Aetiology

Primary alcoholism

Primary alcoholism is where a state of dependence occurs in which continuously drinking too much is not symptomatic of some other mental or personality disorder, but which appears to be due to conditioning; such as can also be brought about in laboratory animals. However, why some become conditioned and others not is not altogether clear. In some subjects *heredity* has now been shown to play a part; in others apparently not. As has already been suggested, custom and social approval of drinking also contribute. Hence there seems to be a statistical relationship between the prevalence of alcoholism in any particular community and total *per capita* consumption. A critical level of alcohol consumption also appears to be important in leading an individual to dependence; this being the equivalent of about 15–16 centilitres of ethanol within a 24–hour period (that is, approximately half a bottle of spirits, 4–7 pints of beer, a bottle and a half of table wine or less of fortified wine, e.g. sherry, etc.). Other factors operative are price in relation to earnings and ease of access. Because of these matters and until it is better known why some become more readily habituated than others, judgements based on generalizations about character and personality which may themselves be damaged by alcoholism are probably best held in reserve. Furthermore, in established alcoholism, even that which has arisen out of normal social drinking, rationalizations and evasions make it increasingly difficult to determine exactly which are the principal factors operative in any particular case.

Until recently it was widely believed that alcoholism was commoner in men than women. Now, however, the female prevalence rate is rising so that currently the rate of cirrhosis in women has, for the first time, exceeded that in men, not because there are as yet more female alcoholics than male, but because women appear to be more liable to alcoholic liver damage. Although in both sexes genetic factors are probably operative, this is not yet universally established, although assortative mating may well play a part. Certain occupations predispose to alcoholism, such as the licensing trade—although it seems likely that here innate predisposition may govern choice of occupation. It should be noted that certain other occupations not directly concerned with catering are at above average risk, according to standardized mortality ratios for cirrhosis of the liver in men aged 15–64. These include actors, musicians and other entertainers, the armed forces, medical practitioners and insurance brokers.

Age is also a factor. Until recently in the United Kingdom, alcoholism was hardly apparent until the fourth decade or later. There is growing evidence, however, that drinking problems are becoming commoner among younger people, even among schoolchildren. Thus it has been estimated that 90 per cent of young people, girls as much as boys, have drunk alcohol by the age of 16. If this trend continues, it seems likely that chronic alcoholism and its various complications may become increasingly prevalent, for there is some evidence of a relationship between prevalence and early established drinking patterns of behaviour.

Secondary alcoholism

Secondary alcoholism is that which can be regarded as a disease within a disease in that excessive drinking may be symptomatic of some other underlying mental disorder. Furthermore, due to some of its complications, alcohol may become the vehicle by which one type of mental disorder may be converted into another. Alcoholism can be a symptom of any mental illness whether latent or overt. Thus in drink the depressive drowns his feeling of despair, the obsessive finds solace from his scruples, and the schizophrenic, a temporary escape from his tormenting perception of reality. It should be emphasized, however, that these cases constitute only the minority of those with alcohol problems. Likewise, where no underlying mental disorder is present, it should not be assumed *a priori* that an alcoholic necessarily suffers from a primary abnormality of personality. This supposition may, indeed, turn out to be no more than a piece of circular reasoning. Also, while in such cases it is often customary to assume that some basic weakness of character is operative, it should be noted that this is largely a moral judgement, having little basis in scientific fact.

Clinical features of chronic alcoholism

Chronic alcoholism develops through a series of stages. Regular heavy drinking gives way, often with a change from long to short drinks, to inability to abstain. An early warning sign is the occurrence of bouts of amnesia (*alcoholic blackouts*) usually covering the drinking spell of the night before. Memory, concentration, judgement and ability to work profitably may all be progressively impaired. Lateness to work on Mondays—the excuse being some vague complaint—following a weekend exacerbation of drinking is an important early sign. Accident proneness and short periods off work on account of vague poorly substantiated ill-health are similar indications. Alteration in the emotional state of the developing alcoholic may soon become readily apparent. This becomes superficial and his reactions labile with outbursts of rage followed by remorse. While he shows considerable bonhomie when with his drinking companions, he may present a very different picture to his family to whom he appears inconsiderate, self-centred, even brutal. His inconsiderateness extends to his sex life so that his sexual approaches to his wife become increasingly uninviting and for her something to be avoided at all costs. Such avoidance tends to cause her alcoholic spouse to project the blame for his increasing impotence upon her rather than upon his drinking. This pattern of behaviour, which is not confined to alcoholism, provides fertile soil for the implantation in his mind of ideas or even delusions of jealousy.

Well before this, *thinking about drink* may become an established pattern of thought—not only the idea of needing a drink but at the same time of promising himself he will resist drinking. Repeated failure and remorse at breaking his own self-promises soon lead him to start taking his very first drink even earlier in the day so that finally he cannot leave the house in the morning or even his bed until his blood alcohol has been raised to the level at which he can still the 'shakes' which overcome him even after such a short period of abstinence as drunken slumber brings. Finally, sacked from his job and deserted by family and friends, he descends into the gutter, almost literally gravitating to that state which in the United States is colourfully called 'Skid Row'. Without money to buy more potable drink he may take to methylated spirits. If he does so fairly gradually, he may work up some degree of immunity to the toxic effects of methyl alcohol, although sooner or later and if his deterioration in behaviour remains unchecked, his physical and mental health may be irretrievably ruined.

In women, the path towards chronic alcoholism is less clear-cut. Whereas the man who drinks heavily may start his alcoholic 'career' in the bar of a public house, women may do their 'tippling' around the house by day. Strong and still fairly cheap sherry appears to be a favourite potion and bottles may be concealed around the house in places where drinks are not normally kept, so-called wardrobe drinking.

Complications. The psychosocial complications of alcoholism, either chronic or acute, hardly need emphasis except in statistical terms when their enormity becomes all the more apparent. Probably the most important are those having domestic consequences. Homicide, whether at home or abroad, commonly occurs under the influence of alcohol. Short of this, in cases of assault such as wife- or baby-battering, drunkenness more often than not plays an essential part. Likewise, alcohol is a powerful determinant of road accidents, particularly among those under 25 year of age, although no age appears to be exempt.

Physical and overt psychiatric complications usually develop between 40 and 50 years, possibly earlier. Physical signs commonly include *suffused facies, tremor, gastritis* and early morning *vomiting. Laryngitis* and *bronchitis*, both either caused or exacerbated by heavy smoking, usual among alcoholics, are frequent. *Peptic ulcers* are common, while *haematemesis* due to *liver cirrhosis* may be a presenting symptom. *Cardiomyopathy* may occur. In the central nervous system alcoholism may give rise to *polyneuritis* or *cerebellar degeneration. Subdural haematoma* is not uncommon because of the alcoholic's ready tendency to fall and hit his head. *Alcoholic epilepsy* may occur during drinking bouts or may herald an attack of *delirium*. Otherwise, fits induced by alcohol differ in no essential way from ordinary *grand mal* epilepsy but are probably precipitated by cerebral irritation and, in the case of heavy beer drinkers, by overhydration.

The principal neuropsychiatric complications of chronic alcoholism are *delirium tremens, Korsakow's syndrome* and *Wernicke's encephalopathy* (see Chapter 9), together with a number of other psychiatric disorders detailed below.

Alcoholic hallucinosis

Hallucinations may succeed an attack of *delirium tremens* or develop insidiously. Usually auditory, they have a persecutory quality and are accompanied by ideas of being watched or followed. The 'voices' may refer to the patient in the third person. The condition occurs in two forms: in the first instance being of a transitory nature only; in the second of longer and more persistent duration. In both forms the hallucinations apparently occur as isolated phenomena and in a setting of clear consciousness.

It is disputable, especially in respect of the second form, whether *alcoholic hallucinosis* is a specific entity caused by alcohol or whether it is an attenuated form of paranoid schizophrenia (*paraphrenia*) released by alcoholism. Where hallucinations and delusions assume an increasingly bizarre quality and thought disorder becomes increasingly evident, the possibility that the disorder is primarily of schizophrenic origin looms larger.

Alcoholic paranoia

It has been suggested that paranoid states occur in chronic alcoholics on a basis of projection of their feelings of guilt and shame. However, as precisely similar delusions may occur in those who are not alcoholic but who suffer, for example, from *diabetes mellitus* or other disorders giving rise to impotence, there are grounds for believing that, in this type of paranoid development as in the case of alcoholic hallucinosis, the true basis may be another kind of psychiatric illness released or complicated by alcoholism.

Dementia

There is some dispute about alcoholism as a cause of dementia *per se*. Although CT scanning has shown that a degree of ventricular enlargement occurs in a proportion of chronic alcoholics, this is not necessarily associated with clinical impairment and may be reversible should the alcoholic decide to mend his ways. There appears, therefore, to be no altogether direct relationship between ventricular enlargement and degree of dementia except in the grossest cases. Dementia or an appearance of it is therefore most likely to be due to damage to subcortical structures such as occurs in Korsakow's syndrome (see p. 157), which although severely mentally incapacitating cannot be defined as dementia in the strictest sense.

Other neuropsychiatric complications of alcoholism include tremor, dysarthria and loss of postural sensation. These may lead erroneously to a suspicion of neurosyphilis (*alcoholic pseudoparesis*). Another early sign is that, owing to central nervous system damage, tolerance may be greatly reduced so that a relatively small amount of alcohol will produce drunkenness. This is also apparent in those who have suffered a head injury and whose tolerance, overall, may be greatly diminished.

Treatment

In the first instance, treatment may demand 'drying-out', sedation and tranquillization being required to cover withdrawal symptoms. Barbiturates and paraldehyde, once popular, should be avoided; phenothiazines, haloperidol or diazepam (Valium) are to be preferred, preferably administered parenterally in the first instance. Chlormethiazole (Heminevrin) is also of value although it is a potential drug of addiction both to alcoholics and others and, in the former instance, should not be given for more than about 7–10 days. Attention should be paid to the patient's general health and nutritional state, both of which are often poor. Parentrovite (a high-dosage vitamin B preparation suitable for intravenous administration) is a useful adjuvant to treatment, especially of delirium tremens and Korsakow's syndrome.

Having dealt with any immediate complications, the next stage consists of examining the patient's current life situation in detail with a view to trying to deal with such personal and other difficulties as seem to have contributed to his alcoholism. The help of his spouse may have to be enlisted, having regard to the fact that an apparent air of willing cooperation may sometimes conceal an opposite even hostile attitude. Some wives or husbands, although complaining bitterly of their partner's habits, undoubtedly connive, paradoxically, by making drink or money more easily available than common sense would seem to dictate. Such partners may be referred to as 'co-alcoholics'!

The psychological treatment of those with alcohol problems demands above all things a willingness to cooperate. Motivation is paramount; without it relapse is inevitable. Individual psychotherapy may be useful for some but the indications are that group therapy is to be preferred. Alcoholics Anonymous can be of great help to many alcoholic patients and most units which treat alcoholics maintain close contact with this organization. Some patients, however, cannot come to terms with AA's somewhat evangelical attitude. Where some kind of mental disorder underlying alcoholism is present this, of course, will require appropriate treatment.

Behavioural modification

This aims to produce in the alcoholic a distaste or disgust for liquor using an aversion technique in which he is given his favourite alcoholic drink together with emetine or apomorphine to make him vomit. Alternatively, electric shocks may be used. The method, while possibly successful in a few cases, appears to be much less so than aversion therapy applied in the treatment of some other conditions (see Behaviour therapy, p. 332).

Antabuse

Disulfiram (*Tetraethylthiuram disulphide*; *Antabuse*) is a chemical substance which blocks the metabolism of alcohol at the acetaldehyde state. This has the effect of causing unpleasant symptoms which occur shortly after ingestion of a small amount of alcohol: congestion of the face and conjunctivae, tachycardia, giddiness, headache and a feeling of general distress. Where large amounts of alcohol have been drunk, a dangerous state of collapse, even death, can occur. In order that a patient so treated should be properly warned of this he will need, after one or two daily doses of 0.5 g, to be given a small tot of spirit, so that he can experience some of the consequences likely to occur should he take a drink unguardedly. It may be wise to repeat this lesson more than once. He may then be instructed to take 200–500 mg of the drug daily over an indefinite period or until he is thought to be able to control his drinking without its assistance. An alternative though similar treatment is citrated calcium carbimide (*Abstem*) which, if the patient does default, produces a milder and less dangerous reaction.

It should be emphasized that these treatments are only indicated in the case of those subjects who are strongly motivated to give up drinking but who require a standby, particularly in the early stages when in risk of relapse. As already emphasized, it is motivation towards cure which surpasses any or all methods of treatment tried; without motivation all will surely fail.

Prognosis

The question of whether the aim should be to prevent the alcoholic from drinking for all time is a vexing one about which there is no universal agreement. To tell a man that as he cannot control his drinking he must give it up for ever is to brand him as an inferior person who cannot hold his liquor. This may lead him to continue to drink in defiance. In view of this it is probably better, in the first instance, to temporize and defer a final decision until the immediate situation is under control, for in some cases it is conceivable that a controlled drinking pattern may ultimately be achieved. In any event, the prognosis of alcoholism is obviously variable and difficult to estimate. One study of 70 alcoholics showed that within two years, 45 had improved, of whom 20 were teetotal whereas the remainder were much the same, the overall mortality rate being about 7 per cent.

Drug dependence and abuse

As with alcohol, the term *dependence* may be preferable to *addiction* for the latter begs the vexed question of whether if a drug is to be considered as addictive, both withdrawal symptoms and increasing tolerance should be present. Drug dependence may be physical or psychological or a combination of the two. In the case of some drugs, dependence of any kind is virtually absent. Here, the term *drug abuse* may be more appropriate.

It is currently in vogue to divide drugs according to some of their effects into 'hard' and 'soft'; this division depending largely on whether the drug-taker suffers from abstinence symptoms if he stops taking his drug. Although this has some validity, it is of limited use in practice simply because most who abuse drugs are often polymorphous in their preferences and tend to switch from one drug to another according to availability. Alcohol is often included.

Narcotics

Those who become dependent on *morphine* usually have easy access, such as doctors, nurses and chemists. Habituation may, however, follow injudicious or long-term therapeutic use of opiates. Likewise, other powerful synthetic analgesics, such as *pethidine* and, among others, *dextromoramide* (Palfium), *dextropropoxyphene* combined with *paracetamol* (Distalgesic), *dihydrocodeine* (DF 118), *dipipanone* (Diconal), *levorphanol* (Dromoran), *methadone* (Physeptone), *pentazocine* (Fortral) and *phenadoxone* (Narphen), may induce dependence. It should be noted, furthermore, that as these drugs are commonly prescribed to control pain their withdrawal may signal a return of pain. This is possibly due to their having a tendency to suppress endorphin or enkephalin activity.

The most pernicious of all such drugs is *heroin* (*di-acetyl morphine*) to which habituation may develop more rapidly than from other opiates. As heroin is little used in therapeutics, most supplies are manufactured and purveyed illicitly. In the Far East, as in Hong Kong, heroin has gained ascendance over opium, especially since the tighter control of opium smoking. In the West, notably in the United States, but also in the United Kingdom and elsewhere, heroin seems to have become the *hard drug* of choice, particularly among adolescents, in whom drug abuse of this kind is a very disturbing phenomenon. The reasons for this seem to be largely subculturally determined, both because of fad and fashion together with a need to experiment. Although by no means all of those who experiment become 'hooked' (drug *argot* is an important aspect of drug subculture), in those who do, it is widely thought that this is due to personality disorder having its roots in a disturbed childhood. This idea, which is difficult to substantiate fully, has already been encountered in discussing alcoholism.

Once dependency has taken hold, its development follows fairly predictable lines. Increasing tolerance demands increasing doses so that lapses, if at all prolonged, cause unpleasant abstinence symptoms which can only be immediately overcome by further resort to the drug. While this is true of all narcotics, it seems to be more so in the case of heroin, especially when administered intravenously ('shooting the main line', 'having a fix', etc.). Although intravenous injection may be pleasurable initially, it soon ceases to delight and merely affords relief against dreaded abstinence symptoms. Thus the life of the addict shortly becomes a journey from one dose to the next with the most miserable prospect of non-arrival.

Abstinence symptoms

1. Coryza with running of the nose and increased salivation.
2. Vomiting, diarrhoea and abdominal colic.
3. Generalized hyperaesthesia, paraesthesiae, neuralgic pains and muscular cramps.
4. Restlessness, insomnia, clouded consciousness and delirium.
5. Utter misery and desperate craving, to the point of inducing suicidal and aggressive impulses.

All these symptoms may be rapidly relieved by an injection of morphine, heroin or by the substitution of methadone.

Withdrawal symptoms apart, a general deterioration of health occurs progressively, for as long as dependence continues. The victim becomes dull, apathetic; anaemic, haggard and cachectic; losing interest both in himself and his environment. He cannot work and has no desire to do so; his intellectual faculties are impaired and his sense of moral values warped. Despite this there is no true dementia, nor do psychoses other than *abstinence delirium* occur. Other physical signs and symptoms include constipation, muscular impairment, tremor of the tongue, face and hands, and small pupils which may be a tell-tale sign. Signs of bodily scarring caused by needle abscesses may be evident.

In some patients—morphine rather than heroin takers—matters do not progress so far. In these patients, dependency may be controlled, so that no increase in dose occurs and the overall effects of habituation are less prominent. There may be a parallel to be drawn here with controlled alcoholism.

Treatment

Initially, treatment must be carried out in hospital. As with alcoholism, it used to be thought that compulsory admission to hospital was almost always necessary, but today many oppose this. As with alcoholism, the success or failure of treatment depends essentially upon motivation rather than upon compulsion in any form. This is all important. Many heroin users, especially those in the earlier stages of their dependency, while professing a desire to be cured, do so in the hope that if admitted for treatment they will be given heroin to combat abstinence symptoms. When they discover that the intention is to withdraw the drug they may become abusive and uncooperative and discharge themselves. Withdrawal, however, is essential and means must be found of overcoming the distress that this may cause. Some form of narcosis is necessary, usually using large doses of tranquillizing drugs, such as diazepam. Intravenous diazepam (Valium) narcosis may help to control withdrawal symptoms. Most authorities advise that withdrawal should be gradual— that is, over several days or a week or two. An alternative method is more sudden withdrawal with the substitution of another narcotic, such as methadone, from which subsequent withdrawal may be easier.

More recently, electro-acupuncture has been advocated as a means of overcoming withdrawal symptoms. While it is too early to assess the final value of such treatment and how it works, the suggestion is that it does so by stimulating CSF met-enkephalin levels previously suppressed, perhaps by addiction to heroin. Treatment following withdrawal will necessarily be psychotherapeutic, with attention to the improvement of the patient's physical condition. As in alcoholism, group as against individual psychotherapy is likely to be more successful. With young addicts successful long-term treatment may demand recourse to all available social agencies geared in any way to dealing with this kind of problem. Those undertaking treatment must be prepared for failure as the relapse rate is high. In some cases modified success in treatment may be achieved by a system of rationing so that dependency, although not cured, is kept within controllable limits.

Hypnotics, Sedatives and Tranquillizers
Barbiturates

Dependency upon barbiturates, which often begins with their use in the treatment of insomnia, has considerably diminished in recent years, probably as a result of propaganda which has led to an alteration in the prescribing habits of family doctors.

The clinical picture of chronic intoxication is like that of drunkenness, the principal symptoms being confusion, clouding of consciousness, ataxia, nystagmus and dysarthria. Tolerance is only slightly increased although where abuse occurs the drug may be taken periodically throughout the day instead of by night only. As withdrawal may lead to fits, even status epilepticus, anticonvulsants should be given.

Other hypnotics

Addiction to paraldehyde, chloral and bromides is now uncommon, once again as a result of a change in prescribing habits. All three may, as a result of chronic overdosage, give rise to various forms of mental disturbance, characterized by alteration of consciousness together with illusions, hallucinations, and other organically induced mental symptoms.

Tranquillizers

Remarkably, major tranquillizing drugs such as chlorpromazine (Largactil) do not appear to give rise to dependency. The position in regard to minor tranquillizers is less clear, there being some evidence of the abuse of such drugs as meprobamate (Equanil, Miltown) and to a certain, although as yet limited, extent, of the benzodiazepines. Continued overdosage with diazepam (Valium) in excess of 40 mg daily or more may, it seems, give rise in some subjects to a condition clinically not too far removed from that induced by barbiturates, having as its main features dullness, confusion, ataxia and withdrawal fits. There is a growing number of reports of dependence upon other drugs in this class, both short as well as long acting.

Stimulants
Cocaine

As cocaine is now seldom used therapeutically, its abuse rarely begins on this basis, if indeed it ever did. Today it is more often taken in conjunction with morphine or heroin, either by injection, sniffed or in mixtures containing other substances. Cocaine allays hunger, removes fatigue and induces a state of euphoria and motor excitability. Taken to excess it may produce delirium with hallucinations which may be visual, auditory or characteristically, it is said, tactile—as if insects were crawling on the skin. Abstinence symptoms include restlessness, insomnia and collapse.

Amphetamine

The effects of amphetamine resemble cocaine though are less powerful. Initially it suppresses appetite, is euphoriant and increases awareness and wakefulness. It has a temporary antidepressive effect although it is of little use in treating depressive illness. Taken in single large doses it is a true hallucinogen. Its abuse is characterized by a remarkable increase in tolerance so that the amphetamine taker may consume up to or even more than 1000 mg daily. After a time this may produce an acute psychotic reaction which while bearing, in some respects, a fairly close resemblance to paranoid schizophrenia tends to be accompanied by clouding of consciousness and visual hallucinations characteristic of delirium. Following withdrawal this reaction usually subsides within 7 to 10 days, although depression and a disturbance of sleep pattern may persist for several weeks.

Although until recently amphetamine preparations, particularly those obtained from illicit sources, were widely abused by young persons ('speed'), following tighter controls amphetamine abuse has considerably diminished. It may also be worth noting that in many cases and on account of its anorexogenic properties, amphetamine dependency once often followed upon its use in the treatment of obesity. The same also applied to *phenmetrazine* (Preludin) and possibly to some other appetite-suppressing agents such as *diethylpropion* (Tenuate, Dospan) which if similarly abused may have similar effects to those of amphetamines. Indeed, it is probably wise to regard all appetite suppressants with suspicion.

Another stimulant drug on which dependence has recently been described is *tranylcypromine* (Parnate), possibly on account of its close structural relationship to amphetamine.

Phantastica

Included under the heading phantastica are those drugs used or abused primarily on account of their hallucinogenic or other special effects. Some have been known for centuries, an early example being the fungus *Amanita muscaria* (Fly agaric) said to be used by the Vikings and the Koryak tribes of Siberia to produce a state of excessive emotion on occasions of festivity. The fungus contains muscarine and myceto-atropine.

Other fungi more recently sought after by 'hippies' and those seemingly in search of some kind of transcendental experience are mushrooms of the genus Psilocybe, the commonest in this country being the Liberty Cap (*Psilocybe semilanceata*). This mushroom and related species contain *psilocybin* and *psilocin*, and are hallucinogenic.

Other substances meriting special consideration include *cannabis*, *mescaline*, *lysergic acid* and *phencyclidine*.

Cannabis Indica

Hashish (Indian Hemp) was first used by the Assyrians as early as the seventh century BC. Since then its use in one form or another has become widespread in Africa and in the East. In the United Kingdom and Europe it is usually smoked in cigarettes ('joints'—'reefers' in the USA) in the form known as marihuana ('pot'). Strictly, marihuana is derived from the American form *cannabis sativa* which, however, appears to be identical in its effects to *cannabis indica*. If taken in sufficient amounts, it may produce vivid dreams or visual hallucinations together with a disorder of the sense of time and space. Increased motor activity, maniacal excitement, aggressive outbursts and schizophrenic symptoms can occur, but such striking effects are not usually to be observed in marihuana smokers in whom the effect of the drug is said to be mildly euphoriant and not dissimilar to alcohol. However, *ganja* and *bhang*, which may contain a much higher concentration of cannabis, may have a more profound effect upon the user. Otherwise, and as cannabis is not addictive in the strict sense and because it seems to be harmless when used in moderation, many believe that its use should no longer be illegal. Others who oppose this hasten to point out that heroin users often begin by smoking marihuana. However, as most persons who smoke marihuana never go further than this, it is likely that even if some do progress to heroin addiction they might otherwise have done so by a different route. A more serious argument against cannabis is that there does appear to be some evidence that long-term use may bring about a state of apathy and inanition.

Mescaline

Mescaline is an alkaloid derived from the cactus *Anahalonium lewinii* (peyotl) native to Mexico. It is a true hallucinogen, producing heightened visual imagery, visual hallucinations and hallucinations in other sensory modalities as well; synaesthesiae, depersonalization and in large doses schizophreniform symptoms.

Lysergic acid diethylamide (LSD 25)

Lysergic acid diethylamide, known colloquially as 'acid', was first synthesized by Stoll and Hofmann in 1938. The discovery that it could produce psychotic symptoms when given in minute amounts initially excited great interest and stimulated a search for a naturally occurring substance with similar properties with which to account for schizophrenia. LSD, like mescaline, produces heightened visual imagery, illusions and sometimes hallucinations. Its more immediate effects are changes in mood varying from giggling euphoria to profound anxiety and depression, and ego disturbances leading to depersonalization, paranoid misinterpretations, confusion and a wide variety of other symptoms. A number of tragedies have arisen from so-called bad trips, one of the more bizarre being a belief by some of the subjects that they can fly which has occasionally had disastrous consequences.

One of the dangers surrounding the indiscriminate use of LSD is that preparations obtained through illicit sources vary widely in the amount of lysergic acid they may contain. This may lead the incautious drug taker to ingest a much larger dose than would normally be considered safe, leading possibly to an acute psychosis of schizophreniform type which may take weeks to subside. Apart from this, it has periodically been observed that certain experiences produced by LSD may recur, well after the immediate effects of the drug have worn off and without further amounts being taken (the so-called flash-back). Furthermore, LSD produces a fairly intense and persistent state of depression in some subjects.

LSD is not a drug of addiction. Its acute immediate effects can usually be countered by the administration of a psychotropic drug such as chlorpromazine. However, in the event of a severe psychotic reaction occurring, a period of more prolonged treatment may be needed. Also, when confronted with an acute reaction to a hallucinogenic drug, the possibility that this may be caused by some substance other than LSD should be considered. Not only does there seem to be a growing number of such substances available, but the subject may be by no means always clear what exactly it is that he or she has taken.

Phencyclidine (PCP, 'angel dust')

Phencyclidine was originally introduced as a dissociative veterinary anaesthetic. After marijuana, it is now said to have become the most widely abused 'street drug' in the United States and there is now some evidence of its use having spread to Britain. Ingestion of phencyclidine produces both neurological and psychiatric symptoms, including a psychosis clinically indistinguishable from schizophrenia.

Inhalants

There is such a large number of substances which can be abused that it seems possible that some subjects may be prepared to try almost anything available. Inhaling nitrous oxide, ether or other anaesthetic agents may occur among dentists and anaesthetists. *Glue-sniffing* or inhaling fumes from various *dopes* used in model making is now frequently recorded, usually among adolescents. Unfortunately these substances contain various organic solvents such as toluene or benzol which, in addition to producing delirium together with presumably sought-after hallucinatory experiences, can also lead to liver failure. Another complication is asphyxia which may be the outcome of using plastic bags to facilitate the sniffing process.

Further reading

Edwards, G. (1982) *The Treatment of Drinking Problems*. Oxford: Blackwell Scientific.

Kessel, N. & Walton, H. (1965) *Alcoholism*. St Albans: Hart-Davis MacGibbon.

Lewin, L. (1931) *Phantastica: Narcotic and Stimulating Drugs*. London: Routledge & Kegan Paul.

12

Abnormal Emotional Reactions

Abnormal emotional (or neurotic) reactions, like personality problems, raise many controversial issues. There is considerable overlap here as most of those manifesting neurotic behaviour are of abnormal personality, and most with evidence of personality disorder will at times suffer neurotic symptoms. As with personality disorders, there are considerable problems with terminology. The term *neurosis* does not imply physical disorder of the nervous system; there is no evidence to support the existence of such disorder.

Definitions

Neurosis is a psychological reaction to acute or continuously perceived stress, expressed in behaviour ultimately inappropriate in dealing with that stress. As this state includes all of us at some time or other, the first major difficulty is to define what is neurosis and what is a normal emotional reaction. This depends on such factors as individual perception of what is an unacceptable symptom and, in its turn, upon social and cultural factors including what sort of help is available and from whom this help comes: doctor, social worker, personnel officer, or priest. The difference between normality and neurosis lies partly in whether the reaction is appropriate in degree and partly whether the behavioural response helps to lessen the source of conflict. Patients with abnormal reactions experience and complain of symptoms continuously and severely at least for a period of time, whilst for the normal person such experience is transient and occurs in response to considerable stress. The neurotic does not achieve a successful adaptation to his symptoms, nor does he cope with further stressful situations, unlike a healthy person. *Neurosis* is not a comprehensive description of a condition like *pneumonia* which one either has or has not. Likewise, it is possible to be minimally neurotic; thus the border between normality and abnormality is arbitrary.

In psychosis there is a qualitative impairment of mental functioning so that insight and reality judgement are affected and thus the subject becomes unable to meet the ordinary demands of life. To account for this some underlying somatic disorder is postulated. However, in neurosis basic personality is preserved, so that the subject does not strike those around him as completely irrational or out of contact with reality (i.e. 'out of his mind'). His condition can be *understood* inasmuch as his anxiety, although seemingly unjustified by the circumstances which have occasioned it, is, nevertheless, an all too familiar experience. Indeed, there appears to be no qualitative difference between *normal* and *morbid* anxiety, only in the circumstances which occasion them. The quality of experience of the psychotic patient is, in contrast, so strange and so unfamiliar that the normal person only approaches it while asleep and dreaming or, if awake, under the most exceptional circumstances, such as when severely exhausted.

It is often very difficult to make a clear-cut distinction between psychoses and abnormal emotional reactions: they may on occasions both be present. It is a mistake to contrast psychoses as serious and causing permanent disability with neuroses as *minor mental disturbances*. Thus a severe obsessional disorder may be so intractable as to be lifelong and far more crippling than two or possibly three or more bouts of relatively short-lived endogenous depression. Much depends on the criteria of illness applied. Similarly, not infrequently sufferers from depressive neurosis kill themselves, and there is also a markedly increased rate of suicide amongst those with personality disorder.

Aetiology

There can be little doubt that both hereditary predisposition and adverse environmental circumstances contribute to the formation of emotional disorders, although most authorities would agree that, here, nurture is of greater importance than nature. There is some evidence that personality type is at least in part inherited and that a genetic influence may determine the type of abnormal emotional reaction manifested. The environmental influences which appear to foster adverse emotional reactions can be summarized into those associated with early life experiences and those developing in the presence of and partly provided by adverse life events or current stresses.

Abnormal emotional reactions as a response to stress may be learnt from parents, just as other behaviour patterns are acquired in the family. Such reactions can also be provoked by conflicts due to family quarrels and arguments which may give rise to split loyalties in the child; adjusting to an absent or delinquent parent or in coping with the rivalries and competing claims of siblings. The importance of the emotional bond between mother and child in the first year of life has been emphasized by Bowlby for the subsequent development of normal emotional responses. Later work has shown that it is not only this earliest period of development when the relationship with mother is crucial; but that the relationship between father and child is also vital for subsequent normal development. Continuing conflict and family disturbance is much more damaging than complete loss of a parent through bereavement. Family atmosphere and the quality of relationships are extremely influential in determining future emotional reactions; they also create the pattern for the home atmosphere and relationships which children will establish when they too become parents.

Psychodynamic theory, as originally propounded by Freud, claimed that neurotic behaviour arose from personal conflicts that remained repressed at an unconscious level since early childhood and could ultimately only find expression in an inappropriate and censored way. Freud considered all such conflicts ultimately to be sexual in nature, and to be established in early childhood usually about the age of three or four. The intolerable emotion, usually of guilt, could not be faced and might therefore be converted into a physical symptom—*conversion hysteria*. Such theories are useful when looking for underlying causes of problems rather than commenting upon the symptom itself; attention has also been drawn to the nature of the relationship between patient and doctor in a helpful way. However, evidence for the universal validity of Freudian theory is lacking.

The immediate cause of neurotic reactions is stress. What is stressful to one person may be stimulating and exciting to another; what is seen by one as a satisfactory, calm way of life may by another be perceived as boring and hence stressful. Stress may refer to the response to a noxious stimulus: also to an experience called *stress* in which certain features of the *general adaptation syndrome* (Selye) occur irrespective of the nature of the stimulus. Stress may be considered to be the circumstances that provoke such a reaction: stressors or *adverse life events*. Perhaps it is best to combine both models and see stress as existing in the relationship between a subject and the way he perceives his environment—at work, at home, or both.

It is part of common experience that unfortunate circumstances or *adverse life events* cause misery and fear, and that such emotions can transcend what can be considered as an appropriate reaction, and become abnormal. The particular categories of life event which are associated with a depressive reaction are those that are undesirable, those that represent *exits from the social field* such as the death of a relative or leaving home for the first time, and events which reveal *interpersonal difficulties* such as family arguments. Adverse life events are prominent at the beginning of many neurotic illnesses.

Abnormal emotional reactions may be seen as *learned behaviour*. One account of how this occurs is the hypothesis of *learned helplessness*, originally described in experimental work carried out with dogs, but subsequently applied to humans in social conditions. The theory is that recurrent exposure to unpleasant situations of suffering or personal failure where the subject is incapable of escape eventually produces a response where no attempt to escape is made even though it is now possible; the victim assumes that activity is hopeless, that everything will inevitably go wrong, and accepts this with resignation. Other learning theory models to explain the development of neurotic reactions include both classical Pavlovian and operant conditioning. The latter is especially appropriate in explaining addictive behaviour.

Classification

The principal forms of emotional disturbance encountered in practice may be conveniently classified under four main headings.

1. *Depressive reactions* (*neurotic depression*; discussed later in this chapter and in Chapter 6).
2. *Anxiety states* (including many *phobic reactions*).
3. *Hysteria* (*dissociative* and *attention-seeking reactions*).
4. *Obsessive–compulsive disorders*.

The last mentioned are dealt with separately and in greater detail in Chapters 14 and 15. These diagnostic divisions are by no means watertight, as many people may show two or more features of neurosis concurrently. Although it is customary to include phobic reactions under the heading of anxiety states, many such reactions veer close to coming within the category of obsessional disorders. Anxiety itself may also be strongly manifest in many cases of obsessional disorder while admixtures of obsessional and hysterical symptoms are not uncommon.

In addition to these principal varieties of emotional reaction there are a number of other possibly less well-defined disorders which require separate consideration.

Acute emotional crises (acute reactions to stress)

Acute emotional crises include more or less short-lived disturbances in behaviour, usually caused quite clearly by an emotionally disturbing experience or trauma, which can be severe enough to justify the attention of a psychiatrist. Bereavement reactions provide a good example. All persons naturally react with grief to the loss of a near relative or with anger to an unprovoked insult. Such emotional reactions are entirely normal, although, when severe, may still bring a patient to the doctor for consolation or sympathetic counsel. There are, however, emotional responses to bereavement which are clearly outside the normal range, leading to an overprolonged reaction which fails to resolve as expected. In such cases an ambivalent relationship between the deceased and the bereaved may often be discovered.

Psychogenic (reactive) depression

Where neurotic disorders are subcategorized it is generally found that neurotic or reactive depression is the commonest form of abnormal emotional reaction. Psychogenic depressions bear a certain resemblance to psychotic depressions as regards the actual mood change and other psychological features, but do not as a rule show such symptoms as early morning waking, the characteristic diurnal variation of mood, loss of weight, or other somatic or so-called biological symptoms. The group considered here includes reactions such as those which occur in mothers who do not wish to continue with an unwanted pregnancy or persons facing a financial or some other crisis. Much of the confusion which surrounds this matter is of semantic origin and bound up with the dual meaning of the term *depression* (see p. 93). In the symptomatic sense, depression of 'normal' or non-endogenous type is familiar to all persons. It is also familiar in this sense as a symptom of an emotional reaction.

For a depression to be truly reactive, Jaspers requires the following three criteria to be fulfilled.

1. The content of the depression must have a comprehensible relationship to the experience.
2. The condition would not have arisen without this experience.
3. The symptoms should disappear on removal of the cause.

Very few reactive depressions fulfil all these requirements, although every now and then a patient is seen suffering from depression apparently wholly precipitated by psychic stress in whom little or no evidence of a constitutional factor can be elicited. Even these patients may on further investigation be found to be suffering basically from some other type of emotional illness.

Mental mechanisms

A considerable part of the terminology used traditionally by psychiatrists to describe the presumed processes occurring in those who show abnormal emotional reactions was derived from psychoanalysis. Such terms should be regarded not as factual entities but as hypothetical working concepts.

Mental mechanisms are modes of irrational or emotionally determined thinking and action. They provide an escape from having to face unpleasant reality which would otherwise occasion anxiety or some other disagreeable affect. They play a part to some extent in everyday mental activity but when they predominate in certain areas of the patient's mental life and modify behaviour to any degree, they may in themselves be regarded as emotionally abnormal (or even in some cases as psychotic symptoms). The difference between ordinary evasion of difficulties and pathological reactions to situations or psychological stresses is one of degree rather than kind.

Compensation is the development of a personal quality to offset a defect or sense of inferiority. Within certain limits, this is a normal, useful process but may be overdone, becoming a matter of *overcompensation*, when it is a reaction to repressed drives. The excessively conscientious and scrupulous individual may be overcompensating for opposite and contrary tendencies.

Conversion is the manifestation of repressed ideas in the form of bodily symptoms. Thus a hysterical paralysis of the legs may represent a crude form of escape from anxiety that might be occasioned if the sufferer were not prevented by his disability from having to go out and about.

Displacement is the shifting of emotion from one object or situation which occasions it to another. This serves as a means of disguising or avoiding unacceptable ideas and tendencies. This is the psycho-dynamic explanation to account for irrational and apparently meaningless fears and phobias, though an alternative hypothesis would regard conditioning as likely to play a greater part, particularly in phobia formation.

Dissociation is a splitting of consciousness whereby inconsistencies in thought and conduct are overlooked. It is also a mechanism which is thought to be operative in hypnosis, in sleep-walking and in hysterical trance states. It also occurs in schizophrenia and accounts for phenomena such as affective incongruity, delusions involving incompatibility and inconsistency in thought.

Fixation is arrest of development of personality to a state short of emotional maturity, even though general intelligence may measure up to average or above average on rating scales. Childish ways of reacting to difficulties, excessive dependence on others and marked egotism are all manifestations of fixation. The Freudian school stresses arrest of psychosexual development as a basis for pathological mental states and, in fact, all inferior adaptations to life situations.

Identification is the conscious or unconscious placing of oneself in the situation of another person and may include the assumption of the characteristics of that person. It is normal for young people to imitate the attitudes and behaviour of older persons whom they may hold in high esteem. However, it is also normal, particularly in the case of adolescents, to try to escape from identification as part of their own search for self-identity. Aping manners involves identification and wishful thinking. Persons drawn together by a common bond of empathy may also identify strongly with one another. In certain delusional states, such as *folie à deux*, such identification may operate at an unconscious level.

Introjection is the turning inwards of aggressive feelings and attitudes towards others which might otherwise give rise to conflict. Thus hostility towards others may be repressed and introjected in the form of suicidal impulses.

Projection is the displacement of personal attitudes on to the environment and thus is the opposite of introjection. It is a way of avoiding self-blame and feelings of guilt. Personal shortcomings and failures are ascribed to 'bad luck' or an unfavourable material or psychological environment, a mechanism seen in an extreme form in delusions of persecution.

Rationalization is another means of self-deception by finding satisfactory socially acceptable reasons for conduct which is really prompted by less worthy or unethical motives.

Regression is a reversion to modes of thought, feeling and behaviour which are more appropriate to an earlier stage of development. Thus an adult may be said to regress to childish petulance and temper tantrums while a physically or mentally handicapped person may regress to a child–mother dependent attitude towards a nurse. So-called regressive behaviour really results from emotional immaturity and fixation.

Repression is the thrusting out of consciousness of ideas and urges to action which are incompatible with ideals, conscience, ethical standards or in general with what is recognized as the right and proper thing to do under the circumstances. It is regarded as an unconscious, involuntary process, in contrast to *suppression* which is a conscious, willed checking or inhibition of thoughts, feelings and actions which conflict with moral standards.

Resistance is the barrier between the unconscious and the conscious, preventing resolution of incompatible elements in mental activity. The patient resists mental exploration, clings to his symptoms and in various ways fails to cooperate in treatment, although he does so unconsciously and not wilfully.

Sublimation is the direction of undesirable or forbidden tendencies into more socially acceptable channels. Childish egocentric conduct should normally, and as a result of increasing maturity, be sublimated into more altruistic social behaviour. Surplus energies may be sublimated into useful channels.

Transference refers to the experience of emotions towards one person which are derived from experience with another. Thus a patient may transfer anxious or hostile feelings which he previously experienced in relation to a harsh dominating parent towards all those whom he later regards as authority figures. This mechanism plays an important part in psychotherapy, where the patient expresses feelings towards the therapist which he has transferred from elsewhere.

Further reading

Freud, S. (1949) *Introductory Lectures on Psychoanalysis*, translated by Joan Riviere, 2nd edn. London: George Allen & Unwin.
Sims, A. C. P. (1983) *Neurosis in Society*. London: Macmillan.

13
Anxiety States

Normal anxiety—that is, anxiety proportionate to the situation which occasions it—is a biologically protective experience. It draws attention to oncoming danger and, unless overwhelming, promotes a state of physical and psychological readiness whereby the subject is able to take appropriate action to protect himself either by flight or fight. Anxiety and pain are analogous: anxiety draws attention to an environmental threat, pain to a threat to some part of the body.

Morbid anxiety is objectless fear, fear disproportionate to that which occasions it or fear displaced on to some relatively neutral object or situation. However, it is not always easy to draw the line between normal and morbid, the matter being one of degree. The quality of anxiety, whether normal or morbid, is, furthermore, of the same order but may vary in degree and duration. Because of this a normal individual can fairly readily understand how a chronically anxious person feels though he may not fully appreciate what that person is anxious about or why he feels as anxious as he does.

Because anxiety, whether real or morbid, is unpleasant and if allowed to persist soon tends to become intolerable, steps must be taken to overcome it. In normal anxiety, fright or flight may provide the answer by separating the source from the subject, but in pathological anxiety, the cause is inappropriate to the degree of anxiety and escape may be impossible.

A state of morbid anxiety may be symptomatic of almost any psychiatric disorder. Anxiety is an integral part of depressive illnesses and, if severe, can give rise to intense agitation, particularly in older patients. In schizophrenia, anxiety is often prominent at the onset of the illness when the patient is bewildered by strange and sometimes terrifying misinterpretations of his environment. In paranoid states, delusions of persecution sometimes lead to panic. Anxiety is also prominent in cerebral arteriosclerosis and even more so in acute organic reactions such as delirium tremens. Where prolonged anxiety occurs in the absence of these conditions, and appears to be the outcome of inability to cope with relatively minor or insignificant day-to-day environmental stresses, this may denote a *primary anxiety state* or *anxiety neurosis*, such a diagnosis being seen as a *reaction* rather than a *disease entity*. Anxiety reactions, apart from those obviously secondary to other psychiatric illnesses such as have been listed, cover several conditions which vary considerably. In some anxiety states, phobic symptoms are marked; in others, obsessional symptoms are more prominent. In a third group, somatic manifestations may be foremost, as for example in 'cardiac neurosis' (*neurocirculatory asthenia* or the *effort syndrome*). What is important about an anxiety state is not the anxiety itself but why the sufferer is anxious and why his anxiety is so severe and prolonged.

Aetiology

Hereditary factors may determine how readily anxiety is evoked by stressful situations. There appears to be an association between proneness to anxiety and an *asthenic* psychophysical constitution. However, the causative influence of socio-environmental factors is more obvious than any physical basis for anxiety. Anxious children are born of anxious parents; undue anxiety in the face of stress may be regarded as a learned response. Feelings of insecurity in children may be greatly enhanced by inconsistent attitudes exhibited by their parents, who may themselves be maladjusted. Such parental inconsistency is probably more damaging than harshness or other negative attitudes for, while defences may be evoked against these, inconsistency by its very nature militates against the establishment of adequate defence mechanisms.

Although as maturity is achieved anxiety tends to lessen, it is prone to recur in later life under the pressures of advancing age. As in the case of childhood, the dependence and insecurity which old age brings often lead to a heightening of anxiety, although this may in due course be dimmed by dementia.

From a psychodynamic viewpoint, it has been postulated that anxiety states and other similar reactions in adult life are the outcome of exposure to psychologically traumatic events during childhood, knowledge of which has been repressed. Such traumatic events were once often thought to be of a sexual nature. Support was lent to this by the uncovering of such incidents in the past history, until it came to be recognized that the accounts given were as often as not fantasy rather than fact. Although it cannot be denied that sexual trauma in childhood may later have harmful psychological consequences, its importance has been exaggerated. Furthermore, it is apparently not so much single incidents which may do harm but those, whether sexual or not (and sometimes in themselves quite minor), constantly repeated which probably do greater damage.

Anxieties leading to phobias may in some cases be an outcome of untoward early life experiences. The more specific the phobia, the more likely this is to be true. While it is thought that a single psychologically traumatic event can, if sufficiently overwhelming, give rise to a phobia, this occurrence is more likely when the subject, having become sensitized by an initial experience, is exposed to a similar trauma before desensitization has occurred, a process known as reinforcement. More diffuse phobic states cannot be so readily explained; some, such as *agoraphobia*, fear of going out into the open (*lit*. fear of the market place), appear to be more in the nature of a secondary defence evolved to protect the patient from social situations or other environmental circumstances with which he or, more often, she cannot cope.

Clinical features

Anxiety states take a variety of forms depending on whether psychological or physical symptoms predominate. Both, however, are always present to some degree.

Psychological symptoms
The presenting complaint may be of anxiety, overtly expressed although not in relation to any particular object or situation, whereupon it may be said to be free floating. There may be a general apprehensiveness over trifles, none specific; a tendency to worry needlessly; or a combination of any or all of these. Fears expressed tend to become attached to any current happening, although often only transiently. Hypochondriacal concern is common; intolerance of strong stimuli, such as bright lights and noise, may lead to minor eccentricities, such as wearing dark glasses in the dimmest kind of winter weather. Irritability is often prominent; due to an extremely common disorder of mood in which there is poor control of impulsive feelings of aggression. Reassurance about all manner of things is often sought so that unduly anxious patients soon become a considerable trial to others. In the Scottish colloquialism: 'They fear for the day they never saw'.

Certain situations in which the patient tends to feel especially inadequate are apt to provoke crises in which psychological and physical symptoms become so dominating as to leave him exhausted. His emotional preoccupation with himself and his anxious feelings may be of such a degree as to cause difficulty in concentration or even to lead to memory lapses. These lapses he all too readily tends to regard as proof positive of mental deterioration and impending insanity. Inquiry should always be made into this as the patient who entertains the fear that he is going mad commonly does not mention the matter in case his fear should be confirmed. If, however, the matter is first brought into the open, reassurance may soon be effected though it may need to be repeated. Sleep is frequently disturbed by anxious dreams or nightmares. Some patients may find difficulty in falling asleep on this account.

Physical symptoms
Physical symptoms are of equal importance and as troublesome as those

which are psychological. They appear to be derived from a disturbance of the equilibrium of the autonomic nervous system; the principal symptoms and signs are pallor, sweating, goose pimples, dry mouth, pupillary dilatation, a sinking feeling in the stomach, frequency of micturition and looseness of the bowels. Panic attacks are discrete episodes of extreme somatic anxiety, whilst in between attacks the person may feel mildly anxious or quite normal. Tachycardia causing palpitations is common, together with a rise in systolic blood pressure. The respiration rate may be raised leading not uncommonly to hyperventilation which may add to already existing feelings of panic by causing feelings of faintness, paraesthesiae and sometimes actual attacks of tetany giving rise to carpopedal spasm (*hyperventilation syndrome*).

Acute panic states (fright reactions)

These may occur in response to sudden severe shocks or threats: after traffic accidents, explosions, mine disasters, under bombardment, during war time and so on. Under such conditions anxiety may be so overwhelming that the sufferer may literally be paralysed with fright (*psychogenic stupor*) or may pass into a fugue state. Alternatively, he may show a panicky type of behaviour with extreme agitation and attempts to run wild. Such reactions often arise in conjunction with a tendency to dissociate under extreme stress and thus may have a markedly hysterical colouring. In less acute states of panic, transient euphoria together with excessive talkativeness may occur.

Phobic states

Phobic anxiety states are of two main types: monophobic and those which are more diffuse. A phobia is an abnormally intense dread of certain objects or specific situations which would not normally have that effect. *Monophobic anxiety states* are of the kind evoked by circumstances which are virtually specific. Animal and some social phobias fall into this class. Thus a patient who may for the most part be untroubled by fears of other kinds may acquire an intense fear of cats, to a degree which can arouse in him a state of panic and lead, whenever cats appear, to a need to take evasive action which in turn may interfere with the normal pursuits of everyday living. Such monophobias must be distinguished from those which are so common as to be considered normal, such as an almost universal fear of snakes, spiders, heights, etc. It is sometimes difficult to decide whether such fears are abnormal or not. Fear of heights is a good case in point. Many otherwise quite normal people might hesitate to approach within a few feet of the edge of a precipice without this being considered as particularly remarkable. A subject, however, who cannot, on account of a phobia of heights, bring himself to climb more than one or two floors upwards in an ordinary office building in pursuit of his everyday occupation, would quite rightly be regarded by most people as in need of treatment. It is in the middle between these extremes where there is difficulty in deciding what is normal and what is not; however, abnormality should only be considered to exist when there is interference with function.

Diffuse phobic anxiety states appear to be much more frequent than monophobias. Typical perhaps is the *agoraphobic* or 'house-bound housewife' syndrome which, of course, is not confined to housewives. However, the clinical picture seems to be fairly consistent. The patient, often female, dependent and immature, perhaps removed some distance by marriage from the home of her parents, with whom her relationship is often highly ambivalent, suddenly starts to develop acute anxiety symptoms whenever she tries to go outside her home for no better reason perhaps than a simple shopping expedition. The condition may first emerge suddenly when she is in a supermarket or some other crowded place. Once in being, it tends to spread to include many other situations. Each fresh experience of panic tends to be self-reinforcing so that all external activities become progressively restricted. Finally, the unhappy woman discovers that she can hardly pass through her front door unaccompanied without being overtaken by feelings of fright and faintness. Her gorge rises, her legs become jelly-like; she panics, palpitates, overbreathes and becomes depersonalized to such a degree that it seems to her that if she does not rapidly regain the security of her home, she will be overtaken by disaster.

Many other related phobic conditions may be encountered, indeed their variability seems almost endless. Some patients panic while in closed places and, even if they can bring themselves to visit the theatre or cinema, must choose an aisle seat or one close to an exit. Others cannot travel by bus or other public transport, for fear of being unable to alight, if need be, while the vehicle is in motion. Other patients have a fear of being caught short and, in planning any kind of outing, even of a relatively minor kind, must plan a route which ensures that toilet facilities are all the time fairly close to hand. This kind of phobic state, as in the case of some others, has an obsessional quality and, indeed, is one of several such examples which seem to bridge the gap between anxiety and obsessive–compulsive states.

Somatic anxiety states

In some anxiety states it is the somatic aspects which loom largest. These have a tendency to become fixed. Because a patient with an anxiety state derived initially from environmental circumstances suffers from palpitations, these may easily come to preoccupy him even more than the original source of his anxiety, so that he begins to fear he may suffer from heart disease. This engenders further anxiety and prolongs his palpitations and other disagreeable related physical symptoms, leading to a vicious circle and the establishment of a 'cardiac neurosis'. Several other somatic anxiety syndromes may arise in a similar way (see also Chapter 12).

Some anxiety states verge upon hysterical conversion reactions. Others are characterized more by doubt and uncertainty and thus veer towards obsessive hypochondriasis in which the sufferer, while not actually convinced that he is physically ill, can never quite accept reassurance that without doubt he is not.

Neurasthenia

Although no longer fashionable, the term *neurasthenia* may still perhaps be appropriately applied to that type of psychological disorder characterized by undue mental and physical fatiguability and bearing a general resemblance to a low-grade anxiety state with depressive features. The patient is usually thin, underweight and sleeps fitfully. Muscle tone is poor with tremor of eyelids, tongue and hands. Cold clammy extremities and hyperhidrosis are common. In addition to the usual visceral and cardiovascular symptoms, gastric discomfort, dyspepsia, flatulence and eructation frequently occur, together with palpitations. There may be a sensation as if a band were drawn tightly round the head or a feeling of pressure on the vertex, often described as numbness and not uncommonly associated with sensations of dizziness or muzziness. Tension in the occipital muscles is common, together with a variety of aches and pains which may occur anywhere in the body. There is marked distractability, lack of attention, inability to concentrate or to sustain any form of prolonged mental or physical effort. The patient is irritable and easily upset and is liable to outbursts and acute emotional crises. He may be given to suicidal ruminations, though not to the same degree as in other depressive disorders. Depersonalization is common together with transient obsessional and hypochondriacal symptoms and attention-seeking behaviour.

Diagnosis

As indicated earlier, anxiety symptoms may occur either as a part of or in association with a wide range of other psychiatric and physical illnesses. It may be necessary, therefore, to exclude any of these, both by thorough physical and mental examination together with all necessary biochemical and other investigations. A neurasthenic state may also be physically determined and is particularly prone to follow infections such as influenza, jaundice, glandular fever, brucellosis, typhoid or any severely debilitating illness, or may be due to some toxic condition the nature of which is not always readily apparent. Head injury is a very common precipitant, although other injuries, particularly of industrial origin in which an element of compensation is involved, may be implicated.

In the presence of an acute anxiety state, the possibility of *thyrotoxicosis* should be considered. Investigation may be needed to clarify this (see p. 259). However, by far the most important disorder to exclude is a *primary depressive illness*. Such illnesses, when mild, so often resemble anxiety states that some authorities are always inclined to regard a diagnosis of anxiety state as suspect. If the illness is relatively circumscribed, has a fairly well-defined onset and occurs in someone not hitherto thought to be particularly disturbed or emotionally immature, then there may be good reasons for suspecting depression, particularly if further inquiry reveals even relatively slight evidence of guilt, self-reproach or an element of despair. Early waking from sleep and diurnal variation, in which the patient's anxious condition is worse in the morning with a tendency to improve as the day goes on, may be useful diagnostic pointers towards a depressive illness.

Treatment

Before symptomatic treatment of anxiety or phobic symptoms is undertaken, a careful assessment of all features relevant to prognosis and management should be carried out. An important consideration here is the distinction between the occurrence of acute anxiety in response to immediate stress or conflict and the presence of chronic anxiety or repeated proneness to anxiety as a continuing trait of personality; knowledge of the duration of symptoms is necessary. Often features of both stress and personality proneness are present. Occasionally it may be possible to help the patient deal with the stress; for instance, a student who is responding to the stress of approaching examinations by panic and consequent inability to study will thereby be increasing his anxiety symptoms. Management will include educational counselling in order to reduce the ever-increasing stress of failing to prepare himself adequately. Acute situational anxiety is much better treated by facing up to it and dealing with the causes, if at all possible, rather than recourse to anxiolytic drugs.

It is important to understand the patient's lifestyle and social situation and it may be possible to modify these and thereby lessen anxiety. Understanding how other people close to the patient view his symptoms may be relevant; for example, it is usual to find the mother of a child who is school phobic to be excessively anxious and quite possibly phobic herself. Effective treatment of the child's anxiety may begin with measures to allay the anxieties of his mother.

Patients who come for treatment of anxiety may have developed ways of coping which may reduce anxiety in the short term but make long-term management more difficult; for example, the official who is frequently off sick on days when he should be making a public statement in the council meeting. Similarly, people may have learnt to cope by using alcohol or drugs not prescribed for them as anxiolytics. It is important to know what the patient's response has been to previous methods of treatment. One also needs to know whether patients obtain any benefit from their symptoms which would therefore tend towards their persistence.

Assessment of the presence and significance of other symptoms is always important. The possibility of physical illness presenting with anxiety should not be overlooked, and appropriate physical examination and investigations need to be carried out. Depression, even if presenting with quite marked additional anxiety, should be treated with antidepressant drugs, for example amitriptyline which has sedative properties in addition to its effect against depression.

Anxiolytic drugs such as the benzodiazepine group are very useful for the treatment of severe short-term symptoms and may be helpful in reducing symptoms to such a level as to enable other methods to be used. The therapeutic efficacy of benzodiazepines probably diminishes after four to six weeks' use, whilst the likelihood of dependence is increased. It is preferable to use one of the drugs with longer duration of action, for example diazepam. All such drugs induce some sedation and there may be a paradoxical effect in some patients, especially the elderly, of increasing rather than diminishing agitation. Suppression of anxiety by drugs, though allowing a short-term escape from symptoms, may prevent a resolution of the causative situation. Beta-adrenergic drugs such as propranolol have been found to be particularly useful in dealing with the somatic symptoms of anxiety.

Detailed discussion of treatment methods is beyond the scope of this chapter, but three methods of psychological management should be mentioned: *dynamic psychotherapy, behavioural modification* and *anxiety control* training.

Dynamic psychotherapy presupposes that the causes of anxiety lie in material that was repressed into the unconscious mind in early childhood and is only able to find expression in an anxious mood that is not associated by the patient with the original, necessarily sexual, cause of the conflict. Treatment involves exploration of this early stage of development using such techniques as *free association*, and concentrating on the nature of the *transference relationship* between patient and doctor.

Behavioural modification is an application of learning theory for the treatment of distressing symptoms. The technique of *systematic desensitization* described by Wolpe has been successfully employed for monophobias. The phobic patient is asked to describe a hierarchy of situations of increasing anxiety involving the object of phobia. Either asking the patient to fantasize each situation and using relaxation, or better still using a real situation, the patient is taken up the hierarchy slowly over several sessions. Therapy never proceeds to the next stage until the patient is able to experience each situation in the hierarchy without anxiety. This technique has often been successful for animal phobias. The alternative technique of *flooding* has been used especially in the treatment of agoraphobia. If the patient is exposed to the worst stress of the anxiety-provoking situation, initial anxiety is very high but gradually wanes, perhaps over a half-hour. The patient is exposed to the stressful situation in this way, on the first few occasions having the support of the therapist with him. This method of treatment is found to be more rapidly successful than desensitization; it is important to maintain practice between treatment sessions.

Anxiety control training has been described by Snaith as a specific symptomatic treatment for pathological anxiety. Using hypnotic techniques, the patient is taught that he can produce the symptoms of anxiety by fantasy in himself, and that he can then bring these symptoms under his own control. The cognitive element of treatment is concerned with the low self-esteem of many such patients and encourages reshaping attitudes towards self and concentrating on situations where the patient has coped successfully. Success of this method also depends upon regular practice between supervised sessions.

The most helpful methods for treatment of anxiety states are therefore psychological. As well as the individual methods of treatment described above, group treatment may also be beneficial, especially when there is a socially phobic element in symptomatology. The relationship between therapist and patient is all important; only when this is firmly established can adequate reassurance be given as to the true nature of his disagreeable and often frightening physical sensations. Even when the roots of a patient's anxiety are uncovered, insight does not necessarily bring about its resolution. This is particularly true when phobias are present. Such anxieties, when established, seem often to persist like habits, even when their source has been removed or has long since disappeared spontaneously, and it is this feature that leads to a need for one of the techniques subsumed under the heading of behaviour therapy.

Further reading

Lader, M. & Marks, I. M. (1971) *Clinical Anxiety*. London: Heinemann Medical.
Marks, I. M. (1969) *Fears and Phobias*. London: Heinemann Medical.
Snaith, P. (1981) *Clinical Neurosis*. London: Oxford University Press.

14
Hysteria

Hysteria is an old-fashioned word describing one of the most complex issues in medicine. While it used to be considered as an exclusively female condition, this, like most other assertions about hysteria, has been disputed. While recently it has been suggested that the term *hysteria* should be rejected altogether, in practice the concept has proved useful and, in the words of Sir Aubrey Lewis, the majority of psychiatrists would be hard put to it if they were no longer able to resort to this diagnosis; and, 'in any case a tough old word like hysteria dies very hard; it tends to outlive its obituarists'.

The International Classification of Diseases (ICD 9), defines hysteria as:

'mental disorder in which motives, of which the patient seems unaware, produce either a restriction of the field of consciousness or disturbances of motor or memory function which may seem to have psychological advantage or symbolic value. It may be characterized by conversion or dissociative phenomena.'

The four implications drawn from this definition are that:

1. the symptoms of hysteria are psychogenic;
2. the cause is unconscious;
3. the symptoms carry some sort of advantage to the patient;
4. they occur via the psychological mechanisms of *conversion* or *dissociation*.

The word conversion implies behaviour appropriate to a physical illness without any organic reason to account for that behaviour. Conversion of an unpleasant effect into a physical symptom must necessarily be unconscious for it to be considered hysterical. Dissociation can be regarded as a narrowing of the field of consciousness serving an unconscious purpose commonly accompanied or followed by selective amnesia; with symptoms which sometimes mimic a patient's concept of mental illness. Perhaps dissociation is best thought of as a form of conversion in which environmental stresses result in illness behaviour in the psychological rather than the physical realm.

The differentiation of hysteria from malingering is always extremely difficult as it is hard to decide how much of the patient's motivation is unconscious. While *secondary gain*—that is, some sort of advantage either actual or expected by the patient himself from his sick role—is often obvious in hysteria, it is, nevertheless, a dangerous diagnostic sign as it is often present in those with organically based symptoms. Hysterical symptoms may be placed at one end of a continuum in which motivation, due to an extreme capacity for the denial of inconvenient reality, is almost entirely hidden from the patient; this probably only applies to a minority of patients. At the other end of the continuum, and once again in the minority of cases, motivation is clear and purposive, amounting to simulation. The majority of hysterical disorders fall somewhere in between. Thus the question is not one of 'either/or' but of 'how much of each?'. If in deceiving himself the hysteric supposes that he can deceive others, at times his belief may be justified, for even the most experienced psychiatrist may err.

Follow-up studies of patients previously diagnosed as suffering from hysteria have cast doubts on its existence as a recognizable condition. In one study, a large proportion of patients had either died or developed serious physical illness or other psychiatric conditions. Only about a fifth of the original sample were without other pathology at the time of follow-up. In another study, over 60 per cent of patients at follow-up showed definite evidence of affective disorder and only 13 per cent a picture consistent with hysteria. It is apparent, therefore, that hysteria has been much overdiagnosed in the past, and that many patients so-diagnosed actually suffer from organic conditions. Likewise, a primary depressive illness may sometimes present in hysterical guise, and failure to recognize this may lead the patient to suicide. Despite these reservations, there undoubtedly appears to be a small minority of patients for whom the diagnosis of hysteria is appropriate.

Aetiology

There is no direct evidence of a genetic contribution to the occurrence of hysteria, although as in other forms of emotional disturbance, an account of a disturbed childhood or of unsatisfactory relationships between parents is common amongst those with hysterical disorders.

The presumptive stresses which provoke hysterical reactions can be very different in their nature and duration. Loss of self-esteem ('loss of face') is usually present but this may either be a short-term affair, such as being charged with a criminal offence, or due to a longer term conflict, as in the case of a wife who knows that her husband is having an affair but cannot take any effective steps to resolve this.

Hysteria is more common amongst those with personality disorder (see Chapter 16). However, a *hysterical reaction* may occur in the absence of personality abnormality. Likewise, the majority of those showing the characteristics of *hysterical personality disorder*, such as histrionic behaviour, shallow affect and an inability to make enduring relationships, never manifest any overt hysterical symptoms. In describing a patient it is best, therefore, to make a clear distinction between hysteria and hysterical personality disorder, although they may occasionally coincide in the same patient.

Epidemic, communicated, or *mass hysteria* has been described for many centuries. It is most likely to occur in closed communities and especially when there is some marked social conflict affecting many members. It spreads by a form of social contagion, and is most likely to affect young girls who are about the age of puberty. The first person affected may have a genuine physical illness. Those who transmit the contagion early on in the epidemic are usually of high social status in their peer group, they are likely to be those who have previously shown instability and are currently going through some personal conflict and from whom the epidemic spreads to more normal girls. Symptoms may include overbreathing, dizziness, fainting, headache, shivering, pins and needles, nausea, pains in the back and abdomen. This condition is an example of socially transmitted abnormal behaviour. There are also some forms of hysteria in which the symptomatology takes a constant form within a distinctive *culture*; identical symptoms may be transmitted to others within the same society. Usually in such situations females again are more commonly affected.

Symptoms

The symptoms of hysteria can occur at any age in either sex; they are considerably influenced by the social group from which the patient comes and also by wider cultural factors. The manifestations of hysteria are legion and tend to adhere to the patient's concept of what a mental or physical disease is like.

It should always be borne in mind that the hysteric is markedly suggestible; hence most scrupulous care must be taken to avoid the creation of fresh symptoms by unnecessarily suggestive questioning or frequently repeated physical examinations which reinforce the patient's conviction of illness. Hysterics can be made as well as born and a heavy responsibility falls on the doctor who is too impatient or gullible to handle wisely those patients who are prone to such symptoms in his practice. Because such patients tend to confuse fantasy with fact, it is often very difficult to get at the truth. It is also common for the hysteric to give a false impression that the home environment is very much better than it actually is.

The symptoms of hysteria can be divided into three main groups: physical, which includes quasi-neurological and less well-defined disorders of the vegetative nervous system; mental; and behavioural eccentricities. The dividing line *is by no means clear cut*. Symptoms of all types may be present in a single case.

Physical symptoms

Although much less common than in times gone by, *quasi-neurological symptoms* include paralyses, contractures, anaesthesiae of 'glove and stocking' type, not corresponding to the known sensory distribution of nervous pathways, hemianaesthesia, ataxia, astasia-abasia, tremors, fits, aphonia, deafness, blindness, tubular vision and many more. These are the symptoms otherwise known as *conversion hysteria*.

Hysterical *fits* may occur which may be confused with those of organic origin. Where the least suspicion of an organic basis exists, a thorough investigation including an electroencephalogram and possibly a CT scan should also be carried out. Differential points, such as atypicality of a seizure, occurrence in the presence of others, histrionic character, apparently purposive nature of movements, manifest motivation, absence of injury, tongue-biting or incontinence, may be of help, although none of these is a certain indicator in itself. During or immediately after an actual fit, the absence of neurological signs such as extensor plantar responses may be of help in differentiating a hysterical from an epileptic seizure. However, these too cannot be relied on in a doubtful case. Real confusion can arise in those patients who have both epileptic and hysterical seizures, this being by no means uncommon. Where there is persistent doubt, it is probably wise to assume, unless proved otherwise, that the patient actually suffers from epilepsy and it is this which gives rise to his associated untoward behaviour.

Vegetative symptoms

Various bodily systems may be involved. For instance, respiratory symptoms such as hyperventilation occur, sometimes to the point where tetanic spasms are induced. Wheezing, which unlike asthma is predominantly inspiratory, may occur.

A wide variety of gastrointestinal symptoms is possible. Dysphagia due to localized oesophageal spasm (*globus hystericus*) may sometimes raise the suspicion of malignant growth. X-ray examination will reveal no structural abnormality. In the abdomen itself, pain is a common complaint. It is usually poorly localized and bears no close relationship to the taking of food. Hysterical abdominal proptosis can occur due to downward pressure of the diaphragm and a lordotic posture which forces the abdominal contents forward. This accounts for the swollen abdomen which occurs in some cases of *pseudocyesis* and occasionally under other circumstances as well.

Hysterical vomiting can be severe. It may succeed the physiological vomiting of the early months of pregnancy and may persist as a result of psychological causes. Hysterical vomiting may also occur in *anorexia nervosa*, particularly in those cases in which the patient, although appearing to eat well, loses weight but conceals the fact that the meal, shortly after being eaten, is vomited into the toilet or in some other convenient place.

In the genitourinary system, dysmenorrhoea is common and may be more disabling than circumstances would appear to justify. Many, though not all, female hysterical patients are sexually frigid and a proportion may suffer from dyspareunia or from vaginismus, often severe and without adequate organic cause. Various urinary symptoms, such as acute retention or gross incontinence, may be hysterical in nature.

Mental symptoms

Some of the mental manifestations of hysteria are remarkable. *Somnambulism*, or sleep-walking, which most commonly occurs in childhood, is an excellent example of dissociation. It can, however, occasionally affect adults. Essentially the patient who sleep-walks resembles one in a hypnotic trance, who may carry out a complicated routine. He may get out of bed, put on his shoes, open the door, go downstairs, doing this, that or the other, while being apparently quite unaware of any of these things. Occasional transient sleep-walking episodes in childhood are of no importance, though, if recurrent, may call for investigation. Related to sleep-walking is the hysterical *fugue*—that is, 'a flight', often from a painful or threatening situation, carried out in a state usually described as a *narrowing of consciousness*, in which the patient is singularly absorbed. Fugues occur also in epileptic and depressive states and possibly are analogous to that degree of intense mental preoccupation in which it is possible to drive a car skilfully through thick traffic, but barely possible to recall details of the journey later.

Hysterical amnesia

In hysterical amnesia, the patient professes to have forgotten long periods in his life, or, alternatively, certain significant episodes. He may appear to have forgotten completely who he is or where he has come from. Interestingly enough, he usually has nothing on his person which might be of help in finding the answers to these questions. Such *global* amnesia, as it is sometimes called, is easily differentiated from memory loss due to organic cerebral disorder by the preservation of other functions. For example, it may be observed how readily he remembers how to use a knife and fork and how his behaviour is in many other essential respects normal; how he finds his way about the ward; is unperturbed by his situation while at the same time giving an impression of wariness. The suspicion of fraud is strong in such states, which not infrequently follow some lapse of conduct. Memory in *hysterical amnesia* usually returns spontaneously within 24 hours or so but, if prolonged, raises the suspicion of malingering. Memory may also sometimes be recovered by hypnosis or under the influence of drugs such as a barbiturate administered intravenously, but these are often unreliable, since a man may lie almost as well when drunk as when sober.

Ganser Syndrome

In its complete form, the Ganser syndrome consists of a disturbance of consciousness, hallucinations, somatic conversion symptoms and, first and foremost, a tendency to give approximate answers (*vorbeireden*) to questions (see under *Pseudodementia*). The syndrome may occur in those in some kind of trouble, such as in remand prisoners or, more commonly, under other circumstances in which the patient is faced with some intolerable situation. It may also be a manifestation of sudden severe depression precipitated by some acutely distressing situation. The Ganser syndrome has to be distinguished from a hysterical reaction heralding schizophrenia. It also bears some resemblance, though it is not identical, to the rather uncommon hebephrenic buffoonery state. Careful examination for neurological symptoms is important as organic brain disease may produce Ganser symptoms.

Pseudodementia

Pseudodementia is allied to, but separate from, the Ganser syndrome in that the change of consciousness (*twilight state*) and other characteristic symptoms are absent. The patient 'simulates' dementia in a more or less stylized way, for example $2 + 2 = 5$; gives the date of the week as the one immediately before or after the actual one; or denies the most elementary knowledge in a childish manner. The observer's impression before very long is that the right answer is really known. Pseudodementia may be seen in mental defectives in trouble. It may also follow head injury. In some instances, it may be difficult to differentiate such behaviour from pure simulation. Even more difficulty is presented by certain elderly patients in whom there is a degree of pseudodementia due often to depression, but which may be superimposed upon true organic memory defect.

Twilight states

Other hysterical twilight states may occur, these being characterized by a dream-like state of consciousness, visual pseudohallucinations and the re-enactment of emotionally charged episodes. Hysterical *stupor* and *hysterical trance states* occasionally occur. Some certainly depend for their development upon the attitudes of those in attendance, who may unwillingly encourage the patient's strange behaviour, either by mistakenly believing it to be that which it is not or paying undue attention to it. Probably a good example is the so-called *multiple personality*, of which several famous cases are on record. In this the patient becomes at times another person, acting differently and sometimes claiming no knowledge of the other 'self'. This state, once much publicized on account of its dramatic quality, is almost certainly an iatrogenic artefact; some more recently published cases betray this clearly.

Compensation neurosis occurs when symptoms are acquired or prolonged unconsciously in association with anticipated compensation. It is, therefore, if it exists at all, a form of illness behaviour with fairly obvious secondary gain. Those who favour this diagnosis consider that it will persist until the subject's claim to compensation is settled and that it will then clear up. However, in a number of cases the disability may persist. Once again the distinction from malingering is both difficult and important.

Behavioural symptoms

The catalogue of hysterical behaviour disorders seems endless. There are some who have a penchant for repeated spurious suicidal attempts. The histrionic character of these betrays their real nature; they are not wholly intended to succeed but are an effort to gain attention. They do, however, occasionally succeed by accident and must be taken seriously on this account. There are those also who are expert at manipulating thermometers in order to produce a spurious impression of fever. Pseudohaemoptysis and pseudohaematemesis can be produced by extracting blood from the lips, gums and pharynx. Particularly troublesome are those patients who slash themselves with pieces of broken glass, razor blades or other sharp objects, even cutlery. Again this is often done to gain attention, as is also the case with those who seek, and are still far too often submitted to, unnecessary surgical operation. The masochistic behaviour of some hysterics surpasses all bounds. Despite the inconvenience caused to all who have to attend to such patients and may be much irritated thereby, it should never be forgotten that underlying their behaviour is some very real problem which needs, if possible, to be solved.

Differential diagnosis

Hysteria is relatively rare in psychiatric practice; even in general hospital psychiatric units serving other medical and surgical specialties, no more than 1–2 per cent of referrals are eventually diagnosed as suffering from hysteria. Hysteria may present to general physicians, to surgeons or to obstetricians; and in a manner characteristic to each specialty. Thus hysterical aphonia may present to the ENT surgeon; or a corkscrew visual defect to an ophthalmologist.

It is important to realize that hysteria is not the only mental mechanism that may result in the appropriation of physical symptoms; indeed, depression with hypochondriacal physical complaints is considerably commoner. Hysterical reactions may also be secondary to other conditions; for instance, amongst known epileptic patients being treated with anti-convulsant drugs, hysterical 'fits' probably occur more commonly than true epileptic fits.

The term *Briquet's syndrome* is widely used in the United States but is not synonymous with the definition of hysteria as used in the ICD 9. Briquet's syndrome refers to polysymptomatic, polysystemic conditions without organic origin; which include many other neurotic conditions in addition to chronic hysteria. Hysteria may affect only one organ or system and in this case does not fulfil the definition of Briquet's syndrome. Similarly, hysterical personality disorder characterized by shallow labile affect, dependence on others, craving for appreciation and attention, suggestibility and theatricality with a combination of sexual frigidity and over-responsiveness to stimuli should also be clearly distinguished from hysteria. The two may coexist but are not identical.

The distinction between hysteria and deliberate disability is extremely difficult. However, it is the aspect of *conscious deliberate dissimulation* which characterizes the latter. *Munchausen syndrome* is one form of deliberate disability in which patients are repeatedly admitted to hospitals with supposed acute physical illness. Such patients, who are perhaps better described as suffering from the *hospital addiction syndrome*, are usually socially isolated, but at the same time highly dependent people. Their behaviour may lead them to undergo a vast number of operations.

The majority of cases of self-poisoning and anorexia nervosa cannot be considered to be hysterical as there is no element of *unconscious conversion*. The desire and the carrying out of the act to endanger one's own life by the ingestion of drugs or by self-starvation can certainly be seen as an abnormal psychogenic reaction, but it is not hysterical in a strict sense. Similarly, there are a number of conditions of physiological malfunction arising from psychological factors such as hyperventilation, cardiac neurosis and aerophagy. Some of these occur as a result of a conversion reaction, others are an automatic response to acute anxiety; they therefore have an affinity with both hysteria and hypochondriasis.

There has always been difficulty in separating the concept of *hypochondriasis* from that of hysteria, and, in fact, in the seventeenth century Thomas Sydenham regarded hypochondriasis as the male equivalent of hysteria in the female. The patient's experience, however, is different in hypochondriasis. There is a preoccupation with bodily functions, the patient is afraid of the symptoms and is convinced that they indicate serious disease despite the lack of objective evidence on the part of the patient or as a result of examination and investigation by the doctor. What hysteria, hypochondriasis, and psychosomatic reactions appear to have in common is that in different ways they manifest *illness behaviour*, or the gains of having taken a sick role unconsciously, to achieve the benefits of such a role in life.

Treatment

An attitude of prejudice or antagonism towards the patient will make effective management impossible. There is a need for a complete and detailed history, not only from the patient but also from a third party who knows the situation well. Particular attention should be paid to personality assessment. Establishment of an appropriate therapeutic relationship is highly important and the beginner should be warned of the tendency of hysterical patients to form neurotic attachments to their physicians. Treatment demands a considerable degree of patience and tolerance, together with a continuing respect for the patient as a sick person, even though the patient's explanation of her symptoms is unacceptable. Both *confrontation* and *collusion* are to be avoided, although there comes a time when confrontation without rejection may be necessary. It is important for the patient to realize that others do not accept sickness behaviour at face value, but still accept the patient as being ill and in need of continuing help. Real change often begins only after an emotional crisis has occurred, after which subterfuge and pretence may be dropped.

It is vital to remember that the patient is ill. Very often the seemingly shallow hysteric has a core of genuineness, this being occasionally bound up with the painful realization of her own inadequacy. On the basis of such self-revelation, modification can begin. Common-sense application of relearning is useful and to achieve this behavioural modification, biofeedback and physiotherapy may be used. Treatment has to recommend itself to the patient as being both reasonable and acceptable, and the patient's notion that there is a serious physical symptom necessitates that the staff use some form of physical treatment. It is very important to build up the patient's feelings of self-respect and esteem. This is achieved by congratulating the patient on successes that occur in the course of treatment and also by encouraging participation in group social activities, and helping her to improve in social skills.

It is often very difficult to deal with hysterical symptoms either as an out-patient or on a general non-psychiatric ward. It may be necessary to admit a patient under the care of a psychiatrist. Instant removal of hysterical symptoms by hypnosis may be dramatic and impressive to junior doctors; however, it is unreliable as a form of treatment; it is difficult to predict in which patients it will be effective, and the same symptoms or others are likely to recur at a later stage.

When embarking upon treatment it is worth formulating jointly with the patient what is expected or hoped for, and for how long this should be attempted. Treatment is based upon the acceptance of a patient as a person genuinely needing help, reassurance that the condition is going to improve, avoidance of collusion in accepting physical aetiology, avoidance of unnecessary confrontation; at the same time working with the patient to try to remove the distresses that have provoked a hysterical reaction. It is important for the patient to feel that both he and his symptoms are accepted by the doctor as real and worth treating.

There should be a thorough physical examination initially to exclude any organic neurological or other disorder; any special investigations should be done as early as possible. Having carried out such procedures, and finding them to be negative, the physical symptoms should then largely be ignored. The next stage draws the patient into cooperation by convincing him that treatment is appropriate and can be effective. Physiotherapy (and biofeedback or other similar techniques) is beneficial at this stage; improvement is strongly rewarded with encouragement; but the mechanism of how physiotherapy is effective is not discussed with the patient. Meanwhile, stresses at home and elsewhere are investigated. The patient is encouraged to work at improving these where possible, and social work aims at minimizing difficult circumstances.

The features of *secondary gain* from the sick role should also be investigated, but not made explicit to the patient. It is important to work out what benefits the patient gains from illness behaviour in order to construct a situation in which the gains from getting better are greater than those from remaining disabled. Such methods of treatment usually involve considerable interdisciplinary cooperation, which of course the hysteric may try to jeopardize by manipulativeness, tending to cause dissension amongst different members of staff.

Drugs and physical methods of treatment alone can never deal with the conversion symptoms. However, anxiolytics may be used in controlling excessive anxiety to enable other methods of treatment to be carried out. Tricyclic antidepressants and also monoamine oxidase inhibitors have been used, chiefly for dealing with associated depressive symptoms. There is no indication for ECT in uncomplicated hysterical conversion reactions and in fact they may be made considerably worse by this treatment.

Prognosis

If the term hysteria is used in the more restricted sense suggested in this chapter, then there will still be some misdiagnosis, and there will still be some patients who subsequently develop serious physical illness or depression. However, the prognosis for a young person with the acute development of a single hysterical symptom in reaction to what she perceives to be a severe stress is generally good; with adequate psychotherapeutic treatment and with remission of the stress, such patients usually make a complete recovery. The prognosis for older patients, for those with chronic disability and especially where there is evidence of marked personality disorder, is very much less favourable. The tendency is for such symptoms to continue and the course of the illness to be interspersed with episodes of reactive depression. There is an increased risk of suicide and also of deaths from accident amongst hysterics. There is an increased likelihood, above the general population, for those having made a recovery from hysterical symptoms to have a second attack either with similar or different symptoms.

The social setting is an important determinant of outcome. Where the provoking situation has been removed, the likelihood of complete recovery is very much greater; where there is clear evidence of secondary gain and the provoking situation continues, then understandably improvement is more difficult to obtain. The more disabling and more apparently permanent a hysterical symptom is, in fact the better is the prognosis: for instance, hysterical blindness has a better prognosis than hysterical attack disorders such as fits or vomiting. At long-term follow-up, although the initial hysterical symptoms may have remitted entirely, there is a tendency for a disproportionate number of patients to show chronic symptoms of anxiety, depression or hypochondriasis.

Further reading

Merskey, H. (1979) *The Analysis of Hysteria*. London: Baillière Tindall.

15

Obsessive–Compulsive Disorders

The central feature of an obsessive–compulsive disorder is the sudden emergence into consciousness of an unwanted thought or train of ideas which is often meaningless and which leads to persistent *rumination*, or an *urge to action* which the subject seeks in vain to dispel, or to some kind of *ritualistic behaviour* he feels compelled to carry out. Attempts to rid himself of obsessive thoughts usually lead to an intense inner struggle which may absorb virtually all available psychic energy. Severe anxiety and tension arise when compulsion towards obsessive–compulsive activity is resisted.

Although the content of an obsessive thought is experienced as alien, it is, nevertheless, always recognized by the subject as coming from within; this distinguishes it from the passivity experience of the schizophrenic who feels that thoughts have been inserted into his mind by some external agency. Likewise, an obsessive idea differs from a delusion in that the latter is accepted with complete certainty, while the sufferer from an obsession recognizes its absurdity and tries to repudiate it, although this is usually an extremely painful mental experience.

The prevalence of obsessional illness is unknown, although obsessional symptoms can occur in almost any setting. They may be unmasked by a depressive illness; or may herald the onset of schizophrenia and become interwoven with its other symptoms. Obsessions may also be engendered by organic disorder such as encephalitis. It may be significant that patients with obsessional symptoms often report a history of head injury. There is, furthermore, some evidence of an association between the later occurrence of some of the severer obsessional disorders and birth trauma.

Mildly obsessive thoughts may transiently disturb those who are otherwise normal, when fatigued or under some kind of emotional stress. They often take the form of a repetitive or meaningless word, catch-phrase or slogan or perhaps a snatch of melody which reverberates irritatingly in the mind. Such happenings cannot be considered as pathological so long as they do not interfere with productive mental activity. In contrast, full-blown persistently repetitive obsessions and compulsions must be regarded as among the most painful and intractable of all psychiatric symptoms.

Aetiology

In the formation of obsessional disorders, heredity, with polygenic mode of inheritance, as well as environmental factors are important. One-third of the relatives of patients suffer from obsessional illnesses or exhibit obsessional traits of varying severity.

Environmental factors such as may form part of a harsh and affectionless upbringing, parental disharmony bringing with it a conflict of loyalties, severe physical or mental illness of one or other parent with whom the patient may have been closely identified, together with demands to assume responsibilities to a degree which exceed a child's capacity to do so are features frequently found in the case histories of obsessional persons. Such people tend to be reared in an atmosphere where approval depends more on conformity to certain standards of behaviour than on love and affection for its own sake. Their intelligence, however, tends to be above average.

Obsessional illnesses are characterized by fluctuations in intensity, in which case the possibility of a link with an underlying primary recurrent affective illness should be considered. The majority, however, seem to arise on the basis of a certain character structure, with insecurity and a feeling of inadequacy as its major foundation.

The obsessional (or anankastic) personality

The term *anankastic*, which has virtually the same meaning as *obsessional*, is discussed in Chapter 16. Transient obsessions which may not necessarily have given rise to real disability are common. Most anankastic symptoms spring from a constant feeling of inner insecurity, anxiety and personal guilt. The sufferer lives in constant dread that he may have done or have omitted to have done something which may have serious consequences for others: for instance, the person who has to get up after going to bed to make sure he has locked the back door or turned the lights off. These are those who often take the dullest but securest jobs, their efforts to obtain security being much more than justifiable prudence. Ritualistic forms of religion may give them strong support. Further, their formality, precision or pedantry, their meticulous attention to dress and detail, their devotion to conformity may all be construed as protective measures; in particular, their perfectionism which has its roots in an effort to overcome what Janet called the *sentiment d'incompletude*. Rigidity and lack of adaptability are the hallmarks of the anankastic personality. Their sexual relations are never entirely normal and are often characterized by polarity and uncertainty of sexual goal and jealousy.

The striking polarity of the anankastic is revealed in all his relationships. The *alternate gratification* which Freud described is a conspicuous and fundamental feature of his behaviour. In trying to escape his instinctual inclinations, he will tend to 'lean over backwards' to do the opposite. Instead of tidying his belongings, his desk may show an almost studied disorderliness. To escape conformism, he may assume mannerisms, such as wearing a monocle or an eccentric form of dress. To escape from rigidity in routine, he may avoid any attempt to coordinate the work of his subordinates. He must either be a slave to a timetable or avoid one completely. Always the one or the other; never the in-between!

That all this can occur indicates a major personality split, which is a feature highly characteristic of the obsessional personality who constantly seeks to repudiate his basic instinctual drives. (This use of the term *personality split* is not to be confused with the concept of schizophrenia which is seen as a fragmentation of mind into its elements.) The patient may describe this split as if he were two entirely different people with differing characters.

The prim, parsimonious, overcorrect and morally censorious demeanour of the obsessional may reflect deep-seated aggressive feelings together with a crude and turbulent sexuality which sometimes receives expression in perverted behaviour of one kind or another. The exhibition of rigid, perfectionistic and unduly scrupulous attitudes may likewise conceal an over-ready tendency to guilt, together with proneness to self-reproach, doubt and indecision. Under stress, symptoms revealing personality disorder such as obsessional ideas, or phobic symptoms occur. These arise out of the all-pervading sense of insecurity and guilt, and may be accompanied by compulsive actions carried out in a fruitless attempt to expiate feelings of failure and inadequacy.

Psychopathology

As with other symptoms, the *form* which an obsession or compulsion takes must be distinguished from its *content*. An obsessional disturbance of thought is in the formal sense, therefore, a primary datum which cannot, as such, be *explained* in terms of its content. Its content can, however, quite often be *understood* in terms of the patient's life experience, without necessarily and in any way explaining why this particular content of thought enters consciousness in an obsessional as against some alternative form such as, for example, a delusion. Although in an obsessional disorder the patient's psyche is split, thus allowing the simultaneous retention of ideas which can be considered as polar opposites, because the one cancels out the other, the essential unity of his ego is maintained. This is why unless and until a psychotic break with reality occurs, as sometimes happens, the obsessional patient never shares the schizophrenic's feelings that his morbid ideas are thrust upon him from outside; indeed, as he tries to contend with his painful thoughts and urges, his awareness of himself as an individual tends, if anything, to be heightened. Thus, recapitulating, the obsessional content of consciousness is always regarded by the sufferer as a foreign although nonetheless familiar body, this being in contrast to a delusion where the morbid content is more or less fully accepted and absorbed into a system of basically irrational thought.

Viewed psychodynamically, obsessions may be regarded as disguised self-reproaches which, according to Freud, are connected with incidents drawn from early life, often having a sexual connotation. Obsessive rituals may also be seen as expiatory ceremonials, allied to magical acts which are intended to keep evil away; evil in this sense springing from the sufferer's awareness and fear of his own primitive instinctual, aggressive and sexual drives which threaten to overwhelm his every effort at self-control. Psychoanalysis strongly suggests that conflict between love and hate towards parents, who interfere with forbidden although pleasurable activities, leads to the state of doubt and indecision which is such a striking symptom of obsessionalism. Thus those subject to the disorder tend to be both overscrupulous and overconscientious, having altruistic aims on the one hand while on the other being drawn towards more childish and primitive pleasures. Sometimes, where childhood upbringing has been fraught by parental conflict and inconsistency of attitude, this very inconsistency is in itself absorbed by the sufferer, which leads him to be divided by conflict. Just as his parents may never have been able to compromise between themselves, so is he unable to compromise within himself.

Symptoms

Normal children often pass through phases in which they exhibit compulsions to count, touch objects (such as running the fingers over passing railings), or step over cracks in the pavement. This kind of behaviour is essentially magical; the obsessional element in childish games bears a very close relationship to superstitious behaviour and to primitive ceremonial ritual. Growing up and exposure to normal social influences lead to their disappearance in the majority of cases. In some, however, especially where the family situation is disturbed, obsessional trends may become more pronounced and troublesome. In rarer cases they may herald the onset of a childhood psychosis. In adults all degrees are met with from an occasional preoccupation with a tune running in the head, a sudden destructive or aggressive impulse usually soon checked, or an unnecessary examination of the gas taps or electric light switches, to more insistent obsessional states which can seriously interfere with comfort and working efficiency.

The patient realizes the nature of his obsessions, regards them as foreign to his personality, and attempts to subdue them. Thus, if told he is silly, he shares this view.

Obsessional thoughts and ruminations

Obsessive–ruminative states often have a metaphysical or philosophical content, in which the sufferer commonly presents himself, as it were, with quite unanswerable questions concerning the nature of God, the Universe, the meaning of life and so on. Not infrequently, elevated and degrading thoughts may occur in contiguity. Thus the appearance of a religious idea may be immediately followed by one which is grossly sexual, to the great distress of the patient (*contrast ideas*). States of doubt and indecision, often associated with depersonalization, may interfere greatly with the patient's activities (*folie de doute*).

Obsessional fears and compulsions

Some obsessional fears and compulsions bear some relationship to, although are probably not identical with, *phobias*. Thus certain obsessional fears may consist of an idea such as that if the patient's hands are unclean he may transmit infection and some other person may come to harm thereby. This may lead to constant *compulsive washing* rituals, wearing gloves and, having removed them, burning them at once, and a whole host of other related behaviour. The variety is endless but the theme remains the same. Again there may be a feeling of compulsion to perform certain acts which the patient realizes are foolish, useless or even dangerous. These ideas may emerge suddenly, accompanied by intense anxiety. A mother may be suddenly afflicted by the thought that she may give way to a desire to injure or even kill one of her children or may do so unknowingly while sleep-walking. This may lead her to lock up all the kitchen knives or cast them through the window into the garden before retiring to bed. When such behaviour extends, as it sometimes does, to the avoidance of any contact with a threatening object or so far as possible with the environment in general, the patient may for all practical purposes become virtually immobilized. Although suicide may be an outcome, it is surprising perhaps that this does not occur more often. Suicide apart, no certain instance of a patient translating his morbid compulsions into action ever appears to have been reported; such is the extraordinary power of control the obsessional has over the turbulent and powerful upsurge of his primitive impulses. Despite this, it has to be said that certain types of deviant sexual behaviour which tend to be recurrent appear to be activated by compulsion by no means altogether dissimilar to that of an obsessional kind.

Rituals

Rituals are legion, varying from a needless compulsion to check and recheck, on retiring for the night, that all doors are doubly locked, all lights are out and all gas and water taps securely turned off, to almost ceaseless rituals concerned with everyday affairs such as dressing and undressing and other matters concerned with toiletry. These simple tasks, normally taking no more than a minute or two, may all too easily become those of the greatest complexity, so that a patient can take three or four hours to prepare for bed and likewise to get himself up in the morning. The left shoe must be removed before the right, likewise the left sock; trousers must be removed before shirt and so on. There are endless possible variations. If in the middle of all this the thought occurs that some sequence has not been performed in its proper order, then all must be done all over again, with of course no absolute certainty of ever getting it right. Just as some obsessional patients search constantly for perfection, so do others search for certainty; both elusive qualities. No compromise can ever satisfy an obsessional patient, which is why he is forced constantly into the futile and repetitive pursuit of making sure of making sure.

Treatment

Obsessional thoughts and compulsive behaviour may be seen as habits which once ingrained do not require a further stimulus to be maintained. Treatment requires relearning normal patterns of behaviour. Behavioural modification, when carried out with a degree of thoroughness and attention to detail, which earns cooperation as seeming appropriate to the obsessional patient, is often beneficial.

It has been found that many obsessional patients feel more anxious after completing their rituals than if they were prevented from carrying them out. In *response prevention*, they are prevented from ritualistic activity by exercising self-control after persuasion, by constant surveillance, by carrying out alternative activity or even, rarely, by force. Response prevention has been successful in compulsive hand-washing by persuading the patient to increase the interval of time between washing his hands and having somebody stay with him while he practises this. For obsessional thoughts, response prevention in fantasy is carried out; this is more difficult for the patient and less often efficacious.

Modelling is of some value in the treatment of compulsions when the therapist demonstrates that the required behaviour is harmless. For example, with compulsive hand-washing there is frequently fear of contamination, and any suspicion of dirt will promptly cause the patient to wash his hands. To combat this fear the therapist will, for example, handle the sole of his own shoe and then carry on with normal activities without washing his hands. This technique is often combined with *confrontation* in which the patient is maintained in the stressful situation in which he is tempted to carry out the compulsive behaviour. With exposure, the anxiety and therefore the stimulus for such behaviour gradually diminish. *Systematic desensitization*, described earlier in the treatment of phobic disorders, has not proved effective in obsessional neuroses.

Drugs have been used mostly as an adjunct when there is associated disturbance of mood in obsessional neurosis. Tricyclic antidepressants, especially clomipramine, have been claimed to be effective; they are most likely to be beneficial when depression of mood is also present. If in doubt about the coexistence of depression, it is worth using an antidepressant drug as it is sometimes unexpectedly successful and, if not, the patient can be reassured that there are other methods of treatment available. With very marked anxiety, a benzodiazepine drug or a small dose of a major tranquillizer may be useful in the short term. Monoamine oxidase inhibitor drugs have been useful on occasions in obsessional states.

Electroplexy (ECT) may be of value in recurrent obsessional episodes but only if the disturbance is manifestly associated with a depressive phase; otherwise it is of little or no value and, indeed, where it fails may have an adverse effect by increasing tension and by suggesting to the patient that his case is hopeless.

For very severe and intractable cases, psychosurgery by some type of stereotactic subcaudate tractotomy is indicated. Disability with extreme incapacity for several years will need to be demonstrated before such a course of action is justifiable. Psychosurgery is only indicated for the most severe degrees of intolerable tension; treatment results may then be highly gratifying.

Occupation is valuable for the obsessional patient under treatment. Whether this is beneficial because it redirects his drives from what would otherwise be pathological behaviour or because achieving something worthwhile improves self-esteem and hence enhances mood is not known; it is probably a combination of both. Attention needs to be given to the type of occupation—work or occupational therapy depending on the treatment setting—that is prescribed; it needs to be absorbing and preferably creative without further facilitating the development of rituals or frustrating the patient because his compulsions prevent his completing anything.

Many patients crave for reassurance, for instance a man who repeatedly asked, 'I haven't got VD, have I?'. However, if given, such reassurance simply reinforces the belief of such patients that they have something to worry about. Support and encouragement given by the doctor are very important, with an emphasis upon the gains made in treatment and the areas of life with which the patient is now able to cope. The doctor's demonstration of his ability to understand and empathize with the tortured psychopathology of obsessive–compulsive disorders is invaluable to the patient in trusting his doctor and knowing that at least there is someone who comprehends what he is describing even if he cannot relieve the symptoms. Of all patients, what the obsessional most needs is a tolerant professional friend who, while prepared to listen to his tale of woe, may encourage him to avoid certain situations which appear to aggravate his obsessional tendencies and to show some resistance to others. Advice concerning sublimatory activities may also be helpful in milder instances.

Prognosis

The prognosis tends to be unfavourable in those with a long-standing history when the onset is insidious rather than acute, and the condition tends unremittingly to worsen over the years. Extraneous circumstances may have some bearing on periods of improvement and aggravation which may occur from time to time. Where an obsessional state develops as a symptom in a depressive phase, remission usually takes place as depression yields to treatment.

Some cases do appear to 'burn themselves out' or possibly the sufferer may achieve some kind of *modus operandi*. Others, perhaps finding treatment of so little avail, no longer seek psychiatric help. However, even in the worst cases, an air of optimism should if possible be maintained. The most remarkable and quite unexpected remissions do sometimes occur. This makes it justifiable and even advisable, perhaps more than in the case of any other psychiatric disorder, to avoid giving too gloomy a prognosis.

Further reading

Beech, H. R. (1974) *Obsessional States*. London: Methuen.

16
Personality Disorders

The matter of personality disorder remains one of the most controversial problems in all psychiatry. Some would abandon the concept altogether; others find it clinically valuable while seeking to improve the reliability of terms used. The standpoint taken in this book largely adheres to that of Schneider who saw personality disorders *not as illnesses* (in the strict medical sense), but as variations of personality in one or several of its traits from a statistical mean though one as yet not mathematically defined. As there is no definable norm, the best is some kind of correspondence with the *average man*—the notional 'man in the street'.

Terminology

Personality may either be considered subjectively, i.e. in terms of what the patient believes and describes about himself as an individual, or objectively in terms of what an observer notices about his more consistent patterns of behaviour. Subjectively then, personality is that unique quality of an individual which he knows to be himself and expresses in terms of his feelings and his aims and goals. Objectively, the characteristic behaviour of an individual is what makes him different from others and allows us to predict how he will act in any particular circumstances. His personality, which includes his prevailing mood, attitudes and opinions, is manifested in social relationships and must be assessed by observing what people actually do in a social context.

In describing personality as 'normal', the word *normal* is used in a statistical sense indicating that various personality traits are present to a broadly normal extent, neither to gross excess nor extreme deficiency. Abnormal personality is, therefore, a variation upon an accepted, yet broadly conceived, range of average personality.

Certain aspects of abnormal personality are clinically important. These characteristics have been collected into typological lists, for example that produced by Schneider or in *The International Classification of Diseases* (ICD 9). This chapter follows the list of types described in this latter classification and which are given later in this chapter. If these characteristics of personality are present to an abnormal extent and this abnormality is such as to cause the person himself or other people to suffer, he may be regarded as having a *personality disorder*. The distinction, however, is not precise, as social setting is all important. Thus a person because of his personality characteristics may be a misfit in one station of life, but when circumstances change, perhaps during war time, he may become a great success as a charismatic leader.

The modern concept of personality disorder has developed from two contradictory ideas. The first is that it is present when any abnormality of personality causes problems either to the patient himself or to others. This is the sense recommended here and used in ICD 9. The other use of the term personality disorder is in a pejorative sense: here, personality disorder implies unacceptable, antisocial behaviour and therefore a person whom we are inclined to dislike and reject; this being enshrined in the word *psychopath*.

These two quite different meanings for personality disorder can be traced through its history. In Greek medicine, individuals were presumed to have a preponderance of different humours which in their turn resulted in a specific temperament, such as *sanguine, choleric, melancholic* and *phlegmatic*. These have subsequently evolved into the *stable/neurotic* and *extravert/introvert* dimensions of personality defined by Eysenck. In the early nineteenth century, Pinel recognized that there were conditions in which reason remained intact, but a person might yet be considered insane because his faculties of emotion and will were disturbed. This he called *manie sans delirie*. Benjamin Rush described *moral derangement* as due to either congenital defect or disease and John Conolly described 'inequalities, weaknesses and peculiarities of human understanding which do not amount to insanity'. The roots of the opprobrious concept of psychopathy have often been ascribed to J. C. Prichard of Bristol, who defined the condition he called 'moral insanity' as:

'. . . madness, consisting of a morbid perversion of the natural feelings, affections, inclinations, temper, habits, moral dispositions and natural impulses without any remarkable disorder or defect of the intellect in knowing or reasoning faculties and particularly without any insane illusion or hallucination.'

Although Prichard equated the word *moral* with *emotional* rather than intending it to have ethical implications, it was with his cases of antisocial or even criminal behaviour that the term *moral insanity* and *moral imbecility* (later *moral defect*) came finally to be associated.

Henderson, in 1939, described the *creative, inadequate* and *aggressive* forms of psychopathy; his contention that psychopathy was a distinct condition becoming enshrined in due course in the Mental Health Act, 1959, where it came to represent the zenith of theories of personality disorder that saw antisocialness as its most important criterion.

More recently, retaining psychopathy as a separate diagnostic category has become increasingly unpopular. The 1983 review of the Mental Health Act, 1959, combines the two different concepts of personality disorder by stating: '*psychopathic disorder* means a persistent disorder or disability (whether or not including significant impairment of intelligence) which results in abnormally aggressive or seriously irresponsible conduct on the part of the person concerned'. (See also Chapter 25.)

It is now accepted that there are a number of different types of abnormal personality that may result in disorder. One such type is the *asocial* or *antisocial personality* which conforms quite closely to the previous description of *psychopathy*. Thus, personality disorder is retained as a term with a much wider meaning than merely in the antisocial or criminal sense.

Reliability of diagnosis

The reliability of diagnosis—that is, the likelihood of the same diagnosis being given to the same subject on subsequent occasions or by two different clinicians—has until now been considered to be very low. Different clinicians tend to concentrate upon different aspects of the patient's personality to the exclusion of others and thereby tend to overdiagnose certain types of personality disorder and ignore others. Likewise, several meanings may be attached to the same term used in personality description, e.g. *hysterical*, thus causing confusion amongst different users. There also is inadequate definition of the variation present amongst normal traits; for instance, how much is *attention-seeking behaviour* to be regarded as normal and at what point does it exceed normal limits? Despite these difficulties, more recent studies, where more precise descriptions of personality types have been used, do show a satisfactory degree of reliability, both when the same rater assesses personality after an interval of 12 months and also between raters. But for this to be achieved the terminology of personality disorder must be used precisely.

Differential diagnosis

The diagnosis of personality disorder needs to be differentiated from *normality* of *personality*, *neurosis*, *criminality*, *affective disorders*, *organic states* and *schizophrenia*. However, personality disorder may, of course, coexist with affective disorders, organic states or schizophrenia, and is very frequently found in association with neurosis. But while neurosis is an inappropriate response to perceived stress which may be acute or prolonged, and is therefore a *reaction*, personality disorder is a long-term effect of constitution and development. Personality disorder is found very much more frequently among sufferers from neurosis than in a normal population.

The distinction from criminality is important; thus all psychopaths are not criminals or vice versa. To distinguish affective personality from an affective disorder it has to be decided whether the abnormality of mood is a temporary state or a lifelong characteristic, the latter pointing to personality disorder.

Various *organic psychosyndromes*, especially *brain damage* following trauma, may result in permanent personality damage and its manifestation in social behaviour. This is recognized in ICD 9 by the term *'specific non-psychotic mental disorders following organic brain damage'*. The contrast between secondary damage to personality with primary constitutional disorder of personality may be compared with the situation affecting intellect where dementia is a secondary effect of illness or injury whilst mental handicap is a primary constitutional impairment of intellect. Simple schizophrenia may be difficult to distinguish from a *schizoid personality disorder* where a person shows callousness, recklessness, shallow affect and a lack of will or drive. In schizophrenia there will usually have been a break at some point of development, as in the case of an adolescent who at some time quite dramatically fails to achieve earlier academic and social expectations. In *residual* or *defect states of schizophrenia*, deterioration of personality is usual.

Aetiology

The aetiology of personality disorders is obscure. Some see them as constitutionally and, therefore, presumably genetically determined; others as being largely if not wholly derived from psychological factors, in particular those operative during early development such as faulty upbringing, emotional deprivation, or undue exposure to parental discord. These views, however, remain theories *only*, for very little is known as yet about the nature of personality and what factors influence its development.

Hereditary factors

There is some evidence that genetic factors determine the type of personality and therefore to some extent whether personality disorder occurs or not. This information comes from family studies and from comparison of monozygotic with dyzgotic twin pairs. It is probable that although personality type is substantially determined genetically, whether or not disorder develops or an abnormal emotional reaction occurs is more likely to be an outcome of environmental influences.

While it is very difficult to unravel the relative contribution of heredity and environment to personality disorder, this is a relatively pointless exercise as usually both factors are present. Even where a child's family environment is clearly unsatisfactory, it may still be impossible to disentangle the influence of this from possible genetic influences derived from parents who are themselves disturbed. What has to be considered is how and to what extent each set of factors interacts. Given *a priori* that heredity must play some part, it becomes a question of how innate predisposition adds to an emotional or personality disorder and likewise how far satisfactory genetic predisposition may counter this development.

Constitutional factors

The views of those who believe that the influence of constitutional factors is preponderant are exemplified by those of Kurt Schneider, which at least have the advantage of clarity and do no violence to everyday clinical experience. Schneider considered what he called 'an anomaly of personality' to be constitutional, in the same way that potential intelligence either below or above average is genetically determined (although whether or not of course this potential is realized may be influenced by environment). However, where defective intelligence is the outcome not of heredity but of disease *in utero* or in early life, Schneider would speak (strictly) not of a deviation but of a disease. Similarly, a personality disorder may also be regarded not merely as a deviation from a *norm*, but a result of acquired cerebral disease giving rise to abnormal and sometimes antisocial behaviour. The effects of frontal lobe damage are a good example.

Where organic influences of this kind are operative, some would prefer the term *pseudopsychopathy*. However, while the influence of adverse environmental factors clearly has the same effect upon those with normal brains as on those with brain damage, in the latter the level of tolerance of adverse factors may be lowered. This is well exemplified by the untoward behaviour sometimes seen in epileptic schoolchildren. While both the nature of their behaviour and the environmental factors which appear to give rise to it are similar to those in non-epileptic children, by reason of their additional disability epileptic children are more prone to react adversely to environmental stress than are their non-epileptic schoolfellows.

Apart from brain damage giving rise to epilepsy and to specific defects which may interfere with learning and, *ipso facto*, emotional and social adjustment, other factors should be borne in mind as causes of abnormal behaviour. For example, an unrecognized attack of encephalitis may possibly account for subsequent personality damage. Also certain personality anomalies may be observed in the near relatives of those with manic–depressive and schizophrenic illnesses. In some cases such anomalies are attenuated forms of the illness or, in the case of schizoid personality, may perhaps be defect states resulting from an earlier mild schizophrenic episode not recognized as such at the time.

Developmental factors

There are many who consider personality disorders to be exclusively or at least predominantly caused by psychological factors derived from the social environment. There are also those who hold an intermediate position and who attempt to give equal weight to all types of aetiological factors. In one such developmental theory, personality disorder is considered to be learned within families or, alternatively, the deprivation of not being brought up in a family so that what is called *personality* simply reflects learned patterns of behaviour in early childhood and through adolescence. Such a behavioural approach seeks to diminish the importance of personality as an independent concept, and prefers to regard behaviour patterns as consistent, while implying that a relearning process properly conducted under appropriate conditions of reinforcement is able to change those patterns. Another seminal influence on the way psychiatrists have viewed personality disorder has been psychoanalysis, in which it is considered that conflicts repressed in early childhood are later manifested as consistent patterns of behaviour then described in terms of personality.

Psychodynamic factors

Fundamentally, psychoanalysis, although never denying the possible role of constitutional factors, construes personality and its disorders as being derived almost wholly from early environmental influences. Psychoanalysis is essentially deterministic in that an individual's conscious thoughts and behaviour, which of course contribute largely to his personality, are seen as something not arising *de novo* but as being determined by mental processes which originate in his 'unconscious'. Behaviour and personality are, therefore, seen as the resultant of a mass of instinctive tendencies together with acquired habits and modes of reaction to the environment. According to Freud, these instinctive tendencies are of an essentially primitive kind and are governed by the *pleasure principle*. Because this principle is at variance with conscious thoughts and activities, and especially with ideas of morality and environmental pressures towards conformity, this has the effect of putting man into conflict with himself. How and at what stage of development these pressures are applied is thought to determine personality. Where development does not proceed normally this, according to psychoanalytic theory, is the result of a fixation in certain stages of psychosexual maturation. From this arise the concepts of *oral* and *anal eroticism* and the *oral, anal* and *genital* types of personality.

Later theorists have seen an association between the psychodynamic oral type of personality and psychopathy; leading to a need for immediate gratification without regard to the long-term consequences. Similarly, the anal type has been equated with the obsessional personality. Such persons experience intense personal emotion, but are unable to express it in anything more than a formal manner. The tendency of obsessional personalities to become collectors (postage stamps, money, ritualistic ways of doing things) is also seen as evidence of an anal retentive type of personality. However, these metaphorical usages of terms about personality should be treated with caution.

Types of personality disorder

The term personality disorder is little more than a descriptive label or perhaps a mere convenience. In the ensuing description the terms are from ICD 9, these having been derived from Schneider's categories. They are *not* separate diagnostic entities, but varieties of abnormal personality which arise out of common groupings of abnormal personality traits according to the degree of intensity of their presence rather than their overall quality. That they are not diagnostic entities is further apparent in that an almost infinite variety of mixtures of combinations of one kind of abnormal personality trait with others may be encountered in practice.

Paranoid personality disorder

People with such a disorder show as a personality trait persistent and conspicuous *self-reference*; they misinterpret the words and actions of others as having special significance for, and being directed against, themselves. They are suspicious of others who they feel to be antagonistic and derogatory. Those more active are often aggressive, quarrelsome, litigious and will go to excessive lengths to defend their rights and redress real or imagined injustice. They are intensely jealous of their own belongings, whether people or objects, and may go to fanatical lengths to avenge themselves. They often have a considerable opinion of their own self-importance.

The more passive type of paranoid personality is less aggressive in achieving his objects. While they know with absolute certainty that others are opposed to them and dislike and despise them, they do nothing about this. They seem to accept as a matter of course that they must suffer from everyone else's ire and greed.

Affective personality disorder

This category includes Schneider's *depressive* and *hyperthymic* personalities. The chronic depressive personality is a gloomy pessimist with a somewhat sceptical outlook who often regards suffering as meritorious. His mood is pronounced and life long; it is therefore a depressive *trait* and not a *state* of depression such as appears in depressive illness. Such persistently *dysthymic* people may be gentle and likeable, although their whole approach to life is tinged with gloom, or they may be hostile, egotistical, morose, cantankerous and spiteful.

Hyperthymic personalities include certain overactive persons whose mood is persistently elevated. They are often thought of as cheerful, kindly disposed, active and possibly overoptimistic, but at the same time may be seen as shallow, superficial, uncritical, happy-go-lucky, cocksure, easily influenced and not very dependable. Although in the main the hyperthymic personality connotes equable temper, it also includes tense, excited, restless people and contentious, querulous individuals having inflated self-esteem; also some shiftless and socially unstable persons who have a tendency to boast and lie. Some persons show a combination of depressive and hyperthymic traits which appear in a cyclical manner and may be referred to as *cyclothymes*. The relation between these personality types and manic-depressive psychoses is still a matter for discussion. Certainly some individuals who suffer from frank attacks of mania exhibit these kinds of premorbid personality.

Schizoid personality disorder
People with this disorder show a disinclination to mix with others, appearing aloof and disinterested. They are not shy or sensitive concerning other people but simply prefer solitary interests with objects rather than people. Their relatives and neighbours find them emotionally cold and detached. Their withdrawal from society may result in a state of callous indifference to the discomfort and sufferings of others.

Explosive personality disorder
The chief characteristic of people with this disorder is a tendency to sudden emotional discharge leading either to sudden impulsive and usually unsuccessful suicidal attempts or to assault on others. Such outbursts may be precipitated by minor frustrations which are quite disproportionate to the reaction which ensues. These are sometimes known as 'short-circuit' reactions. There may be an association with alcoholism, intoxication being a factor which favours explosive outbursts. A previous history of head injury is common.

Anankastic personality disorder
This is a better term than obsessional personality as the latter may be confused with obsessive–compulsive neurosis. Although obsessive–compulsive neurosis and anankastic personality do occur together on occasions, the majority of patients with an obsessional neurosis *are not of* anankastic personality and the majority of people with anankastic personality never develop obsessional neurosis. A person with anankastic personality shows prominent sensitive and perfectionist traits. The term *sensitive personality* denotes heightened impressionability with little power of active expression or capacity for emotional discharge. Such

people tend to ruminate continuously about the possible meaning of any experience and, being insecure, are inclined to look upon themselves as the possible cause of all sorts of unfortunate events. Conflicts over sex are frequent, together with a clash between ethical considerations and sexual and aggressive drives. They have an over-ready tendency to develop sensitive ideas of reference and to believe that others are inclined to regard them askance. The key experience which releases this reaction is some kind of moral defeat; that is, some experience which leads to a feeling of shame or failure.

In order to guard against such defeat the anankast shows meticulous conscientiousness amounting to perfectionism and rigidity in his work and social relationships. He is excessively sensitive to a whisper of criticism which immediately awakens a sense of self-doubt and self-consciousness. The only way he can deal with his chronic sense of insecurity is by always being a little more than correct and less likely therefore to be criticized than other people.

Hysterical personality disorder

Again, it is important to make a clear distinction between hysterical neurosis with conversion and dissociation symptoms and hysterical personality disorder. The two may coincide in the same person but not necessarily so. Histrionic is probably a better description as this most aptly describes the consistent behaviour of these people. They are egocentric and show emotional mobility, excitability and dependency. Although their affect tends to be shallow and labile, and they make excellent superficial relationships, they have considerable difficulty in sustaining long-term exclusive relationships, as in marriage. Attention seeking, appreciation and affection craving are prominent. Theatricality and an air of insincerity typify their social relationships. There is usually a degree of sexual immaturity with flirtatious display in the initial stages of a relationship but rejection and frigidity when the relationship starts to become intense. Hysterical personality disorder is commoner in females and has on occasions been considered to be a female equivalent of the asocial personality disorder.

Asthenic personality disorder

Those with this type of personality appear to succumb to any influence good or bad, the predominant feature being what, in common practice, is usually called weakness of character. They show passive compliance accepting a dominating leadership from another person, for example parent or spouse. They lack vigour when undertaking any activity, especially those requiring determination, and usually establish a life pattern of dependence upon other people. They may only come to psychiatric attention when these dependent relationships break down, for instance separation from spouse, redundancy from employment, discharge from the armed services or other structured organization.

Asocial personality disorder

The antisocial personality, denoted by Schneider as *affectionless* or *feelingless personality*, is characterized mainly by an emotional blunting or complete indifference towards the rights and feelings of others. For such persons, passion, shame and conscience seem to have no meaning. This is what some contemporary writers refer to as '*true*' psychopathy. There is a similarity between this condition and the cold affectionless state of certain schizophrenics, and also a similar state which may appear following brain injury. Such persons are selfish, egocentric, vain and often cruel; they seek primary instinctual gratification with short-term aims and their social adaptation is unsatisfactory or non-existent. The abnormal sexual behaviour of many psychopaths has been compared with that of small children who Freud said were 'potentially polymorphously perverse'.

Whiteley has considered the psychopath to be an individual: (1) who persistently behaves in a way which is not in accord with the accepted social norms in the culture or times in which he lives; (2) who appears to be unaware that his behaviour is seriously at fault; and (3) whose abnormality cannot readily be explained as resulting from the 'madness' we commonly recognize, nor from 'badness' alone.

The core defect in asocial personality disorder is primarily one of empathy. Such a person does not have the ability to understand other people's feelings and especially to understand how others feel about the consequences of his own actions which hurt or offend them. He appears not to experience the shame or psychological pain that prevents normal persons from carrying out unpleasant actions towards other people most of the time. He is unable to put himself into the position of being at the receiving end of such behaviour.

Neurosis and neuroticism

There is clearly an important association between neurosis, an inappropriate reaction to perceived stress, and neuroticism which is the abnormal state of personality in which neurotic behaviour becomes more likely. Very severe stress will provoke a neurotic reaction in a large number of people, perhaps in the majority. A very marked degree of abnormality of personality amounting to personality disorder will predispose an individual to a neurotic reaction with a relatively minor stress. These factors have a marked influence upon prognosis.

Personality is life long; the traits and characteristics manifested by an individual in adolescence are likely to continue throughout life. It is highly likely that a pedantic small boy will develop into a cautious and meticulous middle-aged man and become increasingly perfectionistic, intolerant and rigid in his attitudes as he grows old. Although the basic characteristics of a personality do not change markedly through life, whether these become manifest as a personality disorder is largely determined by the social context. As this changes throughout life there are likely to be modifications of the extent to which personality disorder is shown.

There is an increased likelihood for those with personality disorder to develop alcoholism, drug abuse and other forms of dependent behaviour. Where such dependence is associated with personality disorder the prognosis with appropriate treatment is less optimistic. Those with a personality disorder show an increased likelihood for premature death, especially from suicide and accidental death such as road traffic accidents. Criminal behaviour in those with asocial personality disorder tends to lessen with increasing age, perhaps because of lessening aggression together with diminishing physical strength.

Treatment

In most cases of personality disorder, the patient cannot be brought to treatment unless he is willing. It is important to stress that in discussing treatment all forms of personality disorder need to be considered and not only asocial personality disorder. Treatment is not aimed at altering personality itself, but at the untoward behaviour or unacceptable symptoms resulting from the personality and associated with abnormality.

The most effective form of treatment will combine various types of psychotherapy. Individual psychotherapy, especially of a cognitive type, may be most appropriate for an individual with sensitive or anankastic personality with very marked feelings of low self-esteem and expectation of failure. Between therapy sessions the subject may be encouraged to use his obsessionality to examine and record his thoughts of failure and low self-esteem, and to counter these with rational arguments demonstrating that he did to some extent achieve valuable objectives. This record of his thoughts and counter-arguments is discussed at treatment sessions, working from the assumption that persistent low mood follows depressive thoughts rather than vice versa.

Group therapy is helpful in the treatment of some patients with personality disorder, especially when this is accompanied by social anxiety or fear. The composition of the group is a matter of importance and the theoretical background from which group therapy is carried out will determine the precise nature of sessions and the goals which are important. The aim for the person with the personality disorder is not to change his personality but to help him learn what are the effects of his personality on other people and how to modify his behaviour in a socially appropriate way.

The so-called *therapeutic community* approach has been used to considerable extent in treatment for those with asocial personality disorder or psychopathy. The aim is to help them to learn to take responsibility for their own actions using social pressures derived from the group setting. In such a situation a psychopath will be called by others who may resemble him—in that they too have some of the same or similar problems—to account for his actions and accordingly in so doing to earn social approval or disapproval. The results of this type of treatment are not striking, but they appear somewhat better than other methods that have been used. The social factors operating in a therapeutic community are, according to Rappaport: (1) permissiveness to act in accord with one's feelings without accustomed social inhibitions; (2) communication in sharing of tasks, responsibilities and rewards; (3) democratic decision making; and (4) confrontation of the subject with what he is doing here and now.

The theoretical basis for psychotherapy is different. Dynamic psychotherapy such as psychoanalysis is rarely directly useful in the treatment of personality disorders; however, it has formed a theoretical background to many of the more recently introduced types of therapy. Behavioural modification has been extensively used, for instance with social-skills training where appropriate. Social manipulation is beneficial on occasions; in a different environment the person with an abnormal personality may not cause suffering to himself or to others. Most often, a more eclectic combination of dynamic behavioural and social types of therapy will produce the best environment for the treatment of individuals.

The therapeutic potential of institutions needs to be recognized, also the ways they may hamper the development of a person with abnormal personality. Hospitals and closed therapeutic communities such as certain prison establishments may also be valuable in encouraging a small group atmosphere to develop which enables disordered people to learn about themselves. The disadvantage is that the skills they learn in social interaction may not be relevant to the world outside the institution where different values and attitudes pertain; for instance, it may be quite inappropriate to apply the egalitarian attitudes towards fellow patients and members of staff in a therapeutic community to the much more hierarchical structure operating in a factory. Recently there has been more emphasis on the development of treatment methods in the community such as enforced community projects for those with milder degree of asocial personality.

Physical treatment has relatively little place in the management of personality disorders. However, it may be useful for dealing with specific symptoms. Anxioloytics may on occasions be helpful; antidepressants have also been claimed to have a beneficial effect; major tranquillizers have been used to control explosive outbursts and sometimes small doses have been used prophylactically; lithium is also said to be helpful in reducing aggression, while benperidol and cyproterone acetate have been used to control deviant sexual behaviour.

Those with asocial personality disorder do not fit well in a conventional psychiatric hospital setting. They are at the least a nuisance and on occasions a highly disruptive influence who in their *acting out* may interfere with the welfare and treatment of other patients. They may also present a security risk in the unfortunate situation where no alternatives to treatment exist apart from psychiatric hospital. Such people may require drug therapy to control outbursts of temper. Treatment will normally require to be given under the terms of the Mental Health Act (see Chapter 25).

In general, if the aim is to improve the lot of the patient himself and also those around him, one can be quite optimistic about treatment for personality disorders. There are a number of different options for treatment, but it does require adequate provision locally of a range of different types of therapy. It must be accepted that while the personality is likely to remain unchanged, the aim is to achieve the most appropriate conditions for the individual in which to function.

Further reading

Craft, M. (ed.) (1966) *Psychopathic Disorders*. Oxford: Pergamon Press.

Lion, J. R. (1981) *Personality Disorders; Diagnosis and Management*. Baltimore: Williams & Wilkins.

Schneider, K. (1958) *Psychopathic Personalities*, translated by M. W. Hamilton, 9th edn. London: Cassell.

17

Disturbances of Sexual Behaviour

During the last 15 to 20 years and in the light of increasing knowledge of human sexuality, there have been profound changes in the kinds of sexual problems presenting to the psychiatrist and in the ways in which they are treated. These have included alterations in the public attitude to homosexuality and other sexual deviations; growing physiological and anatomical awareness of the nature of human sexual response and of its malfunctions; more widespread sex education; and the social revolution which in many Westernized countries has led to an improvement in the status of women which, together with the increased availability of effective contraceptive measures, has led them to become more sexually aware and demanding. Together with these changes, many rigid definitions of what is normal or pathological have begun to disappear and are being replaced by a more flexible view of the varieties of human sexual experience. It has indeed now become very difficult to decide what is meant by *normal* sexuality, *normality* being bound up with much more than mere biological response, but subject also to cultural, racial and educational influences which make an all-embracing definition almost impossible.

It is certainly true that there is no form of sexual activity, even including heterosexual intercourse, which has not at some time or other been condemned. Likewise there are possibly no sexual practices (even including incest) which, however occasionally, have not been approved and encouraged. A definition of normal sexuality which might at the present time fit Western culture could therefore well comprise any explicitly sexual act between two people which is acceptable to, and enjoyed by, both and which damages neither, physically or emotionally.

Heterosexual problems

It is only the couple themselves who can decide whether they have a sexual problem or not; there are no absolute standards of sexual performance to which people ought to aspire, although there are probably biological limits beyond which they cannot go. Thus if a couple are contented with their joint sexual practices, however infrequent or bizarre or different these may appear to be to others, providing neither is harmed thereby, then it cannot be said that their sexual behaviour is abnormal. Indeed, help or treatment may only be required if one or both complain of some perceived sexual dysfunction within their relationship. It is most important, therefore, for all who are involved in helping or counselling others not to set standards of human sexual performance, nor should it be implied that if these standards are not attained, there is something wrong with the relationship or perhaps with one or both members of the pair. For example, all women, almost without exception, are biologically capable of achieving orgasm but not all do so during the course of their sexual relationship. Of those who do not, some will see it as a problem and seek help, while others will not feel it to be an essential part of their lives to achieve orgasm.

A couple's decision about whether or not their sexual performance falls short in some way will be bound up not only with their own subjective feelings, which are difficult to measure and standardize, but also with cultural and educational factors and, most importantly, with each partner's expectations. Couples will therefore tend to complain either of a perceptible change in their sexual function or of failing to achieve a desired goal. What for one couple may seem to be a poor sexual performance may, for others, seem completely adequate.

There are no adequate data on the prevalence of sexual dysfunction in the United Kingdom, although it is probably quite high. In the United States it has been estimated that as many as 50 per cent of couples have some difficulties, even in an established sexual relationship. It is important to distinguish between transient difficulties and more severe and permanent forms of the same problem persisting over longer periods of time. Problems of longer standing tend to become secondarily reinforcing, affecting not only the sexual response of each partner, but also the relationships of the couple.

It is usual to distinguish between primary forms of sexual difficulty, where the problem has always existed and continues unabated, and secondary problems, where sexual functioning is initially normal but later deteriorates for some reason or other. Understanding an individual sexual problem also implies understanding the whole person, his upbringing, his character and personality structure and his relationship with his partner overall.

Courtship

As human sexual activity usually starts with courtship, it is here that difficulty may first arise. Some people are so anxious in social situations that they are unable to tolerate any close encounter with a member of the opposite sex. Although they may not present with a sexual problem, their difficulties may prevent a sexual relationship from developing. Some men, indeed, are so inhibited and anxious in the presence of women that they are unable to make the kind of social contact which is necessary to allow a deepening relationship with a woman and may, as a result, be driven by default into a homosexual relationship. These are the so-called *heterophobic homosexuals*.

There are now effective treatments for such difficulties, such as assertive training, the practice of social skills and consequent reduction in anxiety. Some authorities claim that the correct treatment for a person with an intense phobia of approaching the opposite sex and of physical contact with them is a therapeutic sexual relationship with a surrogate partner of the opposite sex. However, a comparison of this type of treatment with more conventional behavioural methods of treating sexual anxiety has never been made. Furthermore, surrogate methods are fraught with such obvious ethical and practical difficulties that they cannot be recommended.

The next stage of development in a sexual relationship is the formation of a close link with just one person of the opposite sex. In most instances, a degree of emotional and physical intimacy is necessary before the sexual act itself can take place, although the speed with which this happens is both culturally and educationally determined, and depends also upon the previous sexual experience of the couple involved. Some people while perfectly at ease socially and capable of the necessary 'chatting-up' skills may still have difficulty with any kind of emotional intimacy such as may lead to the sharing of experiences and having to take responsibility for the feelings of another person. Thus the development of any degree of interdependence may provoke increasing anxiety and lead to a rapid breaking of the relationship. Fears of physical intimacy can also be a barrier to the development of a sexual relationship, particularly in men or women who come from families among whom touching or displaying the body is taboo. The treatment of such problems is usually behavioural, leading to gradual reduction of anxiety.

Difficulties during intercourse

Male dysfunction

In investigating difficulties during intercourse, it is necessary to consider both parties together and to pay due regard to their interaction although, as male and female sexual difficulties show certain distinct differences, it may, in the first instance, be convenient to consider them separately. Those conditions which primarily affect men include erectile difficulties, problems with ejaculation and postcoital difficulties. In impotence or erectile difficulty, either no erection occurs or there is difficulty in sustaining full engorgement for long enough to achieve adequate penetration. Those to whom this happens are liable to become discouraged for, in trying hard to retrieve the situation they soon discover the well-known fact that no man can will himself an erection. Thus fear of failure together with failure itself tend to become self-reinforcing. Apart from this, a man actively engaged in lovemaking may have very little idea of the size of his penis and misinterpret as insufficient what is in effect a perfectly adequate erection.

Some men who may have little or no difficulty in obtaining or sustaining erection may find that just before, during or just after penetration they are unable to control ejaculation and therefore may ejaculate prematurely—*ejaculatio praecox*, or *ejaculatory incompetence*. Other, less common, abnormalities of ejaculation include *coitus reservatus*, in which there is inability to ejaculate after penetration has occurred, *coitus saxonicus* in which retrograde ejaculation occurs into the bladder, and seepage of semen during sexual arousal without experiencing full orgasm.

In the postcoital phase, at its most pathological the situation may be exemplified by the half-drunken male who after a period of clumsy lovemaking or none at all, ejaculates, withdraws, rolls over and starts to snore, leaving his frustrated and disgusted partner sleepless by his side.

Female sexual dysfunction

Frigidity is as pejorative a word as impotence, particularly as it suggests an overall coldness which may well not be present. A better term is *general sexual dysfunction* which, as in men, may be primary or secondary and partial or complete. While the woman with general sexual dysfunction may derive little, if any, erotic or sexual pleasure from sexual stimulation, she may still obtain a great deal of comfort from the warmth and closeness which the relationship brings with it.

The characteristics of general sexual dysfunction include loss of erotic feeling, interest or pleasure; loss of physical response or denial of feeling in the presence of normal physiological responses; or absence of physiological responses but retention of feeling and even orgasm. A woman's educational and cultural expectations of what her sexual response should be are also of importance, as is the reaction of her partner. All these are factors which will determine whether she sees her disability as a problem or not.

Many women with generalized sexual dysfunction do not reach a level of sexual arousal sufficient to reach orgasm and may complain of it. Many, however, who arouse easily and are sexually responsive are unable to achieve orgasm however hard or long they try (*anorgasmia*). This may be the commonest female sexual difficulty. Failure to obtain an orgasm may be primary or secondary and may be situational or with certain partners. Usually this means that she is anorgasmic during sexual intercourse itself but can reach a climax either with her own or her partner's stimulation or by the use of a mechanical aid. Many women who suffer from orgasmic dysfunction are otherwise sexually quite normal.

The other main sexual problem in women is that of vaginal spasm (*vaginismus*) which may or may not be associated with the other difficulties already mentioned. The problem is that during any attempt at penetration of the vagina, there is an intense spasm of the muscles that surround the introitus so that it remains firmly shut. Once spasm has occurred, any attempt at penetration will be painful so that the experience will reinforce the reflex closure of the introitus at any future attempt at penetration. The tight ring of muscles can sometimes be felt by the patient or her partner and may be misinterpreted as a mechanical barrier. Vaginismus is often associated with non-consummation of a marriage, although almost invariably in prolonged non-consummation due to vaginismus the husband will be found to have his own problems as well.

Some women with vaginismus are still able to allow a degree of penetration. Milder degrees of vaginismus in which initial introital pain is experienced but lessens as intercourse proceeds are also common and may reflect the partner's inexperience. The majority of women who describe dyspareunia or pain on intercourse are actually describing vaginismus. Of course, in all cases of female sexual dysfunction gynaecological causes must be excluded.

Effects of ageing

Certain normal ageing changes both in men and women are sometimes mistaken for sexual dysfunction. As a man grows older, certain changes take place in his sexual response cycle, usually from his early forties onwards. It takes him longer to achieve an erection than in his youth and perhaps up to five minutes for a full erection to occur. He tends, however, to be able to retain his erection for longer before ejaculating but may also find he does not ejaculate every time however hard he tries. Following ejaculation, detumescence occurs more rapidly. Likewise the refractory period lengthens so that it may take some hours before an erection can be re-established after ejaculation. Also if an older man loses his erection before ejaculation, he may find it harder to regain it. These are normal ageing changes of no pathological significance although they may be easily misinterpreted by anxious middle-aged men.

If women discontinue sexual activity at the climacteric but later try to resume intercourse, they will find that the normal physiological responses tend to be lost and that the vagina has become dry and atrophic. In order to regain normal sexual responses hormone replacement may be needed. However, if a woman continues to have sexual intercourse during the climacteric, these changes do not occur.

Taking a sexual history

There are many causes of sexual difficulty, although the majority are psychogenic. It is most important to obtain a careful step-by-step account, remembering that the problem may be presented quite differently when the history is taken from each partner separately.

It is necessary to discover when and how the difficulty began and all possibly associated precipitating events. This should be followed by an account of how the problem has progressed until the present time, having regard to the effect of one partner's problem on that of the other. It is not too uncommon to find that the member of a partnership who presents for treatment is not the one with the primary problem. It is also important to investigate other relationships in order to discover whether the complainant's difficulty is one which has been repeated in every relationship, or whether there is something special about the present relationship which relates to the presenting problem.

Other necessary information includes such matters as the time of onset of puberty, how, when and where the subject gained sexual information, masturbatory habits and details of adult sexual activity. Information about basic sexual orientation is often best gained by inquiring about fantasies during masturbation. Inquiry should also be made about the subject's attitudes to all these matters, and how much they have subsequently been modified in the light of experience. An important part of sexual assessment includes the effect upon the subject of the attitudes of his or her parents. It is also necessary to gauge the extent of the patient's sexual knowledge, and that of the partner.

Although normal sexual behaviour is any explicitly sexual act between two people which damages neither, if a man or woman complains of physical difficulty in a heterosexual relationship because of homosexual feelings, or of the need to arouse themselves in such a relationship, by having resort to fetishistic, sadistic, masochistic or other behaviour which is unacceptable to the other partner, then sexual orientation can be said to be abnormal in that particular setting.

Organic dysfunction

The vast majority of sexual problems are psychogenic, the only sexual problem where organic causes are at all common being impotence. Even then, in only about 5 per cent of men with established impotence is this due to some organic cause. Of course, both psychological and organic factors may be of aetiological significance.

In organic impotence, sexual drive is often unimpaired and the onset is usually gradual, with inability to respond to other sexual outlets. *Selective impotence* does not, therefore, occur in organic impotence which may, however, fluctuate in intensity before becoming complete. All aspects of sexual expression are affected so that in addition to impotence, morning erections and nocturnal emissions are absent. In advanced stages of organic impotence the ability to masturbate to an erection and climax will be lost, although it may be retained from purely local genital stimulation if a cortical lesion is responsible. Most organic impotence is progressive and may be associated with changes in bladder and bowel function.

Impotence may follow impairment of sex drive, as in generalized illnesses, liver disease and endocrine disorders, exposure to drugs such as opiates, anti-androgen and some steroid preparations, or physical interference with erection. This occurs with the autonomic neuropathy of *diabetes mellitus* affecting the parasympathetic supply to the penis. The same is true of some cases of *alcoholism* in which autonomic neuropathy may be present although more generalized polyneuropathy may not yet have developed. Impotence associated with alcoholism and sometimes with diabetes also may be projected on to the partner, taking the form of *delusional jealousy*. Other conditions which affect the parasympathetic supply to the penis include some surgical operations such as abdominoperineal resection and radical prostatectomy; neurological diseases such as multiple sclerosis, temporal lobe lesions occasionally, and some drugs such as tricyclic antidepressants and other anticholinergic agents. Tricyclic antidepressants may, however, sometimes have a paradoxical effect by retarding ejaculation where this is premature, thereby improving sexual performance. They cannot, however, be considered as a reliable means of treatment for premature ejaculation. Erection may occasionally be impaired by mechanisms elsewhere such as local penile diseases or by failure of the necessary blood supply to the penis as in the Leriche syndrome or in sickle cell anaemia.

An organic cause for sexual difficulty is very rare in women. Occasionally generalized endocrine or bodily illness may lower libido and impair sexual response. Somewhat more frequently, contraceptive measures may have an influence on female sexual response and there is little doubt that the contraceptive pill may directly impair sexual response in a very small number of women by interfering with the metabolism of testosterone. Testosterone, interestingly enough, is responsible for sexual arousal in women as it is in men.

Depressive illness

Depression is a very common and important cause of impotence, particularly in those who have hitherto had no particular sexual difficulties but who, as they start to become depressed, may suffer a loss of libido together with other characteristic symptoms, namely loss of drive, concentration, appetite and weight. Sometimes when a depressive illness resolves, impotence persists owing to secondary anxiety. It is important, therefore, to emphasize that potency will almost certainly be regained as the patient's condition improves. The treatment in this instance is, of course, the treatment of the underlying depressive state.

Behavioural treatment

Behavioural treatment based on Masters and Johnson's work appears to be the most successful method to date and is largely directed towards correcting the secondary effects of sexual dysfunction such as anxiety arising in a sexual setting. These methods are probably effective because they can be learned relatively quickly and do not need long periods of training before being put into practice.

Discussions are held jointly with the partners until clear goals are agreed between them in terms of treatment aims. Because the initial aim is to deal with the secondary effects of the problem, a ban is imposed on intercourse, or any sexual expression which the therapist may consider it wise to disallow. The couple then begin a series of exercises designed very gradually to reintroduce physical proximity and touching and in such a way that they begin to enjoy physical contact again (*sensate focus*). They are instructed to concentrate on the giving and receiving of pleasure and feedback information to one another about what they are actually feeling, while avoiding setting targets or goals for physical encounter beyond those of giving pleasure. Initially the exchange of touching is entirely non-sexual but gradually, as the exercise progresses, sexual touching is allowed but in a non-demanding way. When the therapist is satisfied that the couple are relaxed in each other's company and enjoy giving and receiving pleasure, while having become less goal directed and watchful, then specific treatment is given for the couple's particular problem.

In men with potency problems and women who are anorgasmic, sensate focus exercises are continued with gradual addition to the repertoire until eventually mounting and penetration occur (during sensate focus, erections almost invariably return). Initially penetration, which does not lead to full orgasm, remains under the control of the female partner. The technique consists therefore of a passive reintroduction of penetration and eventual ejaculation with the man concentrating so much on the pleasure that he is receiving that he stops thinking about the goal. The same approach is used for the anorgasmic female.

Premature ejaculation is helped after the sensate focus by getting the man to concentrate on his ejaculatory feelings. This may be assisted by the *squeeze technique* in which the penis is compressed to prevent ejaculation occurring. Ejaculatory control gradually develops in this way. Retarded ejaculation is treated after sensate focus by vaginal containment during which additional manual stimulation of the penis is carried out by the partner.

Vaginismus is treated by intensive relaxation techniques aimed at teaching the woman vaginal muscle control. During a therapeutic vaginal examination the therapist also directs the woman to examine herself. This part of the treatment may need fairly firm handling to prevent the woman from escaping from confrontation by her own feelings, if vaginismus is severe. There follows graded introduction of vaginal penetration using the partner's finger and a series of dilators. Finally, as part of the sensate focus exercises, the partner's erect penis is used as a dilator by the woman until she has lost her fear of penile penetration. It is at this point that one often discovers the male partner's own difficulties.

The success rate of treatment of problems using this type of behavioural approach is quite high, many clinics averaging an overall 65 to 70 per cent success rate. Certain problems, such as premature ejaculation, vaginismus and secondary impotence, are probably easier to deal with than others. The treatment of primary impotence, anorgasmia and retarded ejaculation is less successful.

Psychotherapy

Psychotherapeutic measures directed at helping the couple to a better relationship, or helping one or both partners to understand better the roots of their difficulties, may be necessary, either on their own or as part of a behavioural approach to the sexual problem. It has been shown, however, that the overall success rate of psychotherapeutic methods of treating sexual problems is, when they are used on their own, quite low.

Physical treatments

Physical treatments are hardly ever necessary. The use of drugs with supposed aphrodisiac properties, drugs which allegedly delay ejaculation or drugs which relieve sexual anxiety should be avoided. There is very occasionally, however, an indication for the use of testosterone, as it may sometimes have a favourable effect on libido, particularly if used in carefully selected cases. In middle-aged men who have not had sexual intercourse for some time, endogenous levels of testosterone are low and exogenous testosterone given during a course of behavioural treatment may, as it were, 'prime the pump'. In men, testosterone must be given by intramuscular depot injections; given orally it is probably useless. Women with low levels of sexual arousal have also been shown to respond favourably to small doses of testosterone, which obviously should be given only for short periods of time. Here sublingual administration may be sufficient. It needs emphasis that testosterone should not be used as a panacea for every case of sexual difficulty but only in those patients whose level of sexual arousal is low due to prolonged cessation of sexual activity.

Masturbation

Masturbation was, in the nineteenth century, believed to produce a variety of signs and symptoms including dyspepsia, epilepsy, blindness, loss of hearing, rickets, acne and, most importantly, insanity! It was even given as a cause of death in American and British mental hospitals. Almost all persons, male and female, masturbate, especially during adolescence, and the realization that this is so has reduced anxiety about this behaviour, so that it is usually only those who are markedly unsophisticated who complain about masturbation as a symptom.

Masturbation becomes a symptom only when it replaces the desire for normal sexual relations when these are otherwise available. Under these circumstances it may be an outcome of a mental or personality disorder. Some who are sexually disturbed may prefer to indulge in abnormal fantasies accompanied by masturbation rather than to attempt a normal heterosexual relationship. Excessive masturbation, sometimes carried out in public, may also occur as a symptom of schizophrenia or mania. In this event it is the underlying psychosis which calls for treatment.

Masturbation does not have any damaging physical effects. The same applies to spontaneous nocturnal emissions which occasionally cause distress. These are common, particularly in those who are sexually abstinent and who may resist conscious masturbation on moral grounds. Women, as well as men, may be troubled by dreams which are accompanied by orgasm. Although these too may be regarded as normal they are thought to be commoner in those who have emotional problems.

Anomalous sexual behaviour

Anomalous sexual behaviour can be defined as persistent behaviour from which a subject obtains sexual satisfaction through some other outlet than that of normal heterosexual intercourse. The word *anomalous* is perhaps to be preferred as carrying rather less moralistic overtones than the more customary terms—*sexual deviation* or *perversion*. This would appear to be appropriate because in no other field of psychiatry has such a rapid change taken place in public and professional attitudes. In recent years there has also been a change in the general attitude towards homosexuality, leading to a much greater tolerance of homosexual behaviour, at least between consenting adults.

Homosexuality

Is homosexuality abnormal or pathological? This is not an easy question to answer. Apart from transient homosexual activity in young animals deprived during the mating season of a partner of the opposite sex, homosexuality as an established pattern of behaviour is not seen in the animal kingdom. On the other hand, it occurs in all races and cultures of mankind and in many is relatively common. Thus about 13 per cent of men will have some kind of homosexual contact leading to orgasm in their lifetime; in women the proportion is probably higher. About 4 to 5 per cent of men and women seem to be exclusively homosexual in that all their sexual relationships are with their own sex. Graduations between complete homosexuality and complete heterosexuality exist, as recognized by Kinsey who divided homosexuals and heterosexuals into seven categories depending on degree. Transient homosexual behaviour in some who are basically heterosexual also occurs in special circumstances such as in prison or on board ship. It is important to distinguish between merely transient behaviour and that of a more persistent kind. This is particularly true in adolescence during which many pass through a homosexual phase.

Until recently, homosexuality was said to be associated almost invariably with a personality disturbance often complicated by a tendency towards alcoholism, suicide, jealousy reaction, spitefulness and blackmail. However, it now seems likely that such reactions were possibly the results of social pressures and the opprobrium under which homosexuals were compelled to live rather than due to the condition itself. Indeed, recent controlled studies have failed to confirm that there is a preponderance of psychiatric problems in those who are established homosexuals, many earlier investigations which drew opposite conclusions being clearly based on biased samples. Homosexual behaviour can probably only be considered as evidence of mental abnormality when it occurs for the first time in a person who was previously strongly heterosexual; this is likely to be indicative of some underlying psychiatric disturbance.

Aetiology

The cause of established homosexuality is still a matter of debate. It is now generally accepted that it arises out of a complex interaction between possible genetic and constitutional factors. Some consideration may also be given to prenatal hormonal environment—including the presence of androgens at critical periods of uterine development which partly determine the future pattern of sexual behaviour—and later, environmental parental and other factors which may lead to reinforcement. There is no evidence, however, that adult endocrine disorders or other physical factors are responsible for adult homosexuality. Any such disorders which may be observed in homosexuals must therefore be considered as secondary or coincidental.

Most of those homosexuals who seek help need counselling in order to help them to adapt to their sexual role. Occasionally, however, they may have a good reason for wishing to change their sexual orientation. This is more likely to be achieved if some heterosexual urges are also present. In an emergency, suppression of sexual drive can be achieved by benperidol or an anti-androgen drug, but such treatment should only be seen as first aid. More permanent results can sometimes be achieved with behaviour therapy. Modern views suggest that it is better to use behavioural techniques to reinforce the heterosexual side of a person's nature rather than adversive measures to suppress the homosexual side. Before embarking on any treatment the therapist should make sure that it is the patient who really wishes to change and that his or her reasons for wanting to do so are valid.

Other sexual anomalies

There is such a wide variety of sexual anomalies that not all will be considered. Apart from homosexuality it should be noted that virtually all sexual anomalies are a male prerogative. Such anomalies may also be homosexually or heterosexually orientated. Thus *paedophilia* is a condition in which adult males interfere sexually with female children and, in the case of *paederasty*, with young boys. In either event, the common factor appears to be an immaturity of personality of such a degree that the subject is unable to relate to those of his own age. Despite this, many child molesters are married and may have children of their own. Treatment, insofar as it is successful, is either by physically suppressing sexual urges using anti-androgen drugs or benperidol, or by trying to help the patient along behavioural lines to develop more adult heterosexual skills. Despite the current pressure for better understanding of men who interfere sexually with children, it is unlikely that society will ever tolerate such behaviour and it is indeed doubtful whether it should.

Exhibitionism

Exhibitionism is one of the commonest of all sexual eccentricities. The subject exposes his genitals to women, often in a park or some relatively secluded spot or in a car parked at the kerbside. The act of indecent exposure may or may not be accompanied by masturbation or ejaculation but is only rarely accompanied by any other overtly sexual act such as indecent assault. Likewise, only very rarely does an exhibitionist attempt to rape his victim. Several different aetiological factors underlie exhibitionism, including an immature form of sexual display, a powerful element of compulsion and occasionally, in older patients, depression, in which it is thought that consciousness of waning libido may play a part. It is important to recognize those patients who are depressed.

Providing they are apprehended, a number who expose themselves do so only once, the subsequent court case being enough to prevent further occurrences. Some, however, continually repeat the offence, in the event of which behavioural methods of treatment aimed at helping the subjects to learn to control their impulses are most favoured at the moment.

Voyeurism (Scoptophilia)

Voyeurism is a form of gratification obtained by observing the sexual and related practices of others. While today there are more commercial outlets to satisfy such appetites, the 'Peeping Tom' may still remain a considerable nuisance.

Transvestism

There are several forms of transvestism. Primary transvestism is an act whereby a person dresses in some or other items of clothing of the opposite sex. Some men, showing this behaviour, masturbate in private and achieve some degree of gratification thereby; others dress themselves up completely and are further excited by parading in public. Such excitement may possibly be enhanced by the risk of being discovered. Many of these patients are married and may have reasonably successful heterosexual relationships with their wives who, however, may not take kindly to their husbands dressing up in their underwear before making love to them. In other instances, female clothing may be obtained by surreptitious means, for instance by stealing underwear from clotheslines. It is uncertain why this widespread phenomenon exists. In most cases it is venial and, by and large, if it does not interfere with her marital relationship, a wife may be encouraged to learn to live with her husband's idiosyncrasy.

Transvestism may also occur amongst passive homosexuals. Here, however, putting on women's clothing is not an end in itself but a piece of play acting which is intended to enhance a homosexual relationship ('in drag'). Transvestism also occurs amongst females. Here again, it is often a homosexual phenomenon but is on the whole more socially acceptable than transvestism in men. Apart from these aspects, dressing up in the clothes of the opposite sex may also be a feature of transsexualism.

Transsexualism

Transsexuals, although physically normal, are convinced inwardly that they are really persons of the opposite sex, believing that by some freak their bodies have developed abnormally and are not in accordance with their real sex. This belief is held with very strong conviction. The condition is distinct from transvestism and probably to some degree from homosexuality, although the fantasy life of these patients is predominantly homosexual. Most transsexuals present not by asking for treatment, but for help in adapting to their chosen sexual identity. The aetiology of the condition remains obscure, but constitutional factors, prenatal hormonal influences, postnatal conditioning and learning factors may be important. No adult endocrine disability is discoverable. There is now evidence that in transsexuals who have lived at ease in their chosen gender, who are emotionally stable and who bear no responsibilities such as may be entailed by a marital relationship, social change of gender such as changing name by deed poll and registration for employment, plastic surgery and endocrinological support may be the treatment of choice. However, as such treatment requires the closest cooperation between surgeon, endocrinologist and psychiatrist, it should never be undertaken lightly.

Fetishism

The phenomenon of fetishism is clearly related to transvestism in that the subject is often sexually aroused by some article of female clothing such as lingerie, stockings, boots or shoes. The range of objects is wide. Some men like their sexual partners to dress in this or that fashion and may be sexually excited thereby. If such excitement is subservient to the satisfactory performance of heterosexual intercourse, it can hardly be described as deviant in that it becomes no more perhaps than one of the trimmings. It all depends on whether the means serves the end or the means becomes an end in itself. Fetishism, like transvestism, probably arises out of conditioning by contact with female clothing at an early age.

Sado-masochism

Sado-masochism demands the infliction of pain, and the offering of restraint or humiliation either to the sexual partner or reciprocally. Once again, in lesser degrees and in the pursuit of heterosexual fulfilment, such indulgence, if carried out only to a minor degree, can hardly be considered pathological, unless it becomes an end in itself. Fully fledged sadists, on the other hand, may be numbered amongst the most dangerous of mentally disturbed patients, as in the case of certain rapists and child stranglers, who may be very hard to apprehend. Masochism can also be a dangerous pursuit, as in the case of adolescents who tie themselves up and carry out hanging and asphyxiation experiments. Minor degrees of pathological sadistic behaviour include clothes-slashing, the making of obscene telephone calls, 'heavy-breathing' and similar pursuits.

Treatment of sexual anomalies

Treatment is difficult and can be disappointing. Conventional psychotherapeutic measures are largely ineffective although in milder cases they may enable a patient to achieve a better level of social adjustment by containing his behaviour at a fantasy level, rather than acting it out. In critical instances with forensic implications, suppression of sexuality by chemical means, either using benperidol or, in severer cases, an anti-androgenic agent such as cyproterone acetate which has the advantage of not giving rise to soreness of the breasts or to gynaecomastia, may be used.

In the case of fetishists, transvestites and some others who may be tempted into untoward sexual behaviour but genuinely wish to be rid of the temptation, behavioural modification appears to offer the best chance of successful cure. An operant conditioning approach can be used with careful attention to the positive and negative reinforcements. A programme is arranged, which must be structured for the individual patient, with careful attention to contingencies so that the advantages of loss of this anomalous form of sexual behaviour with replacement by a more appropriate outlet outweigh the disadvantages. This is difficult as the behavioural patterns are firmly established and treatment results are only moderately encouraging.

Further reading

Bancroft, J. H. J. (1974) *Deviant Sexual Behaviour: Modification and Assessment.* London: Oxford University Press.
Masters, W. H. & Johnson, V. E. (1970) *Human Sexual Inadequacy.* Edinburgh: Churchill Livingstone.
Storr, A. (1970) *Sexual Deviation.* Harmondsworth: Penguin.

18

Psychiatry and Medicine
(Liaison Psychiatry)

Because it is obvious in many instances that psychiatric disturbances are
often a direct sequel of infection, injury, neoplasm or metabolic
disorder, these may well be encountered in patients receiving treatment
in the medical and surgical wards of any general hospital. On this
account, psychiatrists are finding themselves increasingly involved in the
assessment of the psychological problems commonly attendant upon
what may otherwise be regarded as primarily physical disorders (*liaison
psychiatry*). Because these are so many and varied and not all within the
scope of this book, only some will be fully considered. They are included
under several main headings: general medical disorders together with
skin diseases and endocrine disorders; gynaecological disorders and
those associated with pregnancy and the puerperium; postoperative
mental illness; pain, largely of psychogenic origin; and finally attempted
suicide. All of these are conditions which present most often in a general
hospital setting.

It should be noted that these conditions fall roughly into two types:
firstly, those in which psychological problems are inherent in the nature
of the physical disease process itself, for example *myxoedema*, which may
give rise to a depressive seemingly demented state; and, secondly, those
conditions in which such mental symptoms as do occur can be construed
as reactive to pain, disfigurement, fear of outcome, etc., and to which the
premorbid personality of the patient contributes. However, one type of
reaction does not exclude the other so that both may be operative in a
single case.

Psychosomatic illnesses
Recently there has been a considerable diminution in enthusiasm for
psychosomatic hypotheses so that currently the earlier somewhat narrow
definition—physical illnesses primarily of psychogenic origin—has been
widened to include all conditions in which psychiatric investigation may
contribute to the understanding of the aetiology, prevention and
treatment of physical complaints. This more up-to-date approach avoids
entanglement in the body–mind controversy, which surrounded the
psychosomatic medicine of 30 years or so ago. Enthusiasm for the
original concept began to diminish when it became increasingly apparent
that the notion that abnormal mental functioning might give rise to

specific physical lesions was on the wane and that the hypothesis that each psychosomatic illness (for example peptic ulcer, rheumatoid arthritis, ulcerative colitis, etc.) was based on a specific and recognizable personality disorder was proving impossible to sustain.

General medical disorders

Cardiovascular

The presence of actual heart disease may cause profound psychological reactions in some patients. Thus *valvular disease*, or *congenital abnormalities* which limit activity, may interfere with achievement and ambition, leading to frustration and dependency problems. Those who on account of invalidism have become unduly dependent on others may later find difficulty in relinquishing their dependence even if their condition is relieved by cardiac surgery. This goes some way to explaining why, when the result of operation as judged by tests appears to be successful, the overall response of the patient may not be as good as might otherwise be expected.

Myocardial infarction
Although it is uncertain how much psychological stress may contribute to its occurrence, myocardial infarction may, if it does not prove fatal, be little short of a disaster to an active, driving individual. Likewise, in one of obsessional personality an infarct even if mild may lead to undue limitation of activity, invalidism and hypochondriasis.

Hypertension
Whether emotional factors have a role in the production of essential hypertension or not is also a matter of debate. Anxiety and tension can certainly cause a rise of blood pressure, although this is usually transient. However, the possibility that continued frustration for which there is no adequate outlet may play some part cannot be altogether dismissed.

Effort syndrome (da Costa's syndrome, neurocirculatory asthenia or cardiac neurosis)
This, which three or four decades ago used to be a very much commoner condition than it is now, is, in effect, a form of anxiety state in which symptoms which at first sight appear to be cardiac are prominent. The presenting complaint is most often that of pain in the chest—usually on the left side where the patient believes the mass of his heart to be—tenderness, fatigue, dyspnoea and palpitations after exercise or, because of anxiety, at rest. A functional systolic murmur may sometimes be heard, of which the subject may have been made aware of on some previous occasion leading to an increase in his anxiety. Patients with the

effort syndrome are often young men, emotionally immature and of markedly asthenic physical build. The condition was common among conscripts in World War II but today is much less often seen.

Respiratory system

Change in the rate and amplitude of respiration may be a feature of phobic and other anxiety states. *Hyperventilation*, which may give rise to tetany, may be checked by getting the patient to breathe into a bag. Anxiety, frustration and suppressed aggressiveness may precipitate attacks of *asthma* or aggravate an asthmatic response to physical irritants. An asthmatic who develops a psychosis may sometimes be free from attacks as long as the psychosis persists, although the reason for this is not understood.

Chronic obstructive airways disease, particularly in older people, may be an important cause of depressive symptoms in that, like arthritis in the elderly, it may limit mobility and, on this account, lead to a diminution of social contacts.

Alimentary

Anxiety, like depression, may diminish appetite, cause dryness of the mouth and produce a sinking feeling or 'butterflies' in the stomach. If marked, this may constitute a syndrome, *functional dyspepsia*, characterized by vague ill-localized epigastric pain or discomfort bearing no close relationship to meals, eructation from aerophagy, poor appetite and intolerance in particular of fried or fatty foods. Once again the physical constitution of the patient is often markedly asthenic.

Difficulty in swallowing (so-called *globus hystericus*) and spasm of the cardiac sphincter may result from emotional tension. *Peptic ulcers* are certainly aggravated by anxiety but are not, so far as is known, caused solely by emotional factors. *Mucous colitis*, on the other hand, bears a closer relation to emotional instability. Constipation with overflow, diarrhoea and a *spastic* or *irritable colon* may also be in large part due to emotional factors as well as to faulty bowel habits.

Obesity

Although often thought merely to be the result of overeating coupled with restricted physical exercise, a mode of life which may be prompted by boredom and frustration and not merely by self-indulgence, there is much about obesity which is still far from being well understood. There are also some who overeat and gain weight excessively apparently in an effort to keep depression at bay. Attempts at dieting by such persons sometimes result in quite severe depressive reactions. The problem of obesity may have its roots in childhood as a result of overfeeding by anxious mothers whose relationship with their children is insecure. An inordinate appetite (*bulimia*) with increase in weight may follow cerebral trauma, possibly due to a hypothalamic lesion, or may occur following prefrontal leucotomy—also sometimes in dementia (*hyperphagia*).

Anorexia nervosa

This, which is a common condition, appears to be becoming increasingly so, although possibly because earlier cases are now more frequently diagnosed. The condition is usually characterized by marked loss of weight, either from refusal to eat or, if an apparently normal diet is taken, persistent vomiting which is self-induced. A third group may periodically eat enormously ('binges') prior to vomiting and may retain enough food to maintain weight (*bulimia nervosa*). It should be noted that those who starve themselves do not, however, actually lose their appetite, but are able to resist hunger. Paradoxically, many patients with anorexia nervosa, although failing to eat themselves, appear to enjoy cooking and preparing food for others.

The majority of cases occur in adolescent girls more or less soon after puberty (*primary anorexia nervosa*). Some maintain that the condition does not occur in prepubertal children, although a similar condition is occasionally seen in this age group. However, under these circumstances the disorder may be a manifestation of depression in childhood. Another group of cases occurs in adult women, mostly in their twenties, sometimes older. These women are often married and sometimes parous (*secondary anorexia nervosa*). Many bulimics fall into this age group. Primary anorexics outnumber secondary cases in a ratio of about 4 or 5 to 1. A similar condition, or something analogous to it, occurs much more rarely in men.

The loss of weight in some cases is profound and severe enough to cause hunger oedema. The output of faeces may be reduced owing to diminished food intake, or chronic diarrhoea may occur in those patients who deliberately overdose themselves with aperients in order, so they believe, to assist them to lose weight. Although anorexic patients may come to look like concentration camp victims, breast tissue tends to be preserved in all but the most cachectic. Pubic and axillary hair is not lost and there may be an overgrowth of fine downy hair on the back and limbs (*lanugo hair*). Acrocyanosis of the extremities may be present which disappears as the patient gains weight.

Amenorrhoea is an important symptom which is present in nearly every case. It occurs early, often before much weight is lost, and may be prolonged so that frequently even when the patient has regained her lost weight menstruation may not recommence for many months. Until it does so, remission cannot be said to be secure. Even then, relapse can still occur after menstruation has begun again. The duration of anorexia nervosa may easily be five to seven years, rarely much less than two years. In a few patients, the disorder may become chronic so that the sufferer remains for many years in an underweight condition (*anorexia tarda*), but not apparently in a state of undue harm to health. The mortality rate overall has been estimated to be as high as 10 per cent, but should be considerably lower in good hands.

Psychopathology

The underlying psychopathology is complex and often difficult to elicit, particularly in the early stages of the illness. An abnormality of personality is usually present so that the patients are often markedly immature and seem to be trying to resist growing up. Some show obsessional trends or a mixture of these with hysterical or attention-seeking traits. In another group depressive symptoms are prominent. There is also a simple form which follows not infrequently upon a history of overeating and plumpness in childhood about which the patient may have been teased. This may lead to dieting which then gets out of control.

Girls with anorexia nervosa are more liable to come from social classes I, II and III and, less commonly, from social classes IV and V. The reason for this is not entirely clear, but it probably has something to do with the variation in dietary and eating habits among those of differing social class. On close investigation some disturbance of the relationship between anorexic patients and their parents, most often their mothers, may be apparent. In younger girls sexual inhibition and fantasies may be prominent. Fantasies about size are also common so that the majority of patients appear to believe themselves to be much fatter than they actually are. This is often referred to as a disorder of body image, but strictly speaking this is incorrect and a misuse of a neurological concept.

Treatment

This can be both difficult and tedious. Admission to hospital is almost invariably required so that the patient's eating habits can be closely scrutinized. Many favour a regime of *operant conditioning* in which privileges initially removed are restored according to the success of a preplanned programme of weight gain continued up to the point of discharge from hospital. Chlorpromazine may be of help as it stimulates appetite, tends to prevent vomiting and helps to immobilize non-compliant patients. Insulin is dangerous and should be avoided. Psychotherapy is difficult in the early stages and may best be postponed until some degree of symptomatic relief has been achieved, as it is often found that patients with anorexia nervosa become altogether more outgoing and willing to discuss their problems after some weight has been gained. In the early stages, therefore, psychotherapeutic intervention is probably best carried out with relatives, although prolonged psychotherapy with the patient will become necessary sooner or later if recovery is to be at all secure.

Skin diseases

Psychological factors play a prominent part in exacerbating or prolonging a number of skin disorders. This is hardly surprising as the skin itself is an important organ of emotional expression, as is shown by the common phenomena of pallor or blushing as an accompaniment to emotions such as fear, anxiety, embarrassment or guilt. The erotic properties of the skin are also of considerable importance. In addition, as the skin represents the barrier between ego and environment, any conflict between the two and which constitutes, as it were, a 'frontier dispute' is quite likely to be fought out at the barricade.

While such disorders as *atopic eczema, urticaria, lichen planus* and *psoriasis* are almost certainly not of psychogenic origin, there is little doubt that their occurrence soon becomes entangled with the patient's prevailing emotional condition. Where disfigurement (as in *acne*) or irritation is prominent, it clearly exacerbates matters. The undue concern of mothers about eczema in their children leading to excessive cleaning of the skin, the applying of unguents, bandaging and so on tends to bring about an abnormal relationship between mother and child, which the child soon learns to manipulate through the medium of its skin condition.

The origin of *neurodermatitis* is obscure. Commonly although not invariably starting on the hands, it may at first appear to have originated from exposure to oil, grease or some other industrial or household chemical. However, even when these substances are withdrawn, it may persist. Under these conditions infection from scratching and psychological conflicts may be important, the matter being complicated in some cases by the possibility of industrial compensation. Indeed the exploration of such problems may be of much greater value than medication.

Endocrine disorders

Endocrine disorders very commonly give rise to emotional instability and to psychiatric problems which sometimes reach psychotic proportions. While the extent and type of these problems depend to some degree on the patient's premorbid personality, both the severity and rate of change of endocrine function appear to play a part. Where the disorder can be controlled and when this is done in good time, the patient's abnormal mental state is usually reversible.

Thyroid disorders

In *hyperthyroidism*, emotional stress is often thought to be an aetiological factor in that some cases, following upon a period of mental stress, appear to start as anxiety states, progressing later to an actual disorder of thyroid function. However, differentiation in terms of cause and effect can be difficult, for many thyrotoxic patients exhibit emotional symptoms at the earliest stage. These include anxiety, depression, tearfulness, restlessness, emotional instability, tiredness, difficulty in concentration and loss of weight. Tremor tends to be coarse in anxiety states, but fine in thyrotoxicosis. Whereas the pulse rate is raised in both, in anxiety states it slows during sleep to below 80 per minute. The thyrotoxic patient has warm, moist extremities and may have early exophthalmos. The patient with an anxiety state has cold and clammy extremities and exophthalmos is not present, although some lid retraction may occur in very severe and acute cases. In any event tests for thyroid function will establish the diagnosis.

Very severe *thyrotoxicosis*, now rare, may be complicated by more extreme forms of mental disturbance, including manic or acute agitated depressive states, while in a *thyrotoxic crisis*, a post-operative reaction which, these days, should no longer occur, delirium and severe prostration can progress to coma and a fatal outcome.

In *hypothyroidism* the patient may be mentally slow and apathetic with lack of interest and initiative. Memory and other intellectual functions may give rise to a state of apparent dementia which is, however, reversible providing the correct diagnosis is made and treatment not unduly delayed. *Myxoedema* may also cause a paranoid psychosis (so-called *myxoedematous madness*). Milder cases occurring in middle-aged menopausal women may given rise to a depressive state together with fatiguability and a variety of ill-defined bodily discomforts. In such cases and unless considered, the true diagnosis may be overlooked unless appropriate thyroid function tests are performed. In infants hypothyroidism may, if unrecognized, lead to mental subnormality (see *cretinism*, p. 312).

Parathyroid disorders

Some degree of depression may occur in both *primary* and *secondary hyperparathyroidism*, probably largely secondary to the disagreeable nature of the physical symptoms accompanying these disorders which include weakness, anorexia and nausea. These may initially be thought to be of psychogenic origin. In *hypoparathyroidism*, whether postoperative or the much rarer idiopathic form, mental symptoms tend to be more florid and include irritability, depression, emotional lability, memory impairment, and a picture resembling progressive dementia together with epileptic seizures due to tetany. These symptoms, even the apparent dementia, may be reversible if appropriate treatment is instituted in good time. *Pseudohypoparathyroidism*, which presents much the same clinical picture together with some degree of bodily deformity, is usually associated with mental subnormality.

Pituitary disorders

Nearly all pituitary disorders give rise to mental symptoms either as a primary feature or secondary to physical discomfort and disfigurement. Thus patients with *acromegaly* may show a change of character accompanied by loss of initiative, mood changes, impulsiveness and outbursts of violent temper. Bouts of excessive hunger and thirst frequently accompanied by headaches occur. Although libido may be initially increased it is lost subsequently.

Cushing's syndrome, which may be due to a basophil adenoma of the pituitary (*Cushing's disease*) or to some other pituitary anomaly, adrenal adenoma or carcinoma or some other non-endocrine ACTH-secreting tumour, gives rise, apart from the characteristic physical changes, to a wide variety of mental symptoms. These range from severe depression with paranoid features or other schizophreniform symptoms, or a condition with a more organic appearance in which apathy, clouding of consciousness and perceptual disturbances occur, to a more neurotic or seemingly reactive state characterized by anxiety, neurasthenic symptoms and obsessional trends. Psychotic symptoms can likewise be produced by the administration of *steroids* in high dosage or even in moderate amounts in the case of those with some degree of concomitant organic brain disorder such as may be part of *disseminated lupus erythematosus*, although, paradoxically, an increase in steroid dosage may cause the psychosis to resolve.

Panhypopituitarism, of which the commonest cause is postpartum pituitary necrosis (*Sheehan's syndrome*), is followed insidiously by a variety of vague symptoms which may initially lead to a diagnosis of neurosis. These symptoms include dullness, depression, apathy, irritability and loss of libido. While anorexia nervosa is sometimes still included in the differential diagnosis, the two conditions are usually easily distinguished. Sheehan's syndrome most often occurs in parturient women and is characterized by loss of pubic and axillary hair. Cachexia, moreover, is a late phenomenon (see p. 256).

Adrenal disorders

Although tumours of the adrenal cortex may give rise to Cushing's syndrome (see above), both they and *congenital adrenal hyperplasia* may cause *adrenal virilization*. In women this may give rise to profound psychological problems sometimes severe enough to suggest a developing psychosis. How much these problems are a primary manifestation and how much secondary to the startling changes in the patient's appearance, it is difficult to say. A change in sexual interest also occurs with loss of interest in the male sex and occasionally the development of homosexual trends; these changes are reversible if the underlying anomaly can be surgically corrected. Other than this, such patients are frequently depressed and occasionally subject to manic excitement and periods of paranoid confusion. Suicidal contemplation is common and needs to be taken seriously.

Chronic adrenocortical deficiency (Addison's disease) is often associated with asthenia, diminished energy and depression, although states of excitement can occur. Paranoid psychoses and confusional states have been reported as have acute schizophrenic reactions. Apart from specific hormone replacement therapy, such psychotic episodes are said to respond favourably to ECT.

Disorders of pancreatic function

In mild states of *hypoglycaemia* which may follow upon prolonged physical activity with diminished food intake, a sense of emptiness in the epigastrium, associated with an almost imperceptible change of consciousness, tremulousness and an extreme irritability may occur. Judgement may be slightly impaired and it is for this reason undesirable to continue any responsible activity, particularly driving a car, until food has been taken. The condition may and quite often does arise from overdosage of insulin in the treatment of diabetes mellitus or failure to eat after insulin has been taken. More rarely it may result from a *pancreatic adenoma*. In severer cases the condition if untreated will lead through an immediate state of clouded consciousness, often with disturbed behaviour, to *hypoglycaemic coma*. If untreated, serious permanent damage to the brain with characteristic symptoms of a diffuse dementia can occur.

Diabetes mellitus. The majority of diabetics show no abnormality of behaviour but some may become depressed or irritable over dietary and other restrictions. A genetic association of diabetes mellitus with manic-depressive illness is commonly accepted, and there may be a tendency to affective episodes. In *diabetic coma*, delirium with hallucinations and paranoid ideas may occur. Occasionally diabetes may be complicated by dementia due to cerebral arteriopathy.

Miscellaneous

In children *tumours of the pineal gland* may give rise to precocious sexual and mental development. Large tumours may retard the growth of the brain by pressure on the iter and consequent hydrocephalus.

Although *Frolich's disease* was originally thought to be due to a lesion in the anterior pituitary this is no longer the case. Like the *Laurence-Moon-Biedl* syndrome (see p. 261), the primary disturbance appears to be hypothalamic. Both disorders are characterized by adiposity and failure of genital development as well as by apathy, dullness and mental retardation.

Avitaminosis

Attention has already been drawn to vitamin deficiencies in alcoholic states, and also in elderly patients. How far vague ill-health with neurasthenic symptoms such as impaired concentration and fatiguability can be put down to vitamin deficiencies is uncertain, but it is common practice to include vitamins in treatment, probably often unnecessarily, although they may well have a placebo effect.

Pernicious anaemia with or without *subacute combined degeneration* of the cord may be accompanied by paranoid states, depression, clouding of consciousness and ultimately dementia, although most symptoms will respond rapidly to vitamin B12.

Pellagra is common in deprived countries, but has been observed in England particularly in old persons. Nicotinic acid and a diet rich in yeast and liver extracts will usually bring about improvement. The characteristic feature is a symmetrical, exfoliative, erythematous eruption on the backs of the hands, nose, cheeks, and front of neck—parts exposed to the sun. The eruption is associated with intestinal disturbances and sclerosis of the posterolateral columns of the spinal cord. The mental symptoms which are due to an encephalopathy may in milder cases be mistakenly regarded as abnormal emotional reactions. In more severe instances organic signs are obvious. An acute state of delirium can occur with rapid waxing and waning of consciousness together with limb rigidity, grasp and sucking reflexes and a fatal outcome.

Infectious disorders

A large number of infectious disorders, particularly those accompanied by high fever or where the infective organism directly invades the central nervous system giving rise to *encephalitis, meningitis* etc., may produce florid mental disturbances usually of a delirious kind (see Chapter 9). Apart from these, certain virus disorders may be accompanied by mental changes which are probably a result not merely of a direct involvement of the central nervous system but due to some secondary effect, the nature of which is not yet understood. Two prime examples of this are jaundice, due to *virus hepatitis*, and *infectious mononucleosis* (glandular fever). In the latter the sequelae may be prolonged over months. The most common clinical picture is of a mild state of depression together with apathy, irritability, difficulty in concentration, lack of drive and initiative and a general feeling of being 'out of sorts'. Because young adults, for example university students, are often affected, their studies may suffer seriously, and if the true nature of their condition passes unrecognized they may come unjustly to be regarded as academic failures rather than as having a temporary handicap for which due allowance should be made.

Mental complications of medical treatment

Apart from postoperative mental reactions, considered below, certain drugs used in general medical treatment may produce adverse psychiatric reactions. *Sulphonamides* may give rise to depressive states, though this may result in part from the effects of the condition for which they are prescribed. As sulphonamides have now been largely superseded by other antibiotics this is a matter of diminishing importance. *Steroids*, particularly if administered in large doses, may promote severe mental reactions of almost any kind (see Cushing's syndrome, p. 260). More important are the depressive reactions which may occur during treatment with certain antihypertensive drugs, notably *reserpine* and *methyldopa*, and, more rarely, *guanethidine*. The first two are not recommended for use in patients with a history of depression. These reactions present difficulty, for antidepressant drugs, particularly of the tricyclic variety, appear to block the action of antihypertensive drugs although given alone or perhaps together with a diuretic will themselves bring about some fall in blood pressure. In any event and owing to the risk of suicide, it is probably preferable to defer antihypertensive therapy for the time being until any depressive reaction which occurs has been brought under control.

Appetite suppressants such as *fenfluramine* or *diethylpropion*, although less likely than *amphetamine* to cause psychiatric problems, may in some cases produce transient states of confusion and excitement.

Some other drugs which have recently been reported to have caused mental side-effects are *bromocriptine* which may cause visual hallucinations, *propranolol* and some other beta-blockers which may give rise to visual illusions and hallucinations in the hypnagogic state, and *cimetidine* which, in elderly patients having some degree of liver or kidney failure, is prone to give rise to confusional states, disorientation, visual hallucinations etc. This drug is also reported as causing impotence in males.

Gynaecological disorders

Pelvic symptoms in women and low back pain often point to marital difficulties in which incompatibility may be mainly physical and sexual or may involve wider aspects such as mutual interests, care of the children and other interpersonal relationships. Menstrual discomforts are conducive to tension and irritability and may aggravate pre-existing emotional and psychotic symptoms. In older women fibroids may form a basis for *delusions of pregnancy* although much more than this must be evoked by way of explanation. *Amenorrhoea* may occur in the acute stages of a psychosis. The great majority of cases of *dysmenorrhoea* seen in gynaecological practice are psychogenic. Some cases of *leucorrhoea* come into the same category.

The menopause

Although the menopause is still often blamed as a cause of psychiatric problems, the evidence for this is really very slender. Most women in fact pass through this stage in life without the slightest difficulty. In some, while the end of childbearing may be regarded as something of a disappointment, in others it may be one of relief leading to the disappearance of fear of pregnancy and even to an increase in libido. However, it has also to be remembered that the menopause occurs at that time of life when emotional adjustments have to be made, for example to children growing up and leaving home which to some women may be a stressful event. Also the incidence of depression etc., due to quite other causes, tends to rise sharply during the menopausal decade.

Premenstrual tension syndrome

Various psychic disturbances, commonly depression and irritability, not infrequently, but by no means invariably, associated with physical symptoms—headache, swelling of the breasts, feet and abdomen—may occur during the week preceding the onset of menstruation. Although minor degrees are so common that they must be considered normal, within recent years the more severe instances of this disturbance have been elevated into a clinical entity. It has been suggested *inter alia* that a cyclical change in sodium and hence in water metabolism occurs which may be exaggerated and that this change is determined by the level of oestradiol in the tissues, which is regulated in turn by progesterone. This has not yet been confirmed. In unstable women abnormal psychic responses vary from mild emotional upsets to overt psychoses. Similarly, difficult behaviour in adolescent schoolgirls and crimes of violence in women have sometimes been noted to occur immediately prior to menstruation. Despite this, the aetiology of the syndrome is obscure, there being no one-to-one relationship between the occurrence of mental and physical symptoms. Its frequency and importance may, therefore, have been exaggerated.

There is no rational treatment. In some patients some varieties of contraceptive pill may help. In others a minor tranquillizer may be as effective.

Childbearing

In those predisposed, childbearing may precipitate manic-depressive, schizophrenic and other mental illnesses. *Puerperal sepsis* may give rise to delirium and confusional states, although this is now a rare event. About 7 per cent of psychoses in women are said to be associated with pregnancy and the puerperium, but the figures vary widely. Although marital incompatibility, unsuitable housing and other difficult domestic circumstances, exhaustion from too frequent pregnancies, illegitimacy and desertion are stresses which may aggravate emotional instability, there are many women who, nevertheless, state that they never feel better than when with child.

Pregnancy

Capricious behaviour and prolonged *sickness* are not uncommon during pregnancy. *Cravings* are also of frequent occurrence and sometimes *pica* (a craving for inedible substances) occurs. Equally frequent are *aversions* to foods previously liked. Although commonly thought to be so, cravings and aversions are by no means wholly of psychological origin but appear to be caused by changes in the sense of taste and smell which is dulled in pregnancy. *Sleeplessness* and general restlessness may occur either as prodromal symptoms of more serious mental disturbance, or in association with toxaemia or other physical complications. *Depression* is the commonest morbid reaction. Hostility towards husband and whimsical, exacting behaviour in minor degrees may not be of any great significance, unless very persistent. Depressive states developing before the fourth month, if allowed to run a natural course, tend to clear up before full term, while those of later onset persist until after the puerperium. Electroconvulsive therapy may be given without harm to the fetus and may be much less risky than antidepressive drugs or lithium carbonate. Termination may be desirable with clear evidence of aggravation of a psychosis, notably schizophrenia, existing before pregnancy, especially if this fails to respond to treatment. The question of liability to recurrence of a psychosis during pregnancy must be decided from the history with special reference to the likely factors in previous attacks. In general it may be said that termination is practically never indicated on account of a 'true' depressive illness, indeed most abortions are currently carried out on social rather than on purely psychiatric grounds. Furthermore, a psychosis associated with one pregnancy does not indicate that it will recur in another.

The puerperium

Other than puerperal sepsis there is no evidence that eclampsia, obstetric complications or psychosocial factors play any part in the genesis of mental disorders occurring during the puerperium. These, as in other cases, depend upon the patient's premorbid personality, her psychic constitution and her genetic background.

Acute delirium of brief duration may occur during parturition with subsequent amnesia for the event. Mild transient depression and tearfulness—*maternity blues*—are common events during the three or four days immediately following parturition. The prognosis is benign. In other cases there is increasing restlessness with insomnia until about a week or ten days after parturition, when the patient may appear to be confused, possibly losing her previous affection for her child and husband. She may refuse food, show signs of marked apprehensiveness and become hallucinated. Some become deeply depressed and suicidal; infanticide may occur. In others the reaction may be manic. Indeed, virtually any type of psychotic or other emotional disorder can be precipitated by childbirth including schizophrenic reactions which, having an acute onset, tend to resolve fairly rapidly with treatment. Among other symptoms such schizophrenic reactions often contain a confusional element giving rise to a vague bewildered dream-like appearance in which consciousness is clouded—*oneirophrenia*.

Treatment
While it was once the rule, owing to the risk of infanticide, to remove the child and stop lactation, the present fashion and almost certainly more proper form of treatment is to admit both mother and child to hospital and to encourage mothering to continue under supervision. It is now largely believed that depriving a mother of her child at this critical time may lead to feelings of guilt and a further exacerbation of her condition. Apart from this the treatment of so-called puerperal psychoses is similar to that of psychoses unrelated to childbirth.

Postoperative mental disorders

While all major surgical operations may occasionally give rise to mental disturbances these, as in the case of postpartum mental disturbances, appear to be bound up more closely with the personality of the sufferer than with the operative procedure itself. However, on some occasions surgical and anaesthetic complications play a part. In *cardiac surgery* and prolonged 'by-pass' operations, occasional disasters from anoxia, hypotension, air and other embolic phenomena can give rise to brain damage.

Other adverse reactions which result more obviously from psychological factors are more liable to occur with certain types of operations, such as *hysterectomy* in women of childbearing age, amputations and operations for malignancy, such as breast carcinoma. Cardiac operations may be followed by persistent complaints of pain in the chest scar, particularly when the patient has had no prior warning of this possibility.

Marked emotional difficulties may also occur among those undergoing continuing *haemodialysis* on account of chronic renal failure but in whom successful renal transplantation has not yet been carried out. The nature of the procedure is such that it may demand all the emotional resources both of the subject undergoing dialysis and of his relatives. Emotional stability may therefore be numbered among the indications for deciding to start chronic haemodialysis.

Psychogenic pain

Pain of uncertain and possibly of psychogenic origin is among the most difficult of symptoms to evaluate, whether it appears to have no physical basis, or when some possibly relevant physical lesion is evident. Where pain appears to be present in excess of, or to be of a different quality from that which a relevant physical lesion could reasonably be expected to produce, recognizing, of course, that a degree of subjective judgement inevitably enters into the assessment, this difficulty may be greatly increased.

The notion that pain may be of purely mental origin presents some very real conceptual difficulties, despite statements to the effect that because pain is essentially a psychical state there is no reason why its origin should not be psychogenic! This perhaps smacks of Cartesian body–mind dualism, which in its persistence, still seems to be responsible for perpetuating the *organic-as-against functional controversy* which still so strongly blinkers medical thinking; the more so among those primarily concerned with physical illness than among psychiatrists, and giving rise to certain rather quaint old-fashioned notions such as, for example, the deduction that if a patient's symptoms are relieved even temporarily by an injection of distilled water these must necessarily be *functional* in origin. It is the persistence of such dualism which by seeming to ascribe material qualities to mind, almost certainly accounts for much of the difficulty which is encountered when attempts are made to determine the nature of psychogenic pain and to differentiate it from that having a fairly obvious physical basis. Indeed, the concept of psychogenic pain *per se* can be called into question on the basis that all forms of pain are in the last resort a mental experience.

The notion that pain can be imaginary seems, therefore, to be a contradiction in terms for all pain is subjective whatever its origin. Likewise the concept of so-called *hysterical pain* may be called into question. Hallucinatory or illusory pains do not quite fit the bill; if their roots can be traced, they can usually be discovered to have a physical basis. Another possibility is delusional misinterpretation of *normally* occurring bodily discomforts. This may also account for some pain complaints, in that those who are deeply depressed may be led to interpret their bodily sensations in pain terms. Possibly of much greater importance, however, is the idea that certain emotions such as aggressive feelings turned inwards; guilt, shame, remorse and a feeling of need to be punished, may be experienced as 'painful', but in symbolic terms rather than as actual physical sensations. Here there is clearly an equation between pain and suffering which, although commonly associated, are not identical. Nevertheless it may be noted how suffering of almost any kind tends to be communicated in *pain language*. This language draws upon a very extensive glossary of metaphors which clearly express emotions in terms of painful remembered experiences, for example 'hurt feelings', 'a crushing blow to self-esteem', 'the slings and arrows of outrageous fortune', and so on.

Given what has been said, it may be postulated that most so-called psychogenic pain—equated here with *mental pain* or *suffering*—may be differentiated from pain of physical origin largely on the following grounds.

1. It is more diffuse and tends to be poorly localized.

2. It tends to be more persistent and less responsive to analgesics and a variety of familiar measures which usually bring at least some degree of relief to those with physically induced pain other than an initial transient response due probably to a placebo effect.

3. The condition is much more obviously bound up with the emotional state of the sufferer and with difficulties in his or her life situation.

4. Those who suffer from pain thought to be of psychogenic origin usually find great difficulty in giving a satisfactory account of its nature or quality, in every-day more-or-less familiar terms. Failing this they tend to confine their descriptions to its severity or extent, that is, emphasizing how much they suffer rather than being able to say more exactly what it is they actually suffer from, and what their pain is like.

The matter is made much more difficult when both mental suffering and pain of physical origin, particularly that due to some chronic cause, are simultaneously present for, under these circumstances, they soon tend to become inextricably mixed. The same may occur when those whose mental suffering is expressed in physical terms are mistakenly subjected to unnecessary surgical operations, thereby rendering the prognosis immeasurably worse.

Headache

Headache is considered separately because it is probably one of the most common symptoms of psychogenic origin. However, it must be distinguished from other forms of headache, some of which may sometimes have serious underlying causes such as a cerebral tumour. A more difficult differential diagnosis can be that of *migraine* especially where this is atypical and not accompanied by characteristic visual disturbances. The matter may be made more difficult in that it can often be seen that underlying stress factors clearly contribute to many cases of migraine, governing its frequency and the sufferer's response to it, if not its cause. There would also appear to be a significantly frequent occurrence of migraine among those who are somewhat obsessional and overconscientious.

Psychogenic headaches take several different forms. They may be bitemporal and described as 'throbbing' or bilaterally located above the eyebrows. Sometimes they are occipitofrontal in which case they may be the outcome of emotional tension affecting the muscles of the neck and scalp. Another variety is the sensation of a 'cap' on the top of the head, usually described as 'pressure'. Hysterics will sometimes talk of a 'tight band' around the head as if the skull were being squeezed or occasionally, more dramatically, of a knife being plunged into the head. These various forms of headache are often ascribed, *faute de mieux*, to eye-strain, sinusitis and so on, often leading the sufferers to undergo a variety of investigations which, needless to say, bring no real relief.

While the variations are fairly extensive the theme is reasonably constant; the headaches respond poorly and inconsistently to everyday analgesics and indeed on close analysis and, although initially described as painful, can often be discovered as not consisting of actual pain at all, but of sensations of pressure, woolliness and so on. They are furthermore closely bound up with obvious emotional difficulties and problems in living. It is interesting to note, furthermore, how quickly a patient with a psychogenic headache ceases to complain of this as soon as his real problems are brought into the open. Psychogenic headache can often, therefore, be seen as a 'ticket of admission' to the doctor's surgery or the psychiatrist's consulting room (see Chapter 3).

Finally and as usual, *depression* enters into the differential diagnosis of otherwise unexplained headaches and will always need to be excluded.

Attempted suicide (*parasuicide*)

Every general hospital of any size admits annually to its casualty department several hundred patients who have attempted suicide. This subject is, therefore, appropriate to this chapter. Most of these are cases of self-poisoning with hypnotics or with a variety of analgesic, psychotropic, antidepressive or anticonvulsant drugs. Following resuscitation there remains outstanding the problem of assessment of the seriousness of the incident and subsequent disposal of the patient.

Although suicide has been extensively investigated there are many aspects of the problem which are still obscure. It is clear, however, that successful and unsuccessful suicides are phenomena which differ in certain essential respects although the boundary between them is blurred. To give but one example, the peak age of unsuccessful attempts is between 15 and 25 years whereas the incidence of successful suicide rises steadily with advancing age.

In assessing the seriousness of a suicidal attempt or an act of self-poisoning, the following points should be borne in mind.

1. About 5 per cent of those who attempt suicide later successfully commit suicide within three to four years. The longer-term prognosis is unknown. About one-quarter of those who commit suicide have made one or two previously unsuccessful attempts.

2. The method employed is not wholly a safe guide as to the seriousness of the attempt. This particularly applies to drug overdose. An exception can be made in the case of those who experiment with violent methods of self-destruction, such as shooting, hanging, leaping

from a height and so on, which in the majority of instances are successful at the first attempt.

3. The admitted intention of the patient following resuscitation may not indicate the seriousness of the attempt. The commonly made statement that an overdose was taken 'to get a good night's sleep' is often no more than dissimulation. Many of those who attempt suicide profess to be unclear as to their motives at the time.

4. If a clearly definable physical or mental illness such as depression, schizophrenia, epilepsy or alcoholism, is found to be present, and in the absence of a clear precipitating event, the attempt should be regarded as likely to be serious. It should be remembered that where depression is present this may often be temporarily alleviated following a suicidal attempt. Adequate assessment calls therefore for a sufficient period of observation.

5. In the absence of clearly definable physical or mental illness, an attempt at suicide and particularly an act of self-poisoning can often be regarded as a *cry for help* in the face of an intolerable marital or social situation. In these cases an immediate precipitating event, such as a family quarrel, can usually be discovered. Such cases also need to be distinguished from mere histrionic *acting out* by attention-seeking personalities.

6. *Short-circuit* attempts at suicide are often made by those with explosive tendencies. Alcoholic overindulgence immediately prior to the event is frequently a factor. The likelihood of recurrence in these cases is quite high.

These are no more than pointers. It is on the whole unsafe to generalize and each case must be judged on its merits. Investigation should certainly include an interview with relatives or reliable informants. The services of a social worker are often essential.

While until quite recently it was recommended that every case should be referred for psychiatric assessment, this, owing to the sheer weight of numbers, has proved impracticable. In any event, it has now been shown that in most cases assessment can be adequately carried out by other medical staff, even by nurses, and that it is probably only necessary to refer those showing signs and symptoms of overt mental disorder.

Further reading

Farmer, R. D. T. & Hirsch, S. R. (1980) *The Suicide Syndrome*. London: Croom Helm.

Howells, J. G. (ed.) (1972) *Modern Perspectives in Psycho-Obstetrics*. Edinburgh: Oliver & Boyd.

Munro, A. (1973) *Psychosomatic Medicine*. Edinburgh: Churchill Livingstone.

19

The Psychiatry of Old Age

Increasing longevity since the turn of the century and accelerating even more rapidly during recent years has led to the medical, psychiatric and social problems of those growing older becoming ever more apparent. It has been calculated that the size of these problems will continue to grow until the end of the present century so that by the year AD 2000 it is likely that there will be a further increase in the elderly population of England and Wales of approximately quarter-of-a-million persons aged 75–84 years and a similar growth in the number of those aged 85 years and over. These increases will clearly present considerable difficulties for the medical, psychiatric and social services which are already stretched to their limits. Apart from this, the growing number of mentally infirm old people has led to the foundation of a new psychiatric subspecialty, *psychogeriatrics*, a not altogether happy term which suggests that the problems of *geriatric medicine* which some see as being of an essentially *physical* nature are something separate from those which may be regarded as *mental*, when this is so often clearly not the case.

However, in respect, specifically, of the problems of mental ill-health in the aged, virtually all the disorders so far considered in this book are to be encountered in old people, although not necessarily at the same prevalence rates as they occur in those who are younger. While, for example, the incidence of schizophrenia occurring for the first time lessens considerably in older persons—75 per cent of cases at the beginning of a schizophrenic illness are aged between 15 and 30 years—the condition is not unknown at any age. Thus paranoid forms in particular certainly do occur for the first time among those of advancing years. Affective disorders, notably depressive illnesses of various kinds, are much more frequent and are indeed the most commonly occurring form of mental illness among those aged between 60 and 70 years of age. Between 70 and 75 years the numbers of those with affective illnesses and with dementia are about equal, but after the age of 75 the prevalence of dementia rises sharply so that by the time 80 years is attained, about one in five is affected, at least half of them severely. Likewise, manic, neurotic and personality problems are not unknown among those growing old, although in many, if not most, instances these disorders can be viewed as recurrences or late exacerbations which, having run a remitting or relapsing course in earlier life, may manifest themselves once again in a rather more chronic and persistent form than previously. This is commonly thought to be due to organic brain changes supervening which may render further remission less likely.

Aetiology

While the causes of mental disorder in old age may be most conveniently grouped under separate headings—physical, psychological and social— it is the combination and interaction of factors falling under each heading which deserve the closest consideration. Indeed, it has already been suggested that any attempt to deal with them separately should be considered as artificial.

Physical
While all the various physical conditions associated with advancing age—hypertension, heart disease, malignancy, diabetes, etc.—may have psychological and social repercussions for those who suffer from them, some, especially, may lead to increasing isolation and a feeling of impending dissolution. Deafness and failing eyesight may give rise to growing isolation from others; likewise, locomotor disorders consequent upon strokes, arthritis, cardiac failure and respiratory disease may impede an old person's ability to get about and to maintain once well-established contacts.

Psychosocial
Apart from fairly well-defined psychiatric disorders which may be genetically, biochemically or metabolically determined and which may have the same aetiological background in the old as in any other age group, certain factors deserve special consideration as many of these undoubtedly contribute to chronic physical and mental invalidism. They include *retirement* which after a long and active work-life and which in those lacking resourcefulness, hobbies and outside interests can lead to a sense of futility and lack of purpose; likewise, *redundancy*, especially when this is sudden, unexpected and unwanted. Work does not only pass the time or afford the worker the opportunity to earn a living wage, but also serves the purpose of bringing him into daily contact with his fellow workers. In this respect it is a socializing force which may diminish when retirement or redundancy comes.

Another consequence of retirement may be *loss of income* leading to reduction in living standards. Even if retirement is pensionable, the available pension may be eroded by continuing inflation. Where adequate financial provision for old age has not been met so that actual *poverty* occurs, this may result in a further reduction of living standards so that the elderly person, being unable to afford fares etc., loses contact with family and friends. In severer cases, *nutrition* may suffer while, in winter, *hypothermia* tends to occur owing to inability to pay fuel bills, substandard accommodation or from sheer inability to understand how to operate heating apparatus economically or even how to work it at all.

Increasing *social isolation* due to other causes is clearly important. This may follow *widowhood*, perhaps exacerbated by the moving away from the district of sons and daughters and their families or their emigration overseas; *bereavement* following the deaths of other old friends and relatives, and so on. Lack of environmental stimulation which stems largely from the influence of others may well hasten oncoming senility: for the brain (and *ipso facto* the mind) is, like other bodily organs, subject to disuse atrophy. One well-known 'syndrome' is when an elderly couple from, say, the industrial Midlands where their family and friends live, choose to retire to some south-coast resort hoping to enjoy life in a more temperate climate, but in a place where they know nobody well, if at all. Soon after having done so, one or other of them dies leaving the survivor alone and with insufficient social resources, and dementia soon supervenes.

According to current statistics, one-third of those aged 65 years and over live alone; 45 per cent of these are women; 17 per cent men. Seven of 10 live in households with no one else under that age. One in 3 elderly persons cannot do a household job if climbing steps is required; 1 in 10 cannot leave home and walk down the road alone; while 1 in 7 increasing to 1 in 5 of those over 75 years are unable to do their own shopping. On a more positive note, however, the overwhelming majority (6 out of 7) see friends or relatives at least once a week, one-third of them nearly every day (General Household Survey 1980).

Although, while even in the so-called Welfare State the position of many elderly persons must be considered as far from satisfactory, it seems, nonetheless, that a large proportion do get by and are for the most part fairly content. Nevertheless, it should be remembered that old people are often slow to ask for help, even when they need it. Being proud, they tend to accept matters uncomplainingly. But for those who do not, the necessary provision for their care and comfort seems to be continuously falling behind what is required.

The mental disorders of old age

These will be considered in what seems to be the order of their descending importance, although of course such ranking could be a ready subject for debate.

Affective disorders

Depression or *depressive illness*, in the earlier old-age groups (65–75 years), is the most commonly encountered psychiatric disorder, particularly *agitated depression* which may be very severe, although it differs little from *involutional melancholia* which may make its appearance in those somewhat younger. Apart from agitation with accompanying and sometimes severe *restlessness, hypochondriacal ideas* or *delusions* are extremely common. The suicidal risk in these patients is high and should always be borne in mind. However, the results of treatment, especially by ECT, are good, often dramatically so and in patients however old, providing, of course, that there are no signs of marked organic brain changes. If these are present, the longer term results of treatment may be found to be less favourable, there being a decided tendency to relapse and some degree of chronicity to supervene.

The importance of organic brain disorder (e.g. cerebral arteriosclerosis) in giving rise to depression in old age is still a matter of dispute. While it was at one time customary to talk of '*organic depression*', considerable doubt has now been thrown upon this concept as constituting an entity. Also while there is no doubt that depression and dementia may coexist, this, in this age group, does not necessarily indicate a causal relationship and may be no more than coincidence.

Nevertheless, depression, particularly retarded depression, in which there is a considerable degree of inhibition of mental functioning resulting in impairment of memory, concentration and of other intellectual faculties, can give rise to a state easily mistaken for dementia. This condition, which is also often characterized by the giving of approximate answers (see the Ganser syndrome), may resolve completely when the underlying depression is successfully treated or remits spontaneously, whereupon it may be seen to have been not *true* but *pseudodementia*.

As in other age groups, *reactive factors* are of great importance in the depressive illnesses of old age, especially those in which the theme of loss looms large.

Mania. This, which in elderly patients is much less common than depression, also tends to be more atypical than in those younger. Common symptoms include irritability, surliness, paranoid ideas and delusions, together with seemingly organic features. An admixture of depressive ideation is also common.

Dementia

Dementia in old age does not differ in any essential respect from that which affects those who are younger. While most of the various causes listed in Chapter 9 may be operative in old age, the most important appear to be *Alzheimer's disease (senile dementia of Alzheimer type—SDAT)* and *cerebral arteriosclerosis (multiple-stroke syndrome)*. Mixtures of the two are common.

Physical signs

General health is usually impaired, there is loss of weight, atrophic, wrinkled inelastic skin, loss and depigmentation of hair. Movements become weak, clumsy and poorly coordinated. Tremor may be present or displayed by spidery writing. Coarse oscillations of the head, parkinsonism and oral (*tardive*) dyskinesia may be evident. Failing eyesight, increasing deafness and cardiorespiratory embarrassment are all stepping stones on the road to 'sans everything'.

Appetite tends to be capricious, greatly reduced or, alternatively, ravenous. Obstinate constipation ('*obstipation*') and frequency of micturition are often present, together, in men, with difficulties due to prostatic enlargement. In more advanced cases, incontinence of urine or faeces may occur, this from the viewpoint of relatives being the 'last straw' and the factor which most often helps them reduce such guilt feelings as they may experience over the need to seek institutional care for an ageing relative.

Mental symptoms

Memory failure with inability to recall proper names is often the first symptom. This shortly extends to include an ever-growing number of other matters, once more or less readily recalled but now no longer. Lack of adaptability and difficulty in coping with new ideas are soon apparent. Loss of interest in present-day happenings leads to a retreat into the past so that the scenes of childhood are often recalled as if they were yesterday's events. Dotage and 'anecdotage' soon become fused into one. Poverty of ideation, together with *perseveration*, lead to the repetition of platitudes. Inability to empathize with others together with reluctance to recognize his own deficiencies may lead the elderly person to become suspicious, peevish and exacting, while at the same time attempting to exert his authority and pleading for help in his weakness. He may be restless, overactive and interfering or, alternatively, apathetic and somnolent. While the clinical presentation varies, a lack of self-control may result in a sexual offence or a charge of shoplifting. It is important to remember that such an untoward event, seemingly quite out of character, may sometimes be the first sign of organic deterioration, even before overt evidence of intellectual deficit is apparent.

Paranoid and persecutory states

These may be of several different kinds. Some paranoid states which tend to be transient and are associated with chronic brain syndromes may be derived from failing memory. Thus old people who forget where they have hidden their belongings may, being later unable to find them, believe that they have been stolen. Strange hallucinations may contribute; thus an elderly arteriosclerotic widower insisted that 14 persons came into his sitting room and although taking no notice of him, talked among themselves. Another who suffered from *Lilliputian hallucinations* complained that little men in uniform ran over his counterpane and invaded his bed-locker, interfering with his possessions.

Another group showing no evidence of cerebral arteriosclerosis or other organic symptoms may be regarded not only as having paranoid delusions, but other features characteristic of this illness. Thus they may hear voices which comment on their actions and discuss them in the third person. As affective dilapidation appears to be uncommon and thought disorder rare or episodic, it may be appropriate to categorize such patients as suffering from *paraphrenia of late onset*.

Other types of paranoid illnesses may have their roots in a variety of factors. Some subjects are depressed and may recover with treatment. Others include those with sensory defects such as *deafness* and *blindness*. While deafness has been shown to be significantly more common among elderly paranoid persons, this should not be unduly emphasized as there are many deaf old persons who are not paranoid so that if they are, probably more than deafness alone must be invoked. Likewise, blind or partially sighted subjects who suffer from visual hallucinations often recognize the 'imaginary' nature of their experiences and have full insight into their experiences. More serious and intractable perhaps are those who are fundamentally of paranoid personality and who, as they grow older, become increasingly withdrawn, suspicious and cantankerous. Their self-imposed isolation lends further impetus to an already potentially deteriorating situation from which there is ever less likelihood of return.

Neurosis and personality disorders

Neurosis and personality disorders are, on the whole, of less importance in elderly patients than those conditions already discussed. There is indeed a tendency for certain conditions—notably psychopathic personality disorders—to ameliorate with advancing age. The same may be true of those who suffer from obsessive–compulsive disorders which appear to lose 'force' with the passage of time. Nonetheless, anxiety present in those who are younger may increase once more with advancing age. However, the first diagnostic thought when confronted with an anxiety state in those growing old should be concerned with the possibility of a depressive illness of which anxiety is an integral part.

By and large, *senile personality disorders* may almost always be construed as distortions of character traits of lifelong existence and an outcome of inability to 'grow old gracefully'. It is a tragedy that many on growing older do not become better but worse. Senile organic changes do, however, sometimes go some way to disguise this.

Treatment

Quite obviously, all physical defects and deficiencies that can be discovered must be dealt with so far as possible, including such matters as overcoming dietary deficiencies, correcting anaemia, hypothyroidism and other metabolic defects; ameliorating locomotor difficulties by physiotherapy and other appropriate measures.

Apart from attention to general physical health, the treatment of psychiatric illness in old age differs little from that appropriate to those who are younger. In the case of those who are depressed, old age is actually no contraindication to ECT if this is indicated. Antidepressive treatment by drugs should, however, perhaps be approached with greater caution. As a general rule—and this applies not only to antidepressive but to other neuroleptic and tranquillizing drugs— considerably smaller doses should be prescribed for elderly as against younger patients. It should not be forgotten that both neuroleptics and antidepressives can cause both hypotension and hypothermia and that the effect of them on an old person living alone may sometimes have disastrous consequences. Likewise, the effect of barbiturates and benzodiazepines can all too easily add to the confusion to which those who are elderly are prone.

Services for the Aged

As already stated, services for the aged have not kept up with a continuously expanding need. Thus, even in 1975 a Government paper, *Better Services for the Mentally Ill* (Cmnd 6233), noted that critics saw a deficiency in the number of homes, hostels and day centres for the mentally ill (of all ages) as constituting a serious barrier to achieving transfer from hospital to community care, while in 1982 Grundy and Arie observed that the rapid increase in the number of very aged people had not been accompanied by appropriate expansion of local authority facilities.

Although day centres and hostel accommodation are available for old persons, even for some who are mentally disturbed, it would appear that at the present time about six times as many are managed at home as in community care or in mental hospitals where they form a considerable proportion of the 'long-stay' population. In many mental hospitals, about 55 per cent of females and 45–50 per cent of males are aged 65 years and over, although not all are admitted on achieving geriatric status, but have grown old since being admitted to hospital a number of years before.

While caring for elderly mentally ill persons at home seems to be a feature of the British social scene, as compared with parts of

Scandinavia, for example, where community facilities are better developed, home-caring for disturbed old persons is not without its hazards, and in many cases places a considerable strain on the family. In the case of those who are demented, the problem may not be too dissimilar to that of caring for the mentally handicapped child at home; especially as exposure to ordinary domestic hazards places them at considerable risk. This is particularly true of those who live alone, even though fairly frequently visited. Apart from kettles, saucepans of boiling water, and heating apparatus, old people when confused and unsupervised may wander off and be unable to find their way back home. Where this is likely, the lot of those who try to care for them may be considerably relieved by the use of a day centre to which an old person can be taken and there cared for during the day; an even more valuable facility when the carer—a son, daughter or daughter-in-law perhaps—needs to go out each day to work.

It is not merely pejorative but realistic to state that many old people, failing in their faculties, are difficult, demanding and a disturbing influence in a household, especially where there are also young children living, whose boisterousness they may find difficult to tolerate and with whom they may compete for attention. Helping an aged person on the seemingly inevitable journey towards 'sans everything' is no easy task, accompanied as it so often is by a growing feeling of desire for the end of the matter, and conflicting feelings of guilt at the prospect of having to agree that the time has come for him or her to be admitted to a 'mental home', as the local psychiatric hospital is so often euphemistically called. Tragically enough, it is continuing incontinence which often resolves this dilemma; this being a matter with which ordinary domestic resources usually cannot cope.

However, the following principles have recently been enumerated (Rodgers & Muir Gray 1982).

1. No old person should have to live in an institution until comprehensive medical and social assessment has shown that nothing further can be done to reduce the degree of disability and that he or she cannot manage even when the full range of social, health and voluntary domiciliary services are available.

2. If institutional care becomes inevitable, this should be provided as close as possible to a neighbourhood where the old person has friends or relatives.

3. Old people with mental impairment should not be segregated in separate institutions. However, privacy, where desired, and the retention of at least some personal belongings should be assured.

Further reading

General Household Survey (1980) An Interdepartmental Survey, Series GHS 10. London: Central Statistical Office.

Grundy, E. & Arie, T. (1982) Falling rate of provision of residential care for the elderly. *British Medical Journal* 284:799–802.

Pitt, B. M. M. (1974) *Psychogeriatrics: Introduction to the Psychiatry of Old Age.* Edinburgh: Churchill Livingstone.

Post, F. (1965) *The Clinical Psychiatry of Later Life.* Oxford: Pergamon.

Post, F. (1966) *Persistent Persecutory States of the Elderly.* Oxford: Pergamon.

Rodgers, J. S. & Muir Gray, J. A. (1982) Long-stay care for elderly people: its continuing evolution. *British Medical Journal* 285:707–709.

20

Child and Adolescent Psychiatry

Revised by Ian Berg

Classification

Psychiatric syndromes in young people are poorly defined. The two commonest are *emotional* and *conduct disorders*. Emotional disorders include problems such as fearfulness, phobias, tension, misery, obsessional and hysterical symptoms including physical complaints without obvious cause, somewhat similar to neurosis in adult life. Conduct disturbances comprise antisocial behaviour; stealing, lying, truanting, destructiveness and excessive fighting. *Childhood psychoses* are rare; the main one being the *autistic syndrome*. The *hyperkinetic syndrome*, characterized by persistently severe overactivity and distractability in a wide variety of situations, is also uncommon. Other symptoms of disturbed behaviour, such as habits of various sorts and certain interpersonal problems, are not always easy to classify.

There has recently been a tendency to classify psychiatric disorders in childhood by using several different dimensions simultaneously. Thus WHO has promoted a multiaxial classification, the *first* axis specifying just one clinical syndrome of disturbance. However, when symptoms complained of are not severe enough to be regarded as abnormal, a category of *normal variation* is used. If the problem extends beyond this, but does not amount to definite disorder, the child's condition may be classified as an *adaptation reaction*. The *second* axis includes a number of *developmental disorders*, having in common the failure of some function to develop normally. These comprise speech retardation, delayed reading and excessive clumsiness, together with urinary and faecal incontinence (*enuresis* and *encopresis*). The *third* axis specifies intellectual functioning, which falls into five ranges: *normal* (IQ 70 or higher), *mild retardation* (IQ 50 to 69), *moderate retardation* (IQ 35 to 49), *severe retardation* (IQ 20 to 34), and *profound retardation* (IQ less than 20). The *fourth* axis denotes physical illnesses and handicaps; while the *fifth* axis indicates social factors of possible significance. As an example of multiaxial classification, a disturbed child might be classified as having an emotional disorder (Axis 1); delayed onset of speech (Axis 2); mild intellectual retardation (Axis 3); epilepsy (Axis 4); and as coming from a severely discordant family (Axis 5).

Prevalence

While behaviour problems are common in childhood, definite psychiatric disorders affect about 5 to 15 per cent of children, boys being more likely than girls to exhibit conduct and developmental disturbances. Adverse social factors and childhood disorders appear to be related; thus lack of a normal home environment and a disturbed parent tend to be associated with behavioural difficulties. Also those who are intellectually backward or physically handicapped are prone to childhood psychiatric disorders.

Child development
Judgements as to whether particular aspects of behaviour are abnormal or not are more accurate when made by those having detailed knowledge of normal child development. What is normal at one stage of development may be grossly abnormal at another. Thus sound knowledge of physical, intellectual, emotional and social aspects of development is needed to assess abnormal behaviour.

Aetiology

Upsetting Events
A wide variety of events which may affect children severely may lead to persistent psychiatric disorder, such as phobias following some alarming experience, a fear of hospital after medical treatment, dog phobia following a bite, or a terror of cars after a motor accident; hence the truism: 'A burnt child fears the fire'.

Other circumstances which may affect children are *separation experiences*. These involve separation from someone with a close emotional attachment, usually mother; sometimes for only a short time, such as when a child is admitted to hospital. Longer or even permanent separation may follow the death of a parent or break-up of a family. Separation due to hospital admission may be ameliorated by frequent visiting, counselling anxious parents, engaging the child in play, and explaining what is happening. Nevertheless, separation from home and mother of a preschool child for a few days can still have untoward effects, if only in the short term.

Severely upsetting events such as accidents, burns, parental death, family disruption and repeated admissions to hospital are happily not everyday occurrences and not many children become psychiatrically disturbed because of them. However, more commonplace events such as the birth of a sibling or changing school can sometimes lead to problems.

Persisting environmental influences

Isolated events are probably less influential than are the circumstances under which a child lives most of the time. Children not only require reasonable freedom from damaging experiences, such as prolonged exposure to violence between parents, but also a settled existence with affection, interest, protection and, above all, consistency; all of which are part of good parenting. Beneficial experiences at school and with other children are also important. It is hardly surprising that neglect, disruption of family life and periods *in care* lead to psychiatric problems. Social disadvantages such as an unsatisfactory school or living in a deprived neighbourhood are also associated with disturbance in childhood. Separation, divorce, a one-parent family, a step-parent, fostering, adoption or child care, or indeed any anomaly affecting upbringing, carry an added risk.

Subtler factors in parent–child relationships are more difficult to evaluate. Even in seemingly stable homes, interpersonal difficulties may cause problems which are difficult to resolve. Children may not conform to reasonable standards of behaviour at home or at school. Thus stubbornness and wilfulness are often displayed by preschool children and problems involving eating, dressing, toileting, going to bed and difficult behaviour in public are common. In early adolescence, conflict over friends, staying out late, dress and schoolwork may cause difficulty. At all ages, excessive fighting with siblings may create family conflict. Parents may be overprotective, overanxious, vacillating and submissive; or punitive, neglectful or inconsistent. However, it is not yet clear how important these kinds of interpersonal problems are, or indeed to what extent they actually promote disturbances. Nevertheless, attempts to modify the attitudes and behaviour of parents and children who are demonstrably not getting on with each other are often undertaken in the seemingly reasonable belief that increased understanding and sympathy will reduce the effects of problem behaviour, if not the disorder itself.

Constitutional factors

Some of the features of childhood psychiatric disorders may well be due to inherited predisposition or physical factors. Boys in all cultures are more assertive and aggressive than girls. This probably explains their greater tendency towards conduct disorders. More speculatively, the differences between the sexes in language and intellectual function may explain why reading delay occurs predominantly in boys.

Precisely how brain damage due to head injury, encephalitis, meningitis or that associated with epilepsy produces an increased tendency to psychiatric disorder is unknown. One possibility is that environmental changes engendered by physical problems act as a chronic form of stress. Disfigurement constitutes an analogous situation. Thus it has been shown that children of unusual appearance may be rejected by their peers.

Psychiatric disorders are more prevalent in enuretic children; likewise, conduct disturbances often occur with reading backwardness. A positive family history of both suggests that constitutional factors are of importance; although the stress of their occurrence may well give rise to associated neurotic or conduct disorder. Low intelligence, complicated by psychiatric disorder, may well operate in the same way. Temperamental characteristics vary; thus there is evidence, even in infancy, that certain features such as high intensity of emotional response, slowness to adapt to change, irregularity of habits, and negative mood may cause trouble later.

Personality is important; thus in the case of antisocial behaviour it may be difficult to separate personality traits from symptoms. Children who steal, lie, fight, or are destructive often reveal personality attributes in accord with these problems. Those emotionally disturbed are frequently nervous, timid, worriers whose personality characteristics are in keeping with this. Thus a child's character may influence his reaction to stress, so that some are prone to develop antisocial behaviour, while others lean towards emotional disorder. Paradoxically, however, some show emotional disturbance at one time and antisocial behaviour at another. But occasionally such disorders appear to arise 'out of the blue', unrelated to events and seemingly quite out of character.

History taking

History of the present complaint

It is important to allow whoever volunteers information freedom to talk about the problems which cause the child's referral and help them give a clear account of each difficulty, its onset, development, the circumstances under which it occurs and how others react to it.

Past history

This should include previous behaviour difficulties, their nature, severity, duration and treatment; together with an account of physical illnesses and operations. Where possible, information from contemporary medical records should be obtained. Details of gestation and delivery, together with an account of the first few years of life should be included. Obstetric complications occasionally explain early difficulties and retarded development. Problems during infancy may also indicate an abnormal and unresolved relationship between mother and child.

Family history

This should include information about the illnesses of other family members who may have had a significant influence upon a child's development. Their ages and occupations, together with adverse social factors engendered by criminality, alcoholism, violence, inadequacy or other disturbance should be noted. Finding out how a child relates to his parents and siblings is often helpful, as poor adjustment within the family may be an important factor in promoting psychiatric disturbance. An assessment of family attitudes—excessive manifestations of aggression, neglect, and inconsistency on the one hand, or overconcern, overprotection and clinging behaviour on the other—are often relevant both to aetiology and management.

Schooling

Each school attended should be noted. Enquiry should be made as to how the child settled, got on with his teachers and with other children, coped in class and with everyday difficulties. Failure to adjust to school is a major feature of childhood psychiatric disturbance, and frequently contributes to behavioural problems. A child's relationship to his *peer group* is also significant, both in, or irrespective of, school. Inquiry about friends, how long friendships lasted, group activities, play etc., all provide useful evidence about peer group adjustment; likewise, an assessment of the extent to which a child conforms to or deviates from the behavioural patterns of children living nearby.

Examination

While much information about emotional and behaviour problems can be obtained from parents and teachers, it is nevertheless helpful to have a child's own views and to make a direct assessment of any difficulties he may have in communicating, relating or thinking, and which he may reveal in conversation. Indeed, in talking he may be able to give as much information about his problems as adults do. Even if not, both he and his parents may feel that at least some effort has been made to involve him in the effort to help him overcome his problems.

Observation of a child's reaction to members of his family may suggest excessive reliance on or undue attachment to one or other parent, antagonism to a sibling or hostility and lack of affection between, say, mother and child. Timidity and shyness may be apparent, or assertiveness and disinhibited behaviour. Difficulties of speech, intellectual backwardness or psychotic symptoms may be evident. Tics, physical handicaps, obesity, excessive thinness or other physical problems may be apparent; or various emotional difficulties such as fearfulness, worrying, misery, hypochondriacal preoccupations, or obsessional thoughts may emerge. Alternatively, antisocial tendencies, lack of concern, resentment and aggression may predominate.

Talking to children has to be conducted with the greatest tact, so that several sessions may be necessary before the relationship between child and interviewer is such that the child is really able to share his feelings.

Further investigations

Assessment of intelligence and educational achievement by using the Wechsler Intelligence Scale for Children (WISC) and the British Ability Scales (BAS) may be helpful. Such testing is normally carried out by an educational psychologist or, if in a hospital department, by a clinical psychologist. Other tests include the Rutter *A Scale* for completion by parents, the Rutter *B Scale* and Conners' Teachers Questionnaire; and the Self-Administered Dependency Questionnaire (SADQ) which is completed by mothers. Questionnaires concerned with anxiety, depression, hyperactivity and eating behaviour are also available, while a social worker visiting the family at home may be able to provide a detailed report on social conditions. Likewise, school reports are often helpful in defining ability, achievement and maladjustment at school.

Occasionally, under special circumstances such as when non-accidental injury (NAI) is suspected, or when legal proceedings are involved, or because a disorder is very severe, complex and unusual, observation in hospital in a day or in-patient unit may be needed, the child usually spending weekends at home.

Physical investigation can be important. Thus mild cerebral palsy may explain excessive clumsiness. Evidence of self-injury suggests a history of conduct disturbance and institutionalization. Emaciation and weight below the third percentile may indicate anorexia nervosa. Absence of perineal malformation makes it likely that continual daytime wetting is a functional symptom. Distension of the abdomen by hard masses point to faecal retention causing soiling.

Formulation

Formulation should follow assessment. Here the multiaxial classification is useful as it not only covers the major syndrome of disturbance, but other associated features such as developmental and other disorders of intellectual functioning, together with physical and psychosocial factors. A list of the principal difficulties and circumstances which provide the main focus for treatment can be added. The time and effort required to make such an assessment vary from case to case. More difficult problems may require a number of sessions and perhaps a multidisciplinary case conference before satisfactory formulation is achieved.

Special problems

The preschool child

Behaviour problems affecting toddlers may cause much distress to mothers, and are commonly found in play groups and nurseries. As referral of very small children to the psychiatric services is unusual, such problems are commonly dealt with by health visitors, paediatricians and family doctors. They include sleep disturbance, tantrums, attention-seeking behaviour and feeding disorders; fears, timidity, excessive dependence and other symptoms suggesting emotional disorder.

Children are innately fearful of loud noises, being dropped, heights and painful stimuli. In the second six months of life, fear of strangers is often apparent. Toddlers often fear any strange event and run to mother, sometimes clinging to her. The use of mother as a 'secure base' relieves these fears and gives the child confidence to start exploring the environment again.

Fears of dogs, insects, dentists, hospitals, thunder, ghosts and especially of the dark or of being left alone are all very common. *Nightmares* are bad dreams which a child remembers on awakening, in contrast to *night terrors*, when the child is obviously terrified, but has no later recollection of having had a disturbed night. *Sleep-walking* is also common. All these problems are usually mild and due to temporary difficulties in the normal course of development. Occasionally they are severe or persistent enough to cause disruption to family life so that treatment is required. As fears and sleep problems appear to be emotional reactions allied to anxiety and tension, any ways of diminishing these help, such as gradual desensitization.

Aggressive behaviour, excessive fighting, destructiveness and wandering are sometimes severe enough in this age group to warrant consideration as conduct disorders. Such disturbances are more likely to occur along with developmental difficulties such as backwardness in speech or persistent wetting and soiling. Here it can be hard to see the child's behaviour independently from his mother's response, this being complicated by the fact that young mothers tend to suffer from minor psychiatric illness when there are adverse social circumstances.

Management comprises a combination of parental counselling, behavioural methods and, possibly in the case of sleep disorders, drug therapy. Attendance at a play group may help. Sleep problems can be very disruptive, with parents disturbed by crying, calling out, and insistence by the child in coming into their bed. Likewise, the child, fatigued, may be difficult to manage during the day. Here suitable medication may break a vicious circle and give the whole family some rest. Support for mother may help her to be firm about the child going to bed and to resist constant calling out and coming down. Appropriate reinforcement of acceptable behaviour can greatly reduce disruptive night-time activity. A similar approach without using any medication can be used with daytime management problems and feeding difficulties.

Enuresis

This mainly consists of bedwetting, although daytime wetting is not uncommonly associated and may occasionally be the principal or only manifestation. Most children affected have wet continuously from birth. *Enuresis* is, therefore, often classified as a developmental disorder, although it sometimes occurs after a long period of dryness. The majority of infants become dry in their second or third year and enuresis may be said to be present when wetting occurs after the fourth year. It may be associated with daytime frequency and urgency of micturition. As a group, enuretic children produce smaller volumes of urine after drinking fluid and delay emptying as long as possible. Thus their maximum functional bladder capacity is on average smaller than that of normal children.

While there is a definite association between enuresis and psychiatric disturbance, about 50 per cent of enuretic children appear to be well adjusted and free from psychiatric disturbance. Thus it is not clear how enuresis and other behavioural difficulties are connected. Enuresis which comes on following a long period (at least a year) of dryness—so-called *onset enuresis*—may start after some disturbing event in a child's life. Onset enuresis is otherwise similar to that which has continued more or less since infancy. Cases referred to clinics, especially to child psychiatric services, are more likely to be disturbed. Treatment directed towards the bedwetting which is successful often appears to improve a child's behaviour, suggesting that the wetting itself acts as a source of stress through the adverse reaction of other members of the family or possibly teasing by other children.

Enuresis is undoubtedly more prevalent in the poorer socio-economic levels of society. Likewise, psychiatric disorders are commoner under adverse social circumstances. An association between them is, therefore, likely.

Treatment

The use of a *pad* and *bell* may improve bedwetting substantially although using such apparatus to eliminate wetting requires at least a month, often three months or longer. Used properly, about two-thirds of cases will become dry. Relapse may occur but often responds to further treatment. Child and parents require regular counselling to encourage correct use and to overcome problems of failure. The procedure must be followed precisely. Daytime wetting, although much less often severe and troublesome, can be treated by a wetting sensor worn in the underclothes and connected to a small pocket box which emits a noise when wetting occurs. There is some evidence that daywetting may cause urinary tract infections in girls, perhaps because a moist perineum encourages the growth of bacteria.

Imipramine has been found to improve bedwetting whilst the child is actually taking it, but relapse tends to occur later. The dangers of accident of overdose, particularly in syrup, may render its use undesirable.

Enuresis has a high spontaneous remission rate; without any treatment, about a sixth of all cases become dry within a year. Under these circumstances and without proper evaluation, almost any method of management may be successful. Star charts indicating dry nights may often be sufficient or, if not, provide a baseline record for instituting the alarm system when improvement fails to occur. Severe persistent enuresis which fails to respond to out-patient treatment, particularly when cooperation in using the pad and bell is poor, together with associated psychiatric disturbance of some severity, may require admission of the child to a psychiatric in-patient unit.

Encopresis

Faecal incontinence occurring after the fourth birthday for which no physical cause can be found is called *encopresis*. Most children are in fact toilet trained by their second or third year. Encopresis, as a developmental disorder, is much less prevalent than enuresis; however, it is less socially acceptable so that referral for treatment is commoner. Many soilers do not appear to have any other behavioural difficulties. Others, particularly those referred to child psychiatrists, may be psychiatrically disturbed. Encopresis has frequently been present at least episodically all the child's life, but some develop it after a long period of freedom from soiling.

The three main causative factors are *constipation, unsatisfactory toilet habits*, and more *generalized disturbance of behaviour*. Many soilers are found to have a grossly distended lower bowel and are incontinent because of severe faecal retention with overflow. Constipation arises in a variety of ways: some children seem constitutionally prone, others put off going to the toilet—a habit which eventually leads to gross constipation. Infrequent hard bowel motions may also follow an intercurrent illness. Anal fissure which may lead to pain on defaecation may be caused by severe constipation initially—a vicious cycle.

Some soilers fail to develop a normal bowel habit, reaching the age of 7 or 8 years hardly ever having used a toilet appropriately for bowel motions. It is difficult to know whether the toilet is not used because the motions have already been deposited elsewhere or vice versa; for even when the toilet is used, soilers tend to do so with reluctance.

Some soil despite what appears to be a perfectly normal bowel habit and a complete absence of constipation. Soiling of this kind can occur as a reaction to severe stress, for example family disruption and admission to care. However, both failure to use the toilet and holding back from defaecation can also occur as manifestations of a severe resistive behaviour disorder, especially during the preschool period, which may then persist with or without associated behaviour problems of other sorts. These factors are frequently inextricably mixed so that it is often impossible to find out which came first or is the most important. In addition, the reaction of the family and other children is another complicating variable. Punitive attitudes on the part of parents to soiling are common. Teasing by other children causes embarrassment. The hostility of others may lead a soiler to become even more uncooperative and even to smear faeces on the walls, possibly in retaliation.

Treatment

Soiling is most commonly encountered in primary school children, although young teenagers with encopresis are by no means rare. The problem hardly ever persists into later life. Nevertheless, it is important to treat the condition vigorously to avoid the unpleasantness and stress which it causes.

Overadherence to a purely mechanical view has led to the extensive employment of invasive bowel-emptying procedures such as suppositories, enemas and bowel washouts to combat retention. Such procedures may lead to a phobia of hospitals. In fact, they are unnecessary as bowel emptying can be encouraged by increased tolerance and the use of oral laxatives, the main focus of therapy being to encourage the development of a normal bowel habit. This involves both securing the child's cooperation to use the toilet and achieving a more tolerant attitude by parents. A star chart can be used to indicate progress and provide rewards for successful performance. In-patient treatment should be considered if there is failure to improve after three months.

School refusal

Difficulty in going to school due to emotional disorder is called *school refusal* or *school phobia*. It may occur at any age, but most of those involved are young teenagers. Boys and girls are equally affected. No particular social class group predominates. Intelligence is average and educational retardation no more likely than in any other child. The condition may come on quite suddenly, sometimes following prolonged absence due to illness or a long school holiday, or gradually over several weeks. The affected child often finds Monday mornings the most difficult.

Somatic anxiety symptoms may be severe and include anorexia, nausea, vomiting, abdominal pain, frequency of micturition, diarrhoea and headaches. Other symptoms of emotional disturbance include worrying, fearfulness, misery, tension, obsessions, compulsions and hypochondriasis. There may be undue dependence on mother, and clinging in a manner more reminiscent of a toddler than a teenager, together with concern lest harm befall mother when they are separated. Some children show less evidence of fearfulness and more resistiveness, defiance and lack of cooperation when faced with going to school. They may refuse to get up and dress, may lock themselves in the bedroom or even threaten self-injury.

All symptoms are most severe just before the time to leave for school. During school holidays, symptoms improve so that the child may even appear undisturbed. However, problems usually return as the next term approaches. Most school refusers show other evidence of emotional disorder even when they eventually start attending school normally.

As a group, school phobic youngsters tend to be unduly dependent on parents, are reluctant to go far from home on their own and show evidence of emotional disorders even before the onset of the school phobia. Occasionally, physical symptoms are so prominent that the child may be regarded as having an illness such as colitis, glandular fever, migraine or even an acute abdomen. In this way, school refusal may *masquerade* as a physical problem. However, chronic physical illness may also be complicated by the occurrence of school refusal.

As attendance at school is compulsory, persistent absence without good cause may be investigated by the educational welfare service. When absence from school is one manifestation of a conduct disorder, the problem is one of *truancy* not school refusal. Parents of truants are usually unaware of their child's absence until contacted by the school authorities. There are also many children who remain at home whilst their parents are at work or are allowed to do so by parents who do not make strenuous efforts to get them to school. Girls are particularly prone and may be employed in carrying out household tasks. However, there is a fairly clear-cut distinction between the emotionally disordered school refuser and those falling into these other categories.

Parents' attitudes are important in school refusal, as they sometimes seem as anxious as their child about separation, finding it difficult to force the child back into a situation which is perceived by all involved as threatening. A degree of parental collusion may, therefore, be the reason why one child with an emotional disturbance becomes school phobic whilst another does not.

Treatment

The primary goal of treatment is to get the child back to school as soon as possible. Those who continue to stay away often remain severely emotionally upset and sometimes housebound; only when normal attendance is resumed are the secondary effects removed. Even when school-phobic children return to school, associated emotional disturbances often persist and may affect them years later. There is some connection between school refusal in adolescence and neurotic or affective disorders in early adult life; there being an obvious similarity to agoraphobia. In both conditions there is a tendency to emotional disturbance with a need to avoid anxiety-provoking situations.

Immediate return to school requires the agreement of the child, parents and school; it may be necessary for a professional worker to take the child for a few days. If this fails, a more systematic approach using a behavioural technique, desensitization in reality, can be carried out by gradually reintroducing the child into school without causing too much distress, but with sufficient persistence to achieve this aim. Sometimes when all such attempts fail, admission to a psychiatric inpatient unit is required. Although acceptance of admission may prove difficult, after some time in hospital symptoms of disturbance abate so that the child can go home at weekends and return to the unit without too much difficulty. In this way confidence and independence are encouraged. Attendance at the unit school accustoms the child to the classroom so that reintroduction to a day school from home can usually be achieved.

An important aspect of management is to help parents become more consistent and effective in getting the child to accept the need for regular schooling. Very occasionally, when there is little cooperation with treatment, legal means may have to be invoked and either parents or child prosecuted for failure to attend school in order to get effective treatment carried out. Sometimes a change of school to a less demanding school environment or occasionally placement in a residential school for the maladjusted is advisable.

Other school problems

Many children show evidence of psychiatric disturbance only or mainly when in school. Although the usual methods of treatment for behavioural difficulties may help, there is much to be said for focussing treatment on the classroom and counselling teachers. Behavioural methods using reinforcement of approved behaviour are particularly appropriate.

Reading retardation

Reading and intelligence are closely associated; both show a normal distribution in a population of children. *General reading retardation* occurs when a child's ability to read is significantly less than it should be for his years. *Specific reading retardation* is said to be present when reading is poor in comparison with intelligence at a particular age. There is an association between specific reading backwardness and previous difficulties in the development of speech. The family history may be relevant, with other relatives affected. General reading backwardness is more likely to be accompanied by evidence of mild CNS dysfunction. Specific reading backwardness may be associated with adverse social factors such as a disadvantaged family which does little to encourage reading, or a poor school. It is more an educational than a medical problem requiring remedial help, although it is sometimes associated with conduct disorder.

The term *dyslexia* is often used to describe reading backwardness in children of average intelligence from a reasonable home background, but who fail to read satisfactorily, despite adequate schooling. It is an unsatisfactory term, since it only refers to a limited number of children with specific reading retardation and implies the existence of a medical syndrome analogous to parietal lobe disorder affecting adults, without evidence of this.

The hyperkinetic syndrome

There is a small group of children who show persistent overactivity in a variety of different situations who undoubtedly suffer from the hyperkinetic syndrome. There is also considerable overlap between overactivity and proneness to antisocial behaviour and educational retardation. Such children have a short attention span, poor concentration and are easily distracted. There may be a tendency to impulsiveness and outbursts of aggression.

In Britain, it is customary to give greater importance to conduct disorder or to educational difficulties than to overactivity; this being seen as social disinhibition combined with poor concentration and distractability.

In the United States some children who are disturbed are treated with amphetamine-type drugs. Although there is some evidence that this improves symptoms, there are those who consider, in view of side-effects etc., that it is doubtful whether these drugs should ever be prescribed at all. Management, otherwise, includes appropriate educational placement, parental counselling and possibly the use of behavioural techniques to help the child function more appropriately. In any event, overactivity tends to diminish as the child gets older.

Epilepsy

Conduct disorders and emotional disorders often affect children with epilepsy and are related to adverse social factors, as are similar problems in the non-epileptic child. The relationship between fits and psychiatric disturbance is variable. Controlling fits does not necessarily improve associated behaviour problems and may make them worse. Labelling a child as epileptic can in itself have adverse consequences due to the reaction of others leading to overprotection, overanxiety or rejection. Anticonvulsant medication, phenobarbitone especially, may have undesirable side-effects and interfere with the process of learning. Children with temporal lobe epilepsy are often particularly disadvantaged because of lowered intelligence, educational problems, overactivity, and attacks of catastrophic rage. However, the practice of looking for evidence of epilepsy in aggressive children with temper tantrums should be restricted to those children in whom clinically evident fits occur (see also Chapter 10).

Tics and habits

Tics are repetitive, identical, involuntary movements. The face is particularly affected, with blinking, sniffing, grunting and head shaking often being observed. More generalized tics can also occur; rarely, vocalizations and swear words can occur as tics (*Gilles de la Tourette syndrome*).

Tics may occur under stress or when relaxed. They are very common in childhood and variable in severity and persistence. Only occasionally do they present a major psychiatric problem, whereupon they may require treatment in hospital. Apart from a general approach to treatment aimed at reducing stress, particularly that caused by the tics themselves, treatment with haloperidol may sometimes reduce the severity of tics or even eliminate them altogether.

Habits. Apart from tics, habits are very common in childhood and do not usually indicate psychiatric disorder. Thumb sucking, nail biting, picking, hair pulling, eating dirt (*pica*), rocking and masturbation often occur in the normal course of development. Occasionally they are so persistent, so severe, or so inappropriate considering the age of the child that treatment is required. This is particularly the case when other psychiatric disturbance is associated. Behavioural methods of management for habits are probably the most likely to achieve results.

Obsessions and compulsions

These, in a mild and transitory form, are a common manifestation of emotional disturbance, although when severe and persistent may presage later and repeated attacks of obsessive-compulsive neurosis. Rituals involving hand washing, checking, counting or questioning may occur; likewise, various kinds of ruminations. These tend to be relatively short lived and may be improved by reducing stress or, if necessary, relieved by a change of environment by admission to hospital.

Conversion symptoms

These are physical symptoms for which no organic cause can be found, and which may be used to gain some advantage. Thus epileptic children sometimes have hysterical fits as well as true seizures. In others, difficulty in walking due to inexplicable weakness of the legs sometimes occurs, although in some, as is the case with adults, such conversion phenomena may turn out in the end to be manifestations of a physical illness not initially evident.

Depression

Although children often become miserable, weepy and hopeless when faced with difficult circumstances, true depressive illness such as affects adults is uncommon in childhood; likewise mania has never convincingly been described. Misery in childhood, like many other symptoms, is nearly always a response to environmental pressures; there being little evidence of it being relieved by antidepressant medication. Likewise, the fact that many emotional disorders in childhood are recurrent does not mean that they are necessarily due to depressive illness. Adolescents, however, more often complain of a depressed mood and hopelessness than younger children do. Schizophrenia occurring in adolescence not uncommonly presents in depressive guise.

Conduct disorders

A wide variety of conduct disorders occurs in childhood and adolescence so that it often seems somewhat arbitrary whether antisocial behaviour is dealt with by the psychiatric services or by courts, social services, the probation department or the educational welfare service. However, medical treatment is more likely to be sought for problems such as sexual misconduct or where antisocial behaviour affects young people who come from good homes and who have not shown similar behaviour in the past; or where there are obvious personality problems or emotional symptoms in addition to a disorder of conduct.

Conduct disorders do not, however, necessarily bring a child into conflict with the law. Thus aggressive behaviour or antisocial activity which may affect family life and school adjustment does not necessarily lead to prosecution.

Childhood psychosis

Psychosis in childhood is uncommon. As already suggested, *manic–depressive* disturbance before puberty is rare, although possibly not quite so uncommon as some believe. Apart from this, depression in young children tends to manifest itself by psychosomatic symptoms of an ill-defined type or by behaviour disturbance.

The most frequent psychosis of childhood is that known as *early childhood* or *infantile autism*. This is an unusual, but important, condition affecting children. It usually starts within the first two years of life and always within the preschool period. Those affected usually look physically normal. There are two main groups of features. The first is an inability to form normal relationships with people, even parents. This is characteristically shown by *gaze avoidance* and other abnormalities of normal eye-to-eye contact. The second consists of obsessional tendencies, leading to *stereotyped repetitive activities* and a *passion for sameness* and upset if the child's usual regime and environment are disturbed in any way.

Speech only develops in about half of children with this condition, although, if it does so, it usually develops by school age if not later. When it does so it is nearly always very abnormal with *echoing* or *delayed echoing*. The child has difficulty using pronouns such as 'I' or 'me' and shows pronominal reversal. The rhythm of speech is affected so that it sounds mechanical. Intelligence is retarded in three-quarters of cases, although, paradoxically, memory is sometimes particularly good. Unusually good ability for mental arithmetic or a well-developed musical aptitude may occasionally be found.

Preoccupation with stereotyped activities, particular objects or interests is a feature. This may involve collecting items such as keys, or may be manifest in a passionate interest in some esoteric subject, such as in learning railway timetables. Abnormal motor activities include *mannerisms, whole body movements* and *general overactivity*. Eating, sleeping and continence are often disturbed. Fits occur in up to a quarter of cases.

Despite all the characteristic features of early childhood autism, there is no feature which occurs only in this condition. Mentally handicapped children often show mannerisms. Speech may fail to develop or be abnormal for a variety of reasons including deafness. Some children are rather obsessional and others very reserved. Parents with a handicapped child may read about autism and colour their description of the child's behaviour accordingly. It may be possible to conclude that a child has this condition after an out-patient visit, but assessment in a day centre may be necessary before a firm conclusion can be reached. Characteristic features of severe adult mental illness such as delusions and hallucinations do not develop.

Very little is known about causes of this disorder. It affects boys more often girls, and appears to occur more commonly in the children of parents in the professional and managerial classes. There is some evidence that genetic factors may be important.

Outcome is on the whole very poor. Intellectually brighter children do best, thus a testable IQ of over 60 at the age of 5 years indicates a more favourable future. A few autistic children manage in normal school. Some can be educated in special schools for the educationally subnormal; others are so limited that total care is necessary and may have to be provided on a residential basis if parents cannot cope. There are schools specifically for autistic children, some of which are residential and which cater for brighter children who can profit from highly specialist schooling. Parents of autistic children are in need of advice and require a great deal of help and support. Here the National Society for Autistic Children may be of help.

While drug therapy is not usually required, temporary sedation may occasionally be needed where a child is very overactive and disturbed. Behavioural methods are often employed using the technique of reinforcement to encourage more appropriate behaviour with regard to speech, feeding, using the toilet, dressing, going to bed and social interaction. It has been well said that autistic children have to be taught things which others pick up without any instruction. Gaze avoidance and obsessional problems may diminish over a long time, but severe abnormalities of speech, social behaviour and intellectual functioning usually remain so that custodial care is often required. Even those few who are of average intelligence, able to receive a reasonable education, and lead relatively independent lives, remain badly affected by strange personality characteristics and social isolation.

Other psychotic conditions rarely affect children, although they are occasionally symptomatic of degenerative brain disease, such as a lipoidosis. In later childhood and early adolescence, a schizophrenic-like illness sometimes occurs (*late onset psychosis*). This appears to be related to schizophrenia since it occurs in the families of schizophrenics more than would otherwise be the case, which early childhood autism does not.

Adolescent problems

The beginning of adolescence is easier to identify than its end. This is because secondary sexual changes marking the onset of puberty in boys, together with the menarche in girls, identify the point at which it can be said to have begun. The end of adolescence occurs more gradually and within a wide variation of chronological age. Those who develop normally during childhood, without undue physical or psychological problems and within an emotionally secure environment, probably pass through adolescence with relatively little turbulence and mature early. In contrast, children from disturbed families are likely to become disturbed adolescents who may suffer delayed maturity. In any event, adolescence cannot be said to be the most comfortable period of human existence. One reason for this is a growing desire for independence while at the same time having, out of sheer necessity, to remain dependent on parents or parent-surrogates.

The search for identity

One of the adolescent's problems arises out of his need to acquire an identity of his own. Naturally this is to some extent governed by the model which his parents present. 'To be' like father (or mother, of course) 'or not to be' summarizes his dilemma. Even if the parent of the same sex is a *good* model for identification, can the adolescent compete? If not, then to whom should he turn? It is ambivalence which leads the adolescent to identify himself with a series of models often of very varying hue, while uncertainty about his own person leads him into dangerous experimentation—with alcohol, drugs, delinquent and possibly risky behaviour involving motor cycles and a variety of other potentially harmful pursuits—of which he knows his parents would not approve. He seeks to conquer, if only to prove to himself that he can master his environment, at least to his own if not to the satisfaction of others. Failure to do so and the disapproval which his efforts may arouse, may cause him to become morose, sulky, rebellious and depressed.

Sexual problems

The increasing permissiveness of Westernized society towards sexual behaviour and attitudes has probably lessened the tensions which these once produced. Guilt over masturbation has, for example, obviously diminished. Likewise a growing number of schoolchildren now seem to believe that teenage sex is not necessarily to be discouraged and that premarital sexual intercourse is not only permissible but actually desirable. Time alone will prove whether these new attitudes will ultimately benefit those societies in which they are cultivated. Meanwhile, it could be suggested that their more immediate effects, such as the potentially increasing number of illegitimate births, may have been cushioned by factors such as the easier availability of the contraceptive pill and abortion.

Delinquency

The increasing prevalence of vandalism and criminal offences among schoolchildren, in particular among adolescents, and, even more so, crimes involving violence, is understandably a matter of growing concern; the more so perhaps because there is no ready explanation available. Many suggestions have been put forward: the increasing portrayal of violence by the mass media; diminution of religious beliefs leading to a deterioration in moral standards; lack of parental guidance; the glittering temptations of an ever more materialistic society, and so on. As yet, none of these seems a wholly adequate explanation. The only thing which seems certain is that the adolescent's behaviour cannot be judged in isolation, but must be seen as a reflection of the behaviour and standards of the society in which he himself dwells.

Academic pressures

Academic pressures particularly affect sixth-formers and university students. It is necessary among both groups to sort out those whose aspirations are not entirely their own, but have been imposed upon them by others, not only by parents but schoolteachers. There is little doubt that the commonest cause of failure among university students is not mental ill-health but lack of motivation. Prior to coming to university many are unwilling or unable to recognize their lack of motivation, although they may do so during the middle or end of the first year, 'dropping-out' at this point. In some cases this may be a disaster for, if such lack of motivation were recognized much earlier, advice might be given which could lead to the pursuit of a more suitable career.

It should be noted, however, that although lack of motivation may be the commonest reason for the abandonment of university studies, certain illnesses, such as glandular fever and other virus infections prone to occur in this age group, can leave depression and inanition in their wake, often for many months, and yet pass unrecognized as a significant cause of academic failure.

Treatment

Most disorders of childhood and adolescence are managed on an out-patient basis. Only occasionally, when all attempts fail, is attendance at a day unit or in-patient treatment necessary, although rarely certain problems are best assessed and managed from the start by hospital admission. Most child psychiatrists work as members of a multidisciplinary team with social workers and psychologists, while methods of management vary from one to another and few evaluative studies have been carried out. Nevertheless, there is enough common ground to make some general statements about therapy.

Environmental manipulation
It is widely assumed that behaviour problems are responsive to changes in the environment. Advice to move a child into a more appropriate educational setting is an example. Likewise, simple expedients such as making toilets more available by bending school rules or having a child home for lunch may lessen the problem of faecal soiling. Keeping brothers and sisters apart when they are doing their homework may reduce quarrelling. Attendance at a play group may lessen excessive dependence and social isolation in a preschool child. Countless examples of simple remedies can be given which may alleviate psychiatric disturbance in childhood.

Parental counselling
Seeing parents regularly and allowing them to talk about their difficulties may give them emotional support and help them cope more effectively by changing maladaptive attitudes towards their children.

Counselling children and adolescents
Similar considerations apply to encouraging young people to talk about their problems. Play materials and opportunities to draw facilitate

communication. The development of a helpful relationship between child and psychiatrist is an essential therapeutic tool.

Behavioural methods

Techniques derived from experimental psychology and learning theory are increasingly used to deal with childhood behaviour disorders. Reinforcement is centred around reward for desirable behaviour whilst unwanted activities are ignored. Such methods are appropriate in developmental disorders and enable children to learn skills which they have been unable to acquire; speech, reading, toilet training and social skills are good examples.

Behavioural modification may help those intellectually backward to become more self-sufficient and independent. Another group of disorders for which reinforcement techniques are particularly appropriate is conduct disorders. Motivation allows appropriate rewards for conformity contingent upon demonstration of acceptable behaviour. Preschool problems such as sleep disturbance and temper tantrums can be managed in a similar fashion.

Isolated phobias may be treated by desensitization using *reciprocal inhibition*. Thus *school refusal* is commonly dealt with by using behavioural methods.

Drug therapy

In general, drugs have relatively little place in the treatment of psychiatric disorders in childhood. Only rarely in very severe disturbances including psychoses, and when distress is excessive, are the major tranquillizers required. There is little evidence that antidepressant drugs are effective in emotional disorders of childhood, although occasionally they may appear justified in a depressed adolescent. While it is probably true that minor tranquillizers are used extensively, especially by general practitioners to treat childhood psychiatric disorders, until some evidence for their effectiveness is forthcoming their use should be discouraged.

Residential treatment

Placement away from home in special boarding schools for maladjusted, educationally subnormal, epileptic and physically handicapped children is often made because of highly unsatisfactory home circumstances. Many young people go into children's homes and community homes with education on the premises for similar reasons, particularly when they show antisocial behaviour or are exposed to dangers at home. Psychiatric treatment is often provided and all other methods of treatment mentioned. Child-care and teaching staff may, under supervision, use behavioural methods. Likewise, group work with staff may help them to cope more effectively with difficult children in a residential setting. Hospital in-patient units for children or adolescents operate in much the same way, although the emphasis here is usually on short-term treatment rather than long-term care and education. Children away from home, even though spending weekends at home, usually soon respond to efforts directed towards reducing disturbed behaviour, improving their relationships with others and developing appropriate social skills. Such units are particularly helpful in treating previously intransigent problems such as soiling, wetting, eating difficulties or refusal to attend school where close supervision of a child's behaviour is required to achieve success.

Legal procedures

Children and adolescents with psychiatric problems are over-represented among those placed on various court orders because of their social circumstances or other difficulties. Some are supervised by the Social Services Department of a local authority or placed *in care* for a variety of reasons such as *non-accidental injury*, truancy, lack of parental care and control, and moral danger. It is important for those who treat psychiatric problems in young people to be familiar with the law relating to children and to work closely with Social Services Departments, educational welfare and child care establishments such as observation and assessment centres and community homes.

Outcome

Psychiatric disorders in children and young adolescents usually last for several months and may sometimes persist for years while fluctuating in severity. There is a good evidence that antisocial behaviour in adult life is usually preceded by conduct problems in childhood, such as truancy, disruptiveness in school and delinquency. However, most children with conduct disorders do not show severe antisocial behaviour when they grow up. There is also some evidence for a link between emotional disturbances affecting children and neurotic disorders of later life. It would seem that disturbances affecting young adolescents are more likely to persist into adult life than those of young children.

Studies of psychiatric conditions affecting adults have shown that while recurrent obsessional disturbances may first begin in childhood, this is only occasional. Severe animal phobias in women appear to originate in childhood. Schizophrenia may begin in early adolescence or even before. Anorexia nervosa, agoraphobia and manic-depressive psychosis may all start in adolescence. Developmental difficulties affecting children, such as reading delay, wetting and soiling, all tend to improve with time, although a small proportion of these problems persist into adolescence and into adult life.

Further reading

Barker, P. (1979) *Basic Child Psychiatry*, 3rd edn. St Albans: Crosby Lockwood Staples.
Hersov, L. & Berg, I. (eds) (1980) *Out of School*. Chichester: John Wiley.
Rutter, M. & Hersov, L. (eds) (1977) *Child Psychiatry: Modern Approaches*. Oxford: Blackwell Scientific.

21

Mental Handicap (Mental Impairment)

It is only relatively recently that the term *mental subnormality* (*amentia, oligophrenia*) replaced the older more pejorative designation *mental defect*, together with its once popular subcategories, *feeble-minded, idiots* and *imbeciles* which were then used to denote the lower grades of intelligence. In its turn, *mental subnormality* has been superseded by *mental handicap*, although this while referring to 'arrested or incomplete development of mind' was never actually included in the Mental Health Act of 1959. Now, with a new Act currently before Parliament and due to take effect on 30 September 1983, those who are mentally subnormal or handicapped, but who need to be detained under the relevant Section, will be designated as suffering from *mental* or, depending on degree, *severe mental impairment*. This condition is defined as:

'A state of arrested or incomplete development of mind which includes sufficient impairment of intelligence and social functioning and is associated with abnormally aggressive or seriously irresponsible conduct on the part of the person concerned.' (see also Chapter 25).

For those not needing compulsory detention, the term *mental handicap* (or *severe mental handicap*) is retained, the term *impairment* being kept only for those requiring compulsory admission. It should be noted, furthermore, that the qualification '*severe*', whether used in respect of *handicap* or *impairment*, does not relate specifically to intelligence level, intellectual or emotional development or, in the case of handicap, to social competence, but to whether or not the subject can be expected to benefit from special education or training to the extent, in due course, of living a normal life in the community without supervision. Only those who may be deemed to require some form of continuing care or supervision, either in an institution or elsewhere, are likely to be designated as coming within the category '*severe*'.

Finally, by way of introduction, it should be noted that in this chapter the term '*handicap*' rather than '*impairment*' is used. This is because the main focus of interest is on essentially clinical matters rather than on legal implications, which are dealt with separately in Chapter 25.

While the classification of patients into various diagnostic categories is still necessarily incomplete, subdivision into *primary* and *secondary* causes still appears useful. There is also growing awareness that mental handicap is not an *entity*, but has many different origins. This has encouraged research, while looking towards the possibilities for prevention.

An increasing number of conditions have now been shown to be of genetic origin, many of which give rise to inborn errors of metabolism. As fresh discoveries have become almost an everyday occurrence, there appears to be an ever-growing number of these. Currently, some 80 such conditions have been identified. As a result of these disorders, toxic metabolites circulating in the blood may interfere with brain function and lead, among other things, to mental handicap. *Phenylketonuria* affords an excellent example of such a condition which, although genetically determined, may nonetheless be correctable if treatment is begun early enough.

Psychopathology

Intelligence is a function of cognitive capacity and involves the ability to attend, concentrate, perceive and record accurately, to memorize and recall relevant material, to modify behaviour in the light of experience and foresee eventualities. These qualities are to some extent lacking in all mentally handicapped persons, although this is only part of the total picture. *Emotional and motivational factors* are often of equal or greater significance. This is particularly true of marginal cases where such factors may determine whether the patient can remain in the community. Many of those with markedly impaired intelligence but of stable character can fulfil a useful social role; others of higher intelligence, but of lesser stability, may require continuing care. While it is possible to measure intelligence relatively accurately, tests for other qualities of personality are much less reliable.

Severe mental handicap

Because the severely handicapped group covers such a wide range of behavioural characteristics it may be clinically convenient to subdivide those in this category into an upper and lower subgroup.

Those who fall within the lower subgroup exhibit very marked impairment of perception and attention to external stimuli. Their imitative capacity is very limited or non-existent, and they show meagre interest and curiosity. Speech, if present, may be limited to monosyllabic utterances or inarticulate sounds. Response to kindly handling is shown by some, who may be capable of forming some kind of emotional relationship with those who minister to their needs. Others tend to be excitable, non-responsive and destructive. Violence is usually an expression of superadded difficulty, such as psychosis, epilepsy or unenlightened handling, and real rapport may be impossible. Overt masturbation, urinary and faecal incontinence are common, despite active efforts at habit training. Automatic activity such as nodding, rocking and thumb sucking is often seen. Many severely handicapped patients require constant care in order to be fed, dressed, toileted and protected from common domestic dangers.

Patients who are less severely affected may be better equipped for self-preservation and for avoiding common physical hazards. Because their impairment of cognitive abilities is less marked, attention, concentration and more lively perception are possible, particularly if sustained by skilfully offered motivation. Experience has shown that such patients are capable of modified industrial output under sheltered conditions. However, while memory may be good enough for undertaking simple repetitive tasks, more complicated procedures soon reveal its basic weakness. The capacity of these patients for imitation may be good (especially in those with *Down's syndrome*) and speech may be reasonably fluent, although occasionally distorted by echolalia and articulatory defects. While conversation is usually poorly sustained even at a simple level, or may even be irrational, it sometimes reflects a veneer of culture. Elementary reading may be achieved, but comprehension is minimal or much below the level apparently reached. Arithmetic presents a greater problem and few attain even the simplest rudiments. Thus understanding of money is usually confined to coin recognition. Anomalies in physical appearance are dependent upon aetiology. This subgroup contains many patients with easily recognizable clinical syndromes such as *Down's syndrome* and *tuberous sclerosis*.

Mental handicap

More and more of those who are mildly handicapped are currently being trained to become self-supporting and useful members of society. Success, however, is often as dependent upon stability of temperament and a good personality as it is upon the higher level of intelligence which this group possesses, as compared with that of the more severely handicapped.

Perception, attention, concentration, imagination and memory are all underdeveloped. There may be little display of curiosity. As children the subjects soon fall behind their peers and become incapable of competing with them on equal terms. Their mental development is much slower than that of the average child and reaches its maximum earlier so that intellectual disparity becomes more obvious at puberty. Despite this, social and general habit training may still be of considerable benefit in adolescence and in young adults.

Mentally handicapped patients have difficulty in adapting to changing circumstances, are unduly sensitive to the opinion of others and respond badly to direct criticism. Owing to limitations of insight, their sense of humour is poorly developed so that a workmate's joke taken badly may be sufficient to precipitate a situation which may lead to loss of employment. Those of stable disposition may be employed in simple occupations such as labouring, wire-net making, sorting components, soldering electrical apparatus, portering and domestic service. Skilled work which calls for adaptability in performance and consistency of effort tends, however, to be beyond them.

Mental handicap and mental illness

Mentally handicapped patients are less tolerant of alcohol than are normal persons; their threshold to stress is lower. Thus psychosis and personality deviations, whether inherent or reactive, are as frequently found among them as among members of the general population, probably more so. Endogenous psychosis also is probably much commoner among severely handicapped patients than may hitherto have been realized.

Schizophrenia of any variety may occur, but simple and hebephrenic types are most frequently encountered (*propfschizophrenie*). The symptoms differ little from those of persons of average intelligence although a tendency to become apathetic, careless, less accessible and sometimes negativistic may be more marked. Delusions and hallucinatory episodes occur. Instability of temperament and unpredictable aggressive behaviour is common, but catatonic stupor is rare. There is rapid deterioration of already impaired cognitive functions.

Manic-depressive psychosis may give rise to attacks of mania or melancholia but these tend commonly to be of lesser intensity and shorter duration than in those of higher intelligence.

Paranoid states are not infrequent and are often triggered off by the patient's sensitive awareness of his inadequacy.

Anxiety arising from the interaction between external stress and inherent inferiority is common, especially in the upper marginally handicapped group. Unless quickly dealt with, such anxiety may cost the patient his stability, his job and his hard-earned place in the community.

While organized *hysterical* manifestations with physical conversion have been known to occur, *primitive reactions* are commoner, especially in female patients.

Delinquency and criminality

Handicapped patients are suggestible and easily led. Males frequently find themselves charged with minor crimes, committed as part of a gang effort in which the more intelligent leaders may escape retribution. Petty shoplifting is common among females, whereas breaking and entering is typical of the more aggressive male. Indecent exposure and sexual assault, varying in degree of seriousness, are also encountered in males.

Estimates as to the causal relationship, if any, between mental handicap and delinquency vary considerably, but no one now considers this to be a prerequisite of delinquent behaviour. Likewise, criminals are no longer essentially regarded as handicapped. Differences between the IQs of delinquents and non-delinquents may be attributed to *cultural factors* which lower the test scores of the former group. It is also doubtful whether the prevalence of delinquency among mentally handicapped individuals is any higher than in a matched group drawn from the general population. Administrative expediency and common aetiological factors are more likely to determine the relationship between mental handicap and delinquency than any express tendency on the part of the mentally handicapped to break the law (Kirman).

Aetiology

Primary factors are those which depend upon genetic constitution and are therefore potentially operative prior to conception. Two groups are distinguishable.

1. Those with severe intellectual impairment usually accompanied by gross physical disability.

2. Those with minimal intellectual impairment and with only limited, if any, physical disability

The first group comprises those with a *major gene defect* which may be dominant, recessive or sex linked, such as *tuberous sclerosis*, *gargoylism* and certain metabolic and obscure abnormalities of the skeletal system. The second group, which does not follow Mendelian principles, arises from the *additive influence* of a number of genes which in themselves make only a very small individual contribution to the final product. This multifactorial, or polygenic, type of inheritance controls biological traits other than intelligence, such as height and weight. Together with the infantile psychosis group, multifactorial inheritance accounts for the bulk of physically normal-looking cases of mental handicap in which secondary causes can be excluded.

Chromosomal abnormalities are mainly autosomal in type, such as *Down's syndrome* (p. 307). Anomalies of the sex-determining chromosomes are also found, such as *Klinefelter's syndrome* (karyotype multiple X plus Y) and *Turner's syndrome* (karyotype XO), but these patients are not invariably handicapped, although they tend towards low intelligence. In contrast, handicap may be much more likely in rare cases of XXX (*'super-female'*) constitution.

Secondary factors operate after conception and may be classified according to whether they become operative in the antenatal, perinatal or postnatal period, with a range of clinical possibilities including *Rhesus incompatibility*, *toxoplasmosis*, *cytomegalovirus*, *lead poisoning*, *viral encephalitis*, *birth injury* and other diseases. Such cases often show gross physical signs.

The complex interaction which occurs between an individual and his social environment may be decisive in shaping his personality. While the modification of inborn patterns of external stress is fairly commonplace, as the various reactive syndromes encountered in psychiatric practice demonstrate, greater attention is now being paid to the role of the environment as a cause of mental handicap, such as a bad home, parental neglect, emotional trauma, faulty placement, delinquent companions and unsuitable education. While such factors undeniably play a part in influencing the retarded individual, and in particular those less handicapped, their influence is still sometimes overestimated.

Clinical descriptions

Reference has been made above to the twofold grouping of cases of mental handicap into a *pathological* (major gene) group in which physical signs and brain lesions are commonplace, and an *undifferentiated* (polygenic) group bearing few, if any, physical signs or discernible brain abnormality. The conditions to be described below belong to the pathological group. Only the more important or commonplace varieties will be considered, with emphasis also upon some of those conditions which are treatable or may perhaps turn out to be so, or are in some way preventable. For further information reference must be made to more specialized texts.

Mainly primary

Down's syndrome (mongolism)

The incidence of Down's syndrome in Western cultures is 1 in 600–700 births. Progress in cytogenetics now permits classification into two main groups: *trisomy* (95 per cent) and *translocation* (5 per cent). Trisomy mongols, who increase in frequency as a function of advancing maternal age, have trisomy of chromosome 21 and a karyotype showing 47 chromosomes. Translocation mongols, frequently born to younger mothers, with a higher risk of recurrence, giving rise to a familial pattern, have a normal count of 46 chromosomes accompanied by an abnormal chromosome constitution in which the abnormality is cytogenetically masked by a presumptive translocation involving the 21 and the 15–16 group. Such cases occur independently of maternal age. Penrose has drawn attention to the significance of *paternal* age in those characterized by 21:21 or 21:22 chromosomal fusion. He observed that in such cases the mean age of the fathers at the birth of the mongol child was 42.5 years, that is 10.8 years in excess of the mean paternal age in the general population.

Calculation of the *risk* of a second mongol child (which must not be confused with the risk underlying mongol incidence) can only be based upon an investigation of the chromosomes of both parents as well as upon those of the index patient. Where the karyotypes of the parents are normal, and the mongol patient shows trisomy 21 with a count of 47, it can be assumed that non-disjunction occurred during gametogenesis, and that the additional risk in excess of the random risk is a function of maternal age. In the exceedingly rare instance of one parent being chromosomally *mosaic* (that is, possessing an admixture of cells showing a count of 46 and 47 respectively, with minimal or maximal clinical signs of mongolism), the subsequent risk may be as high as 1 in 2. If a translocation defect is shown in the patient, while both parents have normal karyotypes, it may be again assumed that non-disjunction has occurred during gamete formation and that, in young parents, there is no special additional risk. However, where a translocation is shown in either parent, the risk to further children is in the order of 1 in 3, and half the 'normal' children born to such parents will be carriers of the translocation. If reliable facilities for investigations are *not* available, parents who have had one mongol child and have no other close relatives affected may be told that the risk is of the order of 1 or 2 per cent irrespective of maternal age.

Physical signs. The skull is small and round, the face and occiput rather flat. Narrow palpebral fissures slope downwards and inwards. Wide epicanthus is common and the eyes may show speckling of the irises and early cataracts. The ears are small and of simple convolutional pattern. Alopecia, partial or complete, occurs in a minority of cases and is resistive to treatment. The tongue is usually coarse, deeply fissured and the circumvallate papillae are markedly hypertrophied. The hands are short and clumsy in appearance, the little fingers especially so, often showing considerable curving. Anomalies in linear distribution are present on the palms and soles and the palmar pattern may present one simian furrow instead of the usual three lines. A wide cleft characteristically separates the big toe from the others and a short plantar furrow is often present. Congenital deficiencies in the formation of the ribs have been reported. Coarse skin, with a tendency to dermatitis, and a gruff voice may be reminiscent of cretinism. In early differential diagnosis the leading skull signs, together with generalized hypotonia and an iliac index of 60 or less, are valuable signs.

Those with Down's syndrome have a low resistance to infections so that conjunctivitis, blepharitis, rhinitis, bronchitis and broncho-pneumonia are common. Congenital heart disease is present in about 10 per cent of cases, often with dyspnoea on exertion and finger-clubbing. In the blood, abnormality of nuclear lobulation of the polymorphs has been described. Thus a significantly increased risk of concurrence of Down's syndrome and leukaemia has suggested that a locus on chromosome pair 21 may be concerned in leucopoiesis.

Pathology. The brain is simple in type with underdevelopment particularly affecting the frontal lobes, brain-stem and cerebellum. Argentophil plaques and neurofibrillary tangles such as are found in Alzheimer's disease may be evident.

Mental condition. The majority of mongols are severely mentally handicapped, but possess good aptitude for mimicry, rhythm and group training. Rehabilitation and the achievement of simple work status under prescribed and supervised conditions are possible in many cases. Obdurate and temperamentally unstable mongols require close control, especially in situations offering *sibling rivalry* with a younger child.

Prognosis. The former high mortality rate, particularly from respiratory infections, has been reduced by antibiotics, so that the expectation of life at all ages has been correspondingly raised. Death at or before puberty is no longer common among those who survive the neonatal period.

Microcephaly

Many mentally handicapped patients, of diverse type and varying aetiology, show reduction in cranial circumference. Thus the term *microcephaly* best describes a sign rather than a syndrome. Customarily, however, the name is applied to a *genetically* determined, recessive condition, although the condition can result from noxious influences such as exposure to *excessive radiation* either *in utero* or during the immediate postnatal period as at Hiroshima, or to fetal infection by *cytomegalovirus* (see p. 315). Premature synostosis of the bones of the skull, formerly considered to be the causative factor, has been ruled out by cerebral non-response to early craniotomy and other surgical measures aimed at expansion of the cranium.

Physical signs. The head is markedly reduced in size and the circumference in adulthood may be well under 43.2 cm (17 in) with the greatest reduction shown in the height and width of the skull rather than in its length, so giving a very low cephalic index. The forehead recedes, the occiput is flattened and the mandible foreshortened so that, in lateral view, the patient has a bird-like appearance. The scalp tissue is redundant and may assume compensatory folds and corrugations. Physical stature is below average. While a minority suffer from cerebral palsy, ranging in degree from paraplegia to spastic quadriplegia, most patients are ambulant.

Pathology. The brain shows weight reduction corresponding to its underdevelopment in size; this is most pronounced in the temporal, parietal and occipital regions where the convolution pattern is extremely simple and localized areas of microgyria occur. Porencephaly and external hydrocephalus may be present. Microscopically, cortical neurones are scanty and poorly developed.

Mental condition. Most microcephalics are severely mentally handicapped, but as a rule are fond of mimicry, show well-established affection and a possessive interest in toys and other objects of childish admiration. They are incapable of useful work, but respond reasonably well to habit training. As children they tend to be hyperkinetic and so constitute a problem in supervision.

Tuberous or nodular sclerosis (epiloia)

In tuberous sclerosis, neuroglial overgrowth occurs giving rise to nodules varying in size from that of a pea to a walnut. The nodules are pale in appearance, hard and may project above the surface of the brain or into the lateral ventricles, producing a characteristic candle-guttering appearance on air encephalography. Some nodules calcify and may be visible on straight x-ray of the skull. Fibrotic tumours present in other organs, such as the heart, kidneys, spleen, lungs, retina (phakomata) and thyroid. Nodular periosteal thickenings and subungual fibromata may occur in the phalanges. On the skin and in the subcutaneous tissues, café-au-lait spots and 'shagreen' patches are common, the latter showing a predilection for the lumbar, inguinal and forehead regions.

The *triad* of *adenoma sebaceum, epilepsy* and *mental handicap* is characteristic of the syndrome. Adenoma sebaceum is a cutaneous eruption which consists of an overgrowth of the sebaceous glands and capillaries of the cheeks leading to the formation of numerous nodules, the majority of which are smaller in size than a small pea. The colour varies from a bright red to a yellowish or dusky hue, this being dependent on the predominance of the vascular or sebaceous elements, and the formation has a 'butterfly' distribution on the face, although, being progressive, may spread beyond these boundaries. It is not present at birth and usually appears at about 4–6 years of age. The epilepsy is grand mal in type and, in very handicapped patients, may assume status frequency with consequent danger to life. In patients with only a mild degree of mental handicap or occasionally none at all, fits may be infrequent in occurrence, with long intervals between convulsions. Tuberous sclerosis is a developmental disturbance having a close affinity to *neurofibromatosis (Von Recklinghausen's disease)*. Both show an irregular type of dominant inheritance with great variability in genetic manifestation. Mutation is thought to be operative in some cases; in some of these, however, there may be justifiable doubts about paternity.

Treatment. Fits may be controlled by anti-epileptic medication, while in more intelligent patients who may desire it, measures may be taken to minimize the cosmetic effects of epiloia. In female patients the desirability of sterilization should be considered.

Primary and secondary

Disturbances of protein metabolism

Phenylketonuria (phenylpyruvic oligophrenia). This disorder is due to a blockage in the metabolism of phenylalanine to tyrosine, a precursor of melanin, as a result of which *phenylpyruvic acid* appears in the urine where it may be detected by a positive ferric chloride response. The metabolic anomaly is caused by the absence of an essential enzyme, this trait being inherited as a recessive. It occurs in approximately 1 in 12 000 live births. It is usually but not invariably associated with mental handicap, the degree of which *may* be modified by diet. Physically, patients with phenylketonuria are well developed and those of Caucasian origin may have fair hair and delicate skins. Cases have been reported among both Negroes and Asiatics in whom the tissue colouring is again lighter than the racial norm.

Treatment consists of a diet low in phenylalanine, it having been shown that normal mental and physical development is possible when this is begun *within the first three months of life*, and where no other adverse feature is present. Unfortunately, the necessary diet is both expensive and monotonous, and ambulant children require close supervision to forestall attempts at undesirable supplementation. Although the condition is relatively uncommon, routine mass screening of urine at six weeks of age should be carried out and repeated at three months. As, however, a variable response has been demonstrated by urine testing, greater reliance is now placed upon serum phenylalanine levels. Heelprick at about one week after birth is advocated as a screening technique. Carriers of the gene may be detected by their low threshold of tolerance to test doses of ingested phenylalanine.

Other rarer disturbances of protein metabolism, which in due course may conceivably turn out to be correctable, include *maple syrup urine disease* and *Hartnup disease* in which abnormal amino-aciduria is also present.

Disturbances of carbohydrate metabolism

Galactosaemia. In galactosaemia, there is incomplete metabolism of galactose because of the absence of a glycolytic enzyme. Inheritance follows an autosomal recessive pattern. The affected infant vomits persistently, with consequent loss of weight and failure to thrive. Cataracts, jaundice and hepatosplenomegaly develop in untreated cases. Growth is inhibited and deposition of galactose within the neurones leads to progressive mental handicap. Death may be rapid, but amelioration of the condition, compatible with life and average intellectual development, may be achieved through early diagnosis and the institution of a lactose-free diet.

Hypoglycaemia. Familial hypoglycaemia may be genetically determined, leading to cerebral damage, convulsions and mental handicap. Similar hazards may attend insulin overdose in the treatment of young diabetics or in those suffering from pancreatic tumour. A glucose tolerance curve is indicated in any baby showing backwardness and epilepsy. The condition is now considered to be treatable by a restricted leucine diet and the use of ACTH.

Disturbances of lipid metabolism

Cerebromacular degeneration (Tay–Sachs' disease). In this condition, 85 per cent of those affected are of Eastern European Jewish (Ashkenazim) origin. One in 25 is a gene carrier as opposed to 1 in 250 other Jews or non-Jews. If both parents are carriers, there is a 1 in 4 chance of any child born having the disease.

An infant with Tay–Sachs' disease appears normal up to the third month, at which time it becomes weak in the back and its vision starts to fail. At about then, ophthalmoscopic examination reveals the characteristic *cherry-red spot* in the macula surrounded by a whitish-grey area. Progressive weakness ensues and optic atrophy follows leading to complete blindness. In the final stages there is extreme emaciation together with muscular rigidity and spasms. The disease is always fatal and in most cases death occurs within two years. Juvenile cases, showing optic atrophy and pigmentary degeneration of the retina, but without the cherry-red spot, have also been described in non-Jews. The clinical picture is one of slow regression from already established levels of physical and mental attainment. Epilepsy may occur.

There is no specific treatment for either type of disease, although prevention may be possible by termination of pregnancy following the discovery of a deficiency of the enzyme hexosaminadase A in amniotic fluid. Gene carriers can likewise be discovered by a similar, although less marked, deficiency of the enzyme in their blood.

Other disorders of lipid metabolism include *gargoylism* or *Hurler's disease (mucopolysaccharidosis)* and certain familial disorders such as *Gaucher's, Niemann–Pick's* and *Hand–Schüller–Christian's* diseases.

Cretinism (infantile hypothyroidism)

Endemic cretinism is associated with soils poor in iodine content. In Britain most cases are sporadic in type and occur as a result of congenital aplasia, or of biochemical insufficiency of the thyroid gland. The genetics are obscure, but there is some evidence to implicate recessive inheritance. Physical signs may be present at birth, but more usually these appear about the sixth month. The infant ceases to grow and the body, relatively, looks too small for the head. The skin is coarse and dry with an icteric tinge, anaemia develops, the abdomen becomes protuberant. An umbilical hernia is often present and the vocal sounds have a hoarse quality. Weakness of spinal muscles leads to a dorsal kyphosis. The limbs are stunted, and the ligaments of the joints unduly lax. Puffiness of the subcutaneous tissues, especially around the eyes and lips, together with an enlarged tongue, podgy hands, supraclavicular masses, infantile genitalia and stunted growth, constitute a very characteristic picture.

The outstanding feature of the mental state is extreme apathy. The ultimate degree of retardation will depend very much upon early diagnosis and the quality of response to treatment. The *prognosis* for intellectual development should be given cautiously and a watch kept for signs of thyroxine overdose, such as rise in temperature, tachycardia or diarrhoea. Response to therapy may assist diagnosis, but investigations of thyroid function and the effect of thyroid hormones on the blood cholesterol level may be necessary to decide the issue, especially in cases of subclinical thyroid deficiency. Recently, the possibility of screening at birth by using blood from the umbilical vein of neonates has been under consideration. However, blood obtained by heelprick on the sixth day may be used, testing at the same time for phenylketonuria. In older infants, radiographic determinations of bone age may also give useful diagnostic information. The main infantile syndromes from which cretinism must be distinguished are mongolism, gargoylism, achondroplasia and rickets.

Mainly secondary

Cerebral palsy

Lesions in infancy which are severe enough to cause paralysis of one or more limbs are commonly, but not invariably, associated with some degree of mental impairment. They fall into two aetiological subgroups.

1. *Physical trauma.* Injury grave enough to cause mental handicap is rare during the antenatal and postnatal periods. The condition is much more likely to occur during difficult labour or in the course of premature delivery, due to intracranial haemorrhage (gross and punctate) with consequent *cerebral anoxia*.

The clinical picture shows a variable range of intellectual retardation accompanied by spastic paralysis, mainly of the pyramidal, 'clasp-knife' type and with a tendency to unilateral lesions, hemiplegic in distribution. With more widespread neuronal damage, paraplegia and quadriplegia may be associated with recessive inheritance (see below). Epilepsy is a fairly constant feature.

2. *Rhesus factor.* Rhesus incompatibility, if serious enough to produce congenital haemolytic anaemia and kernicterus, may damage intellectual development. The physical lesions tend to have a symmetrical

distribution, especially affecting the extrapyramidal system resulting in *'cog-wheel'* rigidity, *athetosis*, which is worsened by voluntary effort, *muscular tremors, dysarthria* and *torsion spasm* of the neck. Cases showing a predominance of *extrapyramidal* signs require great care in psychometric assessment because, very often, intellectual retardation is minimal compared with the impression gained from the physical signs.

Hydrocephalus

Occlusion of the basal foramina from meningitis, tumour and haemorrhagic debris, or genetically determined narrowing of the ventricular lumen, lead to accumulation of fluid in the lateral ventricles, distension, and pressure atrophy of the cortex. The cranial bones become separated and thinned, so that the skull may be almost translucent. Hydrocephalus may occur before birth, in which case the infant is rarely born alive. A small percentage of cases deteriorate rapidly, becoming emaciated, paralysed, blind and deaf. Others run a more chronic course, or where this is arrested they may survive with varying impairment of their mental and physical faculties. Most hydrocephalics are quiet and tractable, but few are capable of sustained activity. The skull is globular in shape with the greatest circumference in the temporal region. There is no correlation between head size and intelligence. Very early surgical treatment is indicated where hydrocephalus is rapidly progressive, in the hope of preventing further brain damage.

Craniorachischisis

This heading covers a range of malformations varying from *anencephaly*, which is incompatible with life, to *spina bifida occulta* which causes no symptoms and may be discovered accidentally on routine x-ray of the sacral spine. In between lie a variety of neural tube defects. These include *spina bifida cystica* in which a meningocoele or a meningomyelocoele may be present, and which may be associated with the *Arnold–Chiari* malformation which is characterized by herniation of parts of the medulla and cerebellum through the foramen magnum and also with *congenital hydrocephalus* and a number of other deformities. There has been a regrettable tendency in recent years to perform reconstructive operations on patients with severe spina bifida. Although these may prolong life, most of the patients grow up nonetheless to be severely mentally handicapped.

Of greater and more recent interest is the discovery that severe neural tube defects can be discovered before birth by the presence in the serum and in the amniotic fluid of an excess of alpha fetoprotein. Such antenatal diagnosis has possibilities for prevention (see p. 322).

Syphilis

Congenital syphilitics often do not present external evidence of syphilis, although signs of infection (teeth, keratitis, deafness) may develop later.

The condition may be suspected where there is a history of parental syphilis or of snuffles and rashes in the infant. Serological tests are not always positive. Syphilitic subnormals are rarely well developed and mental backwardness is soon apparent. *Juvenile general paralysis* may develop at puberty or in early adult life. Unfortunately the results of antisyphilitic treatment, even when begun early, are disappointing. In view of this, diagnosis and treatment of the mother's condition during pregnancy should be the main aim.

Intrauterine infections and other hazards

Rubella. Virus infections, especially *rubella*, contracted by the mother during the first three months of pregnancy may give rise to deaf-mutism, cataracts, heart malformations and mental handicap in the infant. An expanded rubella syndrome including thrombocytopenia, hepatosplenomegaly and translucency of long bones has been described in a major outbreak in the United States. Bradford Hill considered the fetal risk from rubella to be related to the time of infection—50 per cent in the first month, 25 per cent in the second, and 17 per cent in the third month of pregnancy. Inoculation of girls between 11 and 14 years of age with live rubella vaccine holds out good hope for a further reduction in the incidence of this antenatal hazard.

Toxoplasmosis. This is a protozoal infection which may be transmitted from mother to child, either during pregnancy or in the early stages of neonatal life. The clinical picture in the infant includes subnormality of intelligence, chorioretinitis, miliary intracranial calcification and, sometimes, slight anomalies in brain size. Its incidence is reported to be increasing in Western societies.

Cytomegalovirus. This, which is the commonest fetal infection, may, when congenitally acquired, give rise to hepatosplenomegaly, jaundice, purpura and microcephaly, together with cerebral calcification and chorioretinitis. However, in many cases, infection by the virus is unaccompanied by abnormalities commonly ascribed to it. The clinical manifestations which do occur commonly involve the central nervous system and include blindness, deafness, hypotonia or spastic quadriplegia. The range of mental handicap varies from a minimal degree of abnormality to a non-communicative vegetative state.

Certain chemical substances may damage the fetus, particularly if these have been unsuccessfully used as abortifacients or as contraceptives such as ergot, quinine and aminopterin. The thalidomide tragedy, in which *phocomelia* was the leading sign, further emphasizes the dangers inherent in the administration of certain drugs during early pregnancy.

Lead poisoning. If ultimately established as one of the more widespread causes of mental handicap, *lead* is likely to prove to be a *secondary* or *postnatal* cause affecting the intellectual growth of infants and young children. There is much current argument about the source of high blood-lead levels in these age groups and of the effects of this. While no one now doubts the danger of lead paint, there is argument about the part played by atmospheric lead derived from motor vehicle exhausts, especially among children living in urban areas where traffic is at its heaviest. Tap water contaminated by lead pipes in old houses may be another important source of raised blood-lead levels.

Inflammatory processes

Meningitis and encephalitis in infancy and childhood may be followed by arrest of mental development. Spasticity, epilepsy and hydrocephalus were formerly common sequelae to *pyogenic meningitis*, but antibiotics have very considerably reduced these mental and physical complications. *Tuberculous meningitis* requires very early diagnosis and treatment to minimize psychological sequelae. Modern antibacterial treatment may produce almost complete recovery, but only providing it is begun before the child becomes unconscious. In more advanced cases, some intellectual retardation and neurological damage may be relieved by the early surgical treatment of obstructive hydrocephalus. Personality changes are common following *encephalitis lethargica*.

Epilepsy

A well-marked association exists between major epilepsy and mental handicap, probably because underlying brain lesions commonly predispose to convulsions. Sometimes, reduced intelligence and epilepsy are both due to a common cause, such as meningitis or brain injury. In other cases, epilepsy complicates primary subnormality, and in yet another small group of cases, mental handicap may apparently be produced entirely by epilepsy which recurs in spite of treatment, in some cases giving rise to cerebral anoxia due to uncontrolled *status epilepticus* in infancy. Mentally handicapped epileptics are often stubborn, irritable and prone to outbursts of aggressive behaviour (also see Chapter 10).

Hypsarrhythmia. This causes infantile spasms (*salaam* attacks) which begin shortly after birth and consist of sudden convulsive bending forward from the waist often with arms spread out, during which unconsciousness occurs. *Grand mal* attacks may occur later. The EEG is pathognomic, showing a grossly disorganized recording and widespread epileptic activity. The condition is usually progressive with increasing brain damage, possibly arrested in some cases by ACTH.

Sensory deprivation (isolation oligophrenia)

Acute infections, trauma, haemorrhage or genetic predisposition may give rise to loss of the use of one or more of the special senses, especially sight and hearing. The brain is then cut off, to a greater or lesser degree, from environmental stimuli and, in consequence, may suffer a lack of development.

Children unable to hear high-frequency sounds which are important for the proper development of speech are also likely to suffer in their educational progress. Although of average or above average intelligence, they may develop defects of articulation and appear backward at school, although they are not deaf in the ordinary sense. Antisocial conduct, as a form of unconscious compensation, may occur. In the absence of adequate audiometric screening and extensive psychometric investigation, therefore, these children may be regarded as maladjusted or even as mentally handicapped. Considerable therapeutic help is now available in the form of specially adapted hearing aids, speech therapy and modified educational curricula. The celebrated cases of Laura Bridgeman and Helen Keller demonstrate how much can be achieved by special care and training. Most progressive local education authorities now initially identify suspect children by group audiometry, and subsequently determine the exact degree of disability by serial audiometric and specialist examination of individual pupils.

Examination of cases of mental handicap

An approximate idea of the mental development of a schoolchild may be obtained by ascertaining the standard reached and by asking him to read, write and to answer questions in mental arithmetic. A more accurate result may be forthcoming through the measure of one area of achievement, such as verbal development, where he is asked to name and describe objects, name colours, carry out commands and to define short words which are in common use. However, such tests cover only limited areas of intelligence and are often markedly affected by other factors such as physical illness, high-frequency deafness, unhappy home life and truancy.

To overcome this problem, various standardized tests of intelligence have been devised, based upon both verbal and non-verbal responses. Some batteries include examples of both types of response with an overall bias towards the verbal type. Chief among these are the Terman-Merrill revision of the Stanford–Binet series and the Wechsler tests. Examples of non-verbal tests are Alexander's Passalong, Kohs' Blocks, Porteus Mazes and Raven's Matrices, the last two being non-manipulative rather than involving performance in construction. When all the rules of application are obeyed, such tests may give a worthwhile assessment of the subject's mental ability, and may indicate particular weaknesses which have an influence upon his achievement.

To assess how far scholastic achievement measures up to innate ability and as a guide to learning problems, tests involving the use of the three 'Rs' also should be given, such as Burt's or Schonell's tests. Reading should always be measured in terms of comprehension. All mental tests have their critics and while it is generally agreed that Wechsler is superior to the Stanford–Binet for use with mentally handicapped adults, recently even the former has been criticized in respect of its validity.

The *intelligence quotient* is the ratio of the *mental* to the *real* age of the child, expressed as a percentage. For example, a child of 10 with a mental age of 5, has an intelligence quotient (IQ) of 5/10 × 100 = 50. If the chronological age is 16 or over, the denominator, in all cases, is taken as 16 in making the calculation. In the third revision (1960; composite form 'L' and 'M') of the Stanford–Binet test, the denominator was raised to 18 years. In approximate terms, those with lesser grades of mental handicap have an IQ of 50 to 75, and those severely handicapped one of under 50. It should be remembered, however, that an IQ is only one relatively minor aspect of total personality and that temperamental and emotional factors must always be taken into account when making a diagnosis.

Diagnosis of mental handicap

Whereas mental handicap may be first encountered at any age, the possibility is raised most commonly during infancy, school life, or in the immediate postschool years.

Infants

The techniques advocated by Illingworth for developmental assessment in infancy should be studied by everyone with an interest in this aspect of diagnosis. Where mental handicap is present at birth, the child is backward in all fields of development. Children who fall victims to some intercurrent hazard after a period of normal growth, develop signs consistent with interruption of, or regression from, the developmental stage already reached. Possible signs of mental retardation include lack of interest and concentration, lateness in smiling, taking notice, following with eyes, response to sound and chewing, together with persistence of slobbering, taking objects into the mouth, reciprocal kick and hand regard. Illingworth also emphasized the importance of serial measurements of skull circumference which, in comparison with norms, give early indication of microcephaly or macrocephaly.

It is essential to carry out a thorough overhaul to exclude systematic conditions including malnutrition, avitaminosis, haemopoietic disease, otitis, tuberculosis, inflammations of the central nervous system, alimentary disorders and subclinical hypothyroidism. Radiographic examination of the skull and long bones, urinary examination for reducing substances and chromatography may prove invaluable aids to diagnosis, but even following the most thorough examination, the diagnosis of mental handicap in infancy is not always easy, and the value of intellectual findings may be difficult to evaluate from the point of view of prognosis.

Schoolchildren

Mental handicap may be suspected where there is a history of failure to maintain satisfactory progress from the time of admission to school, irrespective of whether there is also a superimposed behaviour problem. Handicap of varying degree *may be* the result of physical ill-health, special sense defects, emotional instability, irregular attendance, frequent changes of domicile, faulty parental management or adverse parent– or teacher–child relationships. Scholastic backwardness and inefficiency in themselves must be distinguished from true mental handicap. Problems of this kind require active collaboration between psychiatrist, paediatrician and psychologist for their proper elucidation; thus, before any child is recommended for a special school, his case should be reviewed by a psychiatrist with a special interest in such matters.

Adults

The diagnosis of mental handicap presents little difficulty in the case of severely affected patients, or in those whose physical make-up gives evidence of some clinical syndrome, such as Down's syndrome. With minimally affected subjects, the position is entirely different and doubts may arise in respect of the contribution to aetiology of any superadded, or even underlying mental illness.

Mental handicap may, however, be suspected when a patient, in the absence of serious physical disability, or of mental deterioration due to schizophrenia, juvenile taboparesis or some demyelinating disease, regularly displays a poor record of economic efficiency and drifts from job to job. Some males come under notice for the first time on account of criminality, being less capable of evading detection than their more intelligent peers. The Mental Health Act of 1959 made it clear that promiscuity, or other immoral conduct *alone*, should not be construed as implying that a person should be dealt with under the Act as suffering from any form of mental disorder. Nevertheless, amongst women the frequent bearing of illegitimate children and prostitution may call for an examination of mental development, and also of other personality factors. Mentally handicapped persons are not immune from depressive and paranoid episodes, which often appear as reactions to some easily detected special stress. They are also prone to persistent hypochondriacal symptoms. In marginal cases, diagnosis is supported by evidence of retarded mental development and by a poor scholastic record.

In addition to an accurate assessment of intelligence, the following procedures should be adopted in each case.

1. Consider factors other than those which are purely cognitive, so

providing a broader estimate of the individual's personality, for example his emotional stability and drive.

2. Assess his personality in relation to the environmental background, which must contain facts from the past as well as from the present, for example what use has he made of his scholastic and work opportunities and how much has his culture contributed? Records from the local health and welfare authorities are invaluable in this respect.

3. Review his state of health and physical development. What has either of these factors contributed to scholastic deprivation, to poor work record or to any antisocial behaviour?

4. Exclude rare sensory defects, such as high-frequency deafness or defects in colour vision.

5. Consider the effect of any psychosomatic variables, such as those due to drugs, epilepsy, cerebral disasters and subclinical hypothyroidism.

A diagnosis of mental handicap or mental impairment is justified only when the findings indicate, beyond any reasonable doubt, that the individual conforms to the requirements of the definitions laid down in the Mental Health Act.

Treatment

The Royal Commission on the Law relating to Mental Illness and Mental Deficiency (1957) advocated 'a reorientation of the Mental Health Services towards Community Care and away from Hospital Care, except where the special facilities of the hospital service are needed'.

In the case of mentally handicapped individuals, treatment and training are not synonymous, but are complementary in their application. Local authorities have wide powers and responsibilities in connection with the care and aftercare of handicapped people, principal among which are the provision of educational establishments such as adult training centres, courses at colleges of further education, work orientation and work experience schemes, non-vocational courses, sheltered employment and sheltered work groups in open industry. The establishment of activity community programmes such as these is considerably reducing the population of hospitals and helping health authorities better to fulfil their specialized function: namely, the provision of an adequate service with sufficient beds and other facilities. In this respect and having regard to the notion that hospitals, in future, should not be regarded as a necessary long-term provision for any mentally handicapped person and should instead, provide specialized facilities for those who cannot either temporarily or permanently live elsewhere, the services provided should include the following.

1. Nursing care for those in need.

2. Active treatment for mentally handicapped persons whose condition is complicated by psychotic or personality breakdown, and training for those requiring in-patient care.

3. The provision of short-term care, either in hospital or local authority hostels, thus allowing families who normally care for their mentally handicapped relatives to go on holiday every now and then.

4. Day hospital and other day-care facilities as and where required on account of psychiatric state or social circumstances.

5. Establishment of out-patient clinics for preliminary diagnosis, community treatment and counselling. Such treatment should be carried out in cooperation with other specialists and with general practitioners. Counselling may be family and social in type, or genetic in respect of the index case and the prospects of pathology in any future children.

6. Promotion of research.

Adults

All progressive hospitals, other residential accommodation and day services for the mentally handicapped should offer an extensive variety of therapeutic facilities. These need to be graded according to the age, physical state, mental level, stability and interest of the patients, and should include occupational, social and industrial therapy, general and special domestic training, home management, applied civics, further education for late-maturing adults, and training in a variety of pursuits suitable to the case of those patients who may have industrial potential in sheltered employment. Physical training may be useful in developing physique and in promoting group cooperation. Physiotherapy, orthopaedic surgery and speech therapy often produce worthwhile results. Social clubs, especially those democratically conducted by the members themselves, are of value, together with 'Outward Bound' movements aimed at providing experience in group relationships with a high standard of social conduct, and in appreciation of the attitudes and feelings of others. Discussion sessions, in which patients and staff take part, can serve a familiar purpose. Mixing the sexes both socially and at work should be encouraged within the limitations of supervisory responsibility. Swimming and other outdoor sports are also of use in promoting social contacts.

Likewise, a psychiatrically orientated rehabilitation programme consisting of medical and training elements should be drawn up and modified from time to time in the light of individual needs. In this, emphasis placed upon the inculcation of satisfactory work habits, self-discipline, standards of conduct and social 'know-how' is likely to be of greater use than the acquisition of specific skills.

For long-stay hospital patients who, for a variety of reasons, cannot be returned to the community, the object should be to provide as happy and as full a life as is possible. In the case of very severely handicapped adults, who may be incapable of the simplest tasks, the major emphasis should be upon protective care, feeding, toileting and habit training. Good results have been obtained in resocialization with groups of manageable proportions, and where staffing ratios permit repetitive application.

Children

By statutory enactment, all children, irrespective of their degree of handicap, are now the teaching responsibility of the education authority. This applies whether the child remains in the community, attends a special residential school, or is admitted to hospital in pursuance of his particular needs. Decisions of the last kind will be based upon psychiatric, medical or nursing requirements, and education within the hospital will be supplementary to such basic therapeutic demands. This administrative change has now re-integrated hospital teachers with the mainstream of educational practice and, at the same time, ensured that the pupils concerned have the advantage of modern techniques in teaching practice.

Mentally handicapped children require constant stimulation to promote their maximum possible development and encouragement should be given freely in response to constructive effort. The general aim should be directed towards the *socialization* of the child, this being attempted by providing creative outlets which are stimulating to his imagination and to his intelligence. While academic subjects are of secondary importance, those children who are capable of benefiting should receive instruction in the three 'Rs'. Efforts should be made to ensure, as far as may be possible, that comprehension of meaning keeps pace with the ability to read mechanically. Practical examples are necessary in teaching a child to handle money and to perform simple calculations. The acquisition of the three 'Rs' should be utilitarian in purpose with the object of providing a small number of visual clues which promote the patient's ability to write his name, produce a simple message, handle money, read notices of social importance (such as 'Danger', 'Keep out', 'Toilet') and the understanding of transport destinations. The skilled teacher will avoid making the mentally handicapped child unduly anxious, by ensuring that the curriculum is broadly based and that it provides elements variable in proportion to the needs of the pupil concerned, such as music, plasticine modelling, eurhythmics, handwork, nature study, free and controlled play, listening to the radio, story-telling, painting and drawing and so on. It may be necessary to try several forms of occupation until something is found in which the child takes an interest, or for which he displays some aptitude.

Prevention

Throughout this chapter certain possibilities for prevention of mental handicap have been mentioned. Although so far these are not very great, there clearly have been advances and with the passage of time there are likely to be many more.

Primary prevention includes such procedures as inoculating schoolgirls against rubella and diagnosing and treating syphilis in mothers at an early stage of pregnancy.

Secondary prevention is exemplified by termination of pregnancy in those women who, following amniocentesis, can be shown to be bearing a child with Down's syndrome, Tay–Sachs' disease or one having a severe neural tube defect. In the case of the former, amniocentesis is indicated in those who have already borne one mongol child and where either parent can be shown to be a carrier of the translocation defect or, even more rarely, to be chromosomally mosaic. A defect in the unborn child may be revealed by chromosomal examination of the amniotic fluid.

Neural tube defects are particularly likely to occur in children born to a mother who has already given birth to an anencephalic fetus. A raised alpha-fetoprotein in the amniotic fluid may be indicative of a fetus having spina bifida cystica or some allied deformity. Because the serum alpha-fetoprotein is also raised, the possibility of screening all pregnant women is currently being considered, it having been suggested that those in which it is raised should be subjected to amniocentesis. However, there are difficulties. Amniocentesis is not without risk to the fetus and, furthermore, neural tube defects are not alone in causing a raised alpha-fetoprotein which can be due, for example, to normal twin pregnancy. For this reason ultrasonic screening is also required, but this facility is not yet universally available.

Other forms of secondary prevention include the early identification of infantile hypothyroidism (possibly by placental blood), phenylketonuria, galactosaemia and certain other inborn errors of metabolism which may be corrected by early treatment. No doubt, and as more becomes known, other such disorders will also be shown to be treatable and mental handicap thereby prevented.

Further reading

Heaton-Ward, A. W. (1975) *Mental Subnormality*. Bristol: John Wright.
Reid, A. H. (1982) *The Psychiatry of Mental Handicaps*. Oxford: Blackwell Scientific.

22

Treatment I: Psychological

In the next three chapters, psychological, social and physical aspects of treatment are considered. These distinctions, while arbitrary, are a convenience. Many patients will require all three: thus a person requiring antidepressant drug treatment will also need attention to social and psychological considerations. Similarly, while psychotropic drugs may be used in conjunction with psychotherapy, attention to social relationships, work problems and difficulties at home are nearly always important, whatever the condition being treated.

A primary consideration in psychological methods of treatment, unlike surgery or pharmacotherapy, is that the patients' own psyche is both the recipient of therapeutic endeavour and also an agent in carrying this out. The patient can never be merely a recipient, but must always contribute to change, it being important to give him insight as to how he can change himself and some confidence that this is possible. This can be achieved by helping him see that small successes in daily living are possible and that these can be built on to make progress in more difficult areas of life. Patterns of behaviour can be shown to be comprised of constituent parts and, if attention is given to these, behaviour can be changed.

Deciding what are appropriate goals of treatment is not always easy. In psychiatry there are few physical signs against which to gauge efficacy. Subjective improvement described by the patient is not always reliable and is difficult to quantify. The aims of treatment are to relieve specific symptoms, to produce an overall improvement in the patient's condition and to optimize the capacity for independent action despite residual disability.

Most important in any type of psychological treatment are the personal qualities of the therapist. His skill and training should determine how complex are the cases which he takes on for treatment. While some are intrinsically helpful in personal relationships, they are, without further training, unlikely to be able to judge the limitations for improvement in a particular patient and are ignorant of the potential damage they may do. A satisfactory knowledge of psychiatry is important for the therapist in order for him to avoid using psychological methods when these are not indicated. While intensive training in a particular technique of psychotherapy is very valuable, there seems to be some movement towards the position where ideally a therapist will use different techniques according to the differing symptoms and needs of his patients.

Where the characteristics of effective therapists have been studied, such qualities as *non-possessive warmth*, a capacity for *empathy*, and *genuineness* have been found to be valuable. It is possible that such qualities can to a certain extent be cultivated. Those involved in psychological treatment—nurses, occupational therapists, trainee psychiatrists, etc.—will inevitably become role models to their patients, so that the latter will tend to imitate their behaviour and fantasize about their private lives. As this situation cannot altogether be avoided, modelling must be recognized and used as an aspect of treatment; clearly this has important implications for the recruitment of staff. Thus in the selection or self-selection of those undertaking psychotherapy, those who become involved with patients in order to solve their own problems should be excluded; they are likely to become overinvolved and more destructive than helpful.

General principles of psychological management

Inevitably, the doctor will need to give some direction as to what is the likely goal of treatment. He cannot be completely *non-directive*. At the same time it is important for patient and doctor to agree on what is possible and therefore what is worth aiming at; a treatment contract should be established which may even be worth putting in writing. Considerable attention should also be paid to helping patients develop methods of coping, for often during the course of a psychiatric illness *demoralization* occurs in which the patient may feel he cannot handle problems which others expect him to. This tends to increase lack of self-esteem and feelings of alienation from others. Treatment should, therefore, concentrate upon goals which are well within a patient's capacity to achieve whilst supported by his therapist, so that he learns that more of his behaviour than he previously believed possible is actually under his own control.

Insight is important in that a patient needs to see how his *problem* relates to other aspects of his behaviour or personality. He also needs to realize how other people respond and how this affects his relationships. Arising from this, he may be able to take on new attitudes and change his behaviour, although in practice behaviour change may have to precede change of attitude.

A general principle of treatment is to help a patient gain insight and relief from symptoms while avoiding *collusion* and *confrontation*. A patient showing *illness behaviour* with physical symptoms resulting from a psychological cause usually wishes to believe that the cause of his condition is physical. In treatment this belief must be resisted in such a way that he does not feel rejected. While there are times when confrontation is helpful, it may be best avoided whilst the therapeutic relationship is being established. A vital part of psychological treatment is the need for patients to *internalize*, to make the effects of treatment their own by repeated practice of what they have learnt between treatment sessions. A large part, for example, of the value of behaviour therapy accrues from such practice.

Psychotherapy

Psychotherapy in the widest sense is the basis of all psychiatric treatment and certainly, in one form or another, the oldest. Psychological measures also play a profound part in the treatment of many physical disorders whether deliberately or unconsciously applied. The manner in which a drug is prescribed and administered in part determines its efficacy. The more non-specific the remedy, the more likely is this to be true. The same may be said of many other treatment procedures. Religious and magical healing appear to depend on psychotherapeutic processes for their efficacy. Three essential features stand out.

The first is the *relationship* between the patient, the client, or the analysand (the name varying according to the situation in which the relationship is established) and the doctor, social worker, priest, healer or psychotherapist.

The second is *insight*. Arising out of the relationships with the therapist, the patient arrives at a fresh understanding of how he got into his present difficulties, how he himself played a part in producing his own problems, how his personality tends to determine his behaviour, and how other people react to him. He may not make all these discoveries at once; enlightenment may only dawn very slowly and even then he may not be able to put it into words. However, to be beneficial insight must be more than intellectual; the patient must understand how his emotions and will are involved. *Knowing* must be accompanied by *feeling*. Indeed, of the two, the latter is much the more important. It is for this reason, perhaps, that some of the forms of rational psychotherapy in vogue during the last century and even up to a few decades ago—moral treatment, explanation, persuasion and re-education—met only with very limited success.

The third stage is *incorporation*. It is not enough that the patient relates well to his therapist and begins to understand how his symptoms developed; he also needs to learn how to develop more appropriate behaviour, both during therapeutic sessions and between, so that this becomes an intrinsic part of himself. Whether the theoretical basis of treatment is psychodynamic, cognitive or behavioural, such incorporation is essential.

It is often asked whether psychotherapy really works; one of the problems being the extreme difficulty of carrying out adequately controlled studies which might demonstrate its efficacy or otherwise. There are many who clearly think that it is effective, otherwise so many hours would not be spent on its practice. Although perhaps no confidently expressed opinion of the matter can yet be given, what can be said is that even if psychotherapy does not cure, at least it comforts.

Hypnosis

Hypnosis, a special technique producing heightened suggestibility, has had a long history though it has waxed and waned in popularity. More recently, it has found favour both as a method of treatment and as a research tool. Although its application in treatment of psychiatric disorders is not wide, it is sometimes of value when applied early in certain hysterical states such as paralyses, aphonias and amnesias following psychological trauma. However, it is *unwise* to apply hypnosis to the mere removal of symptoms, without a thorough prior exploration leading to some knowledge of their cause. Failing this, at best the effect may be temporary only, with a return of symptoms in the same or other form; at worst, the patient, deprived of his defences and unable to cope with his basic problem may become severely depressed, even suicidal. Most authorities regard hypnosis as useless in obsessional states and in those with psychotic disorders who, in any event, are difficult if not impossible to hypnotize.

Hypnosis is, perhaps, most useful in certain psychosomatic states, such as skin conditions, in which it may be effective in controlling itching, and in gastrointestinal and other disorders where relief of emotional tension may be of benefit. Hypnosis can also be used in chronic painful conditions, even when these are due to some demonstrably organic cause. It may also be used to considerable effect to induce relaxation before and during parturition. Adequate training for this can be given in the antenatal clinic where group hypnosis can be applied to save time. This technique has more uses for conditions that are not psychiatric in nature than in psychiatry, for example in dentistry or for burns dressings.

Some favour *hypnoanalysis* during the course of psychotherapy to uncover material which is repressed in the fully conscious state. This method was originally used by Breuer and Freud, though later abandoned in favour of *free association*. In suitable subjects the induction of hypnosis does not present undue difficulty providing both patient and doctor have confidence in the procedure. For details of the technique, special manuals on the subject should be consulted. Lesser forms of relaxation, not amounting to deep hypnosis, are extremely useful in *anxiety control training*. In *autogenic training*, the patient is taught how to produce relaxation for himself. An important part of such treatment is the practice that takes place between therapy sessions.

Psychoanalysis

Psychoanalysis as a method of treatment embodies techniques designed to explore, to interpret and in due course to modify unconscious mental processes which may have given rise to symptoms or to abnormal behaviour. Psychoanalysis makes considerable use of *free association*, as well as *dream interpretation* and the use of other material derived as much from fantasy as from fact. An important part of the procedure is dealing with *unconscious resistances* and in interpreting *transference* relationships towards the analyst. The ultimate aim of psychoanalysis is not only to give the patient insight into his problems and to free him from his emotional entanglement with these, but also to release him from any dependence he may develop towards the analyst or that which he may already have towards other authoritative or overprotecting persons so that he is able to feel on terms of equality with them and to conduct his life according to an ideal or model without any sense of inferiority. It is also concerned with the way a person preserves the present state of equilibrium using *ego-defence* mechanisms such as *projection* or *denial*.

One difficulty about psychoanalysis as a method of treatment is that it is extremely time consuming both for analyst and patient. Orthodox psychoanalysis may take up to five hours weekly and be of several years' duration. Because of this, economic considerations, both of time and money, may be of paramount importance. In any event, by no means all patients are suitable for this form of treatment, the principal criteria being that the patient must be reasonably young (preferably less than 40–45 years of age), of at least average or higher intelligence, strongly motivated and of good ego strength. Opinions vary as to the types of condition best suited to psychoanalytic therapy. Whereas most authorities seem to be agreed that patients with emotional and personality disorders do best, success or not may well be determined more by the personality of the patient than by primary diagnostic considerations.

Brief psychotherapy

Brief psychotherapy derives from psychoanalysis in that it utilizes many of its theoretical concepts. In an attempt to cut short the procedure, the classical technique and use of the couch is, however, abandoned, and therapy is usually carried out face to face for periods varying from 30 to 50 minutes, two or three times weekly and for a period of three months or so. It is sometimes thought appropriate to put at least a provisional limit on the duration of treatment before this is begun. Much greater use is made of interpretation almost from the very beginning and the rapid analysis of transference relationships as these arise and alter. As will be gathered, the therapist plays a very much more active role in this form of treatment than in orthodox psychoanalysis.

Brief psychotherapy on analytic–interpretative lines has obvious advantages in that it can be made available for a much larger number of patients. Also, if it proves unsuccessful, much less time and effort are wasted. It can furthermore be used as a test procedure to help determine the suitability of a patient for subsequent psychoanalysis.

Group psychotherapy

Man is a social species who lives in families, works with others and often finds recreation in companionable ways. Because relationships are often the primary basis of psychological symptoms, group therapy is particularly useful where symptoms manifest themselves in a social setting. Also, because individual therapy is very expensive of time and money, group treatment of about eight people may commend itself as economical. A session of treatment lasts about one-and-a-half hours and may take place once or twice a week.

Various insights can be learnt and more appropriate patterns of behaviour may be better rehearsed in a group setting. A group member learning how others react to one another may be helped to understand how natural *groups* such as his family interact. In seeing other patients resolve their difficulties, he begins to learn how improvement can occur and how his own involvement is necessary. While some patients are unable to benefit from group therapy, many do surprisingly well, often better than in individual therapy, in the course of which transference relationships and dependency problems may impede progress. Some patients, however, benefit from group therapy after first undergoing a short period of individual treatment; others may start in a group immediately following initial diagnostic assessment. Groups may be open, receiving new members and discharging those improved as appropriate, or closed in which all the members start, continue and finish in treatment together. The composition of the groups requires considerable care; mixed sex groups of roughly equal proportions are said to do best.

Group therapy is particularly suitable for those suffering from emotional or personality disorders. Those who are depressed are often unsuitable, but some not too deteriorated schizophrenic patients may benefit. It is important to realize that, like other potent forms of treatment, groups can be harmful as well as beneficial if used for the wrong patient or conducted with an inappropriate style of leadership.

Often therapeutic groups are too verbal and intellectual to suit the majority of patients referred by family doctors. A combination of group therapy technique with role playing or *psychodrama* is sometimes helpful. Here the members of the group take a situation of conflict for one of them and role play the drama by representing the characters involved and trying to explore their probable states of mind. Insight may be more readily achieved in this setting than in an orthodox group.

Family therapy

Family therapy is based on the observation that the patient who presents for treatment is not necessarily the most disturbed member of the family from which he comes. Indeed, when a family constellation is thoroughly explored, it may be perceived that the patient has, in effect, become a 'whipping-boy' and that the emotional stability of one or more of the other family members is only preserved at his expense. It is, in fact, axiomatic that no psychiatric patient can be successfully studied *in vacuo*. If treatment, therefore, is to be effective, it may be necessary to involve the family as a whole, or at least those amongst whom there is a significant disturbance of interpersonal relationships.

Following an analysis of processes and interactions when the whole family is together, a family *taken as a whole* may be considered to be *healthy* or, indeed, merely getting them together, either in the consulting room or at home, often indicates only too clearly where the trouble really lies and allows the application of a better remedy than can be offered to the 'patient' alone. As the technique of handling a family group is difficult and demands much tact and skill, it is often beneficial to have more than one member of staff involved (co-therapist).

Joint marital therapy

As with family therapy, dealing with two marital partners together may produce better results. While one or other is likely to be referred initially as *the patient*, it is important to interview the other to corroborate the story, assess the conflicts within the marriage, find out how the spouse evaluates the patient, assess the personality and resources of the spouse, and following this decide upon a treatment plan taking both partners into account.

In some cases the best plan may be for the therapist to see husband and wife together; in others it may be preferable to involve a second therapist so that neither partner feels that he or she is under attack from an alliance of his/her spouse and therapist. Joint interviews are only likely to be successful when both parties wish to make the marriage work and are prepared to make some concessions. If one or both partners intend to separate, joint interviews are unlikely to be beneficial, although here there may be a need for supportive psychotherapy for the partner who does not wish the marriage to end. Such therapy may be invaluable in helping a patient through an acute crisis such as the break-up of marriage. The *ego defences* the patient uses, rather than being challenged as might occur in psychoanalysis, are accepted and used to maintain feelings of self-esteem. A danger of such treatment is that it may reinforce the patient in his position of being a patient and therefore *sick*, rather than encouraging a more positive attitude to treatment aimed at recovery from the underlying causes of disability.

Supportive psychotherapy

Psychotherapy which is palliative rather than analytically orientated is usually referred to as supportive. Thus many anxious persons and other patients with abnormal personality reactions, especially those who consult their doctors on account of somatic symptoms of emotional origin, can often be helped by relatively few and often infrequent psychotherapeutic interviews. Once a preliminary examination has been completed, the patient may be given an opportunity to talk about himself and his problems rather than about his bodily discomforts. Under informal conditions a patient may feel more inclined to get matters 'off his chest', with considerable relief. The art of being a good listener is essential for success in psychotherapy.

Behaviour therapy

Behaviour therapy includes several varieties of treatment, some of which actually have a very long history although they have begun to gain some degree of scientific respectability only relatively recently. The principles underlying modern behaviour therapy techniques are largely based on learning theory. Treatment is aimed at the removal of symptoms rather than at their underlying cause, the symptom being regarded as an inadvertently conditioned *response* which may be removed by appropriate learning. Long-established techniques of common-sense learning have been systematized to produce improved treatment results. Behavioural modification has the great advantage of being less demanding of time than analytic forms of treatment.

The following are some of the main behaviour therapy techniques in current use.

Desensitization (reciprocal inhibition). The basis of desensitization is Wolpe's deduction that anxiety aroused by a specific anxiety-producing situation can be suppressed by the simultaneous evocation of other physiologically antagonistic responses. In essence, the procedure involves training in progressive relaxation to a point where presentation of the anxiety-producing stimulus or imagining it ceases to arouse anxiety. This is achieved by constructing a hierarchy which grades, from the least to the most disturbing, those stimuli or circumstances which cause the patient to become increasingly anxious. Either using imagery or in a real-life situation, the patient starts at the bottom and, as he becomes able during each session to overcome his anxiety at each step of the hierarchy, he progresses gradually up the scale. The treatment appears to be particularly successful in monophobic states and less so where phobic anxiety is more diffuse, as in agoraphobia.

Operant conditioning is a term introduced by Skinner. It involves the systematic manipulation of environmental events to produce desired objectives by the skilled use of reinforcement. The subject's behaviour is altered by the use of contingencies, for example social praise of a desirable action on the part of the subject is likely to result in the repetition of that act. The principles of operant conditioning have been successfully applied to the rehabilitation of the chronically mentally ill and in training the mentally handicapped.

Flooding involves the exposure of the patient to the phobic situation in full force until he feels anxious no longer. For agoraphobia it is both more effective and quicker than desensitization. The patient will be taken by the therapist into the most anxiety-provoking situation, for instance a supermarket, and they remain there until the patient's anxiety subsides. While it may be a quick and effective method of treatment in those patients who feel able to cooperate, in others it may be contraindicated because of the painfully high level of anxiety evoked.

Aversion therapy is a technique whereby a subject is adversely conditioned to a situation to which he is attracted but would prefer to be able to avoid. Considerable success has been claimed for the method in the treatment of sexual deviations such as fetishism or transvestism. Basically, the method consists of getting the patient to indulge in either fact or fantasy in the deviant behaviour of his choice while at the same time administering a series of unpleasant stimuli, usually in the form of electric shocks. Some degree of automation of the process appears possible.

Response prevention has been used with success in patients with obsessive–compulsive symptoms. For example, a ritual hand-washer is prevented from washing his hands for increasingly long intervals after carrying out activity which he regards as contaminating. Anxiety gradually subsides although initially it is intense.

Social skills training uses behavioural modification to improve functioning of socially phobic patients. It is best carried out in a group with reinforcement, usually in the form of approval from other group members, being given for successful behaviour in improving relationships or with specific social tasks.

Token economy is a method of behaviour therapy used, for example, in long-stay psychiatric wards in order to modify antisocial behaviour. Approved forms of behaviour (such as getting out of bed in the morning at a prescribed time) are rewarded immediately with tokens which can later be exchanged for goods (money, bars of chocolate) or privileges.

Behaviour therapy of one sort or another may also be of value in the treatment of non-organic tics and habit spasms, stuttering, some cases of impotence and frigidity and experimentally in a wide variety of other conditions.

Biofeedback is a technique whereby subjects are taught to control physiological responses either mediated by the voluntary or the autonomic nervous system. Specially designed electronic apparatus is used to give the subject information he can use about certain of his bodily reactions. The method is still very much in its experimental stages and awaits evaluation of its clinical application. There appears to be some evidence of the effectiveness of the method in the treatment of migraine and possibly hypertension also, although in the latter condition the results obtained appear to be transient.

Further reading

Balint, M. & Balint, E. (1961) *Psychotherapeutic Techniques*. London: Tavistock.

Bloch, S. (ed.) (1979) *An Introduction to the Psychotherapies*. London: Oxford University Press.

Eysenck, H. J. (ed.) (1976) *Case Studies in Behaviour Therapy*. London: Routledge & Kegan Paul.

Foulkes, S. H. & Anthony, E. J. (1973) *Group Psychotherapy*. Harmondsworth: Penguin.

Malan, D. H. (1963) *A Study of Brief Psychotherapy*. London: Tavistock.

Rachman, S. (1971) *The Effects of Psychotherapy*. Oxford: Pergamon.

Storr, A. (1979) *The Art of Psychotherapy*. London: Secker & Warburg.

23

Treatment II: Social

Britain's most distinctive contribution to the care of the mentally ill has
been in the development of *social psychiatry*, starting at the beginning of
the nineteenth century with the humane practices of the four generations
of Tukes at the York Retreat and culminating with the provision for
psychiatric patients by the National Health Service. *Moral* methods of
treating insanity include careful attention to environmental factors and
the establishment of a *therapeutic milieu*. In mental hospitals there has
been continuing advancement towards liberal and more humane
management and, since World War II, a much greater part played by the
social services. This has been facilitated by a number of significant pieces
of legislation such as the National Health Service Act 1946; the Mental
Health Act 1959 (recently revised); and the Local Authority Social
Services Act 1970. *Mental disorder*, as defined in the Mental Health Act
1959, includes mental illness, handicap and certain inadequate and
aggressive behaviour disorders considered to be amenable to medical
treatment and designated as 'psychopathic disorder'.

It should be noted that the distinctions drawn between the *medical* and
social aspects of psychiatry are more apparent in theory than in practice
and that there is much overlap.

The statutory health and social services

By operation of the National Health Service Act 1946, a mentally ill
person, in his capacity as a citizen, is entitled to a general practitioner
service, a hospital in-, out-, and day-patient service and, under certain
conditions, a consultant domiciliary service. Also, where need is shown,
he is entitled to other services from his local health authority, such as
ambulance, home nursing and health visiting. In addition he may have
the counsel and support of specially appointed social workers of the local
authority. Following the implementation of the Local Authority Social
Services Act 1970, local authorities have unified their personal social
services under a single committee working through a Director of Social
Services specially appointed for this purpose. The responsibilities of the
Social Services Committee include:

   1. the services of the former children's department;

2. the former welfare services for the elderly, homeless, disabled or handicapped;

3. the home help service, mental health social work services, the social work services and day nurseries, all of which were formerly provided by local authority health departments.

The probation service remains outside the social services department.

Local authority social services departments are organized on a sectorized basis with sector teams of social workers. The aim is to provide a community-based and family-orientated service. Social workers employed in these departments are mostly *generic*, although some specialization, such as in mental health, child care and so on, exists at a higher administrative or consultant level.

There is currently an increasing movement towards community care. This is in line with the Department of Health and Social Security's policy to run down extensively the number of mental hospital beds and to substitute smaller psychiatric units based on district general hospitals. The number of existing psychiatric beds varies from about 1.0 to 2.5 per 1000 population, but with satisfactory facilities for community care 0.5 acute adult psychiatric beds per 1000 in-patient and 0.65 per 1000 day-hospital places or even fewer should be adequate. However, the attainment of this norm or anything approaching it will only be possible if sufficient in-patient accommodation is made available for geriatric patients, who currently occupy 50 per cent or more of mental hospital beds, particularly those suffering from dementia, and also if adequate provision is made for local authority community care. Most local authorities, however, still lack sufficient funds for the purpose. Until they do, it must be strongly emphasized that not only will community care facilities such as hostels and day centres be sadly lacking in many places, but such facilities as do exist will be very unevenly distributed. Staffing is also far from uniform.

Social and administrative aspects of treatment

Where to treat the mentally ill

The social aspects of treatment are perhaps more obviously apparent in psychiatry than in other medical disciplines. The first consideration, then, is often not so much how but where a mentally ill patient should be treated. Thus at the turn of the century the treatment of mental disorders was largely limited to the care and control in institutions of persons unfitted to be at large. Sedation took its place with seclusion, often in a padded room, when sedation did not prove wholly effective. Up to then, psychiatric treatment meant compulsory admission to an asylum, voluntary treatment being impossible until the passage of the Mental Treatment Act of 1930.

There were few psychiatric out-patient facilities. Then, during World War I, interest in psychotic illnesses and emotional disorders among members of the Forces and the alleviation of abnormal personality reactions by psychotherapy fostered the hope that more could be done if both soldiers and civilians were seen sufficiently early and possibly well before hospital admission became necessary. This led to the establishment of clinics for the diagnosis, investigation and treatment of mental and nervous disorders.

While initially these provided accommodation for out-patients only, following World War II in-patient units began to be established in general hospitals. Although their number is not yet large and their size, in most cases, limited, their development has now become official policy. While originally only patients with emotional disorders and the milder forms of psychotic illness were treated in general hospital units, experience has shown that given proper facilities and a sufficient number of medical and nursing staff, most acutely ill psychiatric patients can be adequately treated. In contrast, longer stay patients require special occupational, recreational and rehabilitation facilities which a general hospital unit may find it impossible to provide. While the day of the mental hospital is by no means dead, and probably never will be, general hospital units seem particularly well suited to the admission of acutely mentally ill patients, a further advantage being that the often artificial dichotomy between mental and physical illness is blurred.

Another important development has been the establishment of day hospitals where patients attend for up to five days per week on a 'nine-to-five' basis. The first of these was established in 1946 by Bierer. Many types of physical, psychological and especially social treatment can be carried out on a day basis, provided that the patients are not so disturbed as to require 24-hour supervision and can readily travel to and from their homes, preferably without the expensive use of ambulance services. Apart from this, such services have the advantage of being relatively economical and of allowing patients to keep in close touch with their families, thus tending to prevent institutionalism. They appear to be particularly well suited to the treatment of those who suffer from emotional difficulties and milder forms of psychosis. Day treatment is also useful in promoting rehabilitation when in-patient treatment is no longer necessary, although fairly close supervision may still be required, prior to overall discharge.

Likewise, units for children and, separately, for adolescents have been established, it being thought undesirable to mingle these with adults. All else apart, special facilities for their education and recreation are needed.

Principles of psychiatric care

The first consideration is often whether admission to hospital is necessary or desirable.

If the patient is acutely disturbed, is suicidal or a risk to others, there may clearly be no alternative. If the patient will not accept informal admission—it is surprising how many do if tactfully handled—some form of compulsory admission may be required (see Chapter 25), although currently about 85 per cent of patients are admitted informally. Much depends on the patient's degree of insight. Thus some depressed patients regard themselves as wicked or sinful, protesting that they are undeserving of care and attention. They can, however, usually be persuaded. Manic and paranoid patients can be much more difficult to handle. Those who are confused or delirious or out of touch with the environment cannot make their intentions known. Even then, compulsory admission may not be necessary. Being physically ill, they can usually be dealt with as such. Other reasons for admission (though not compulsorily) may be unsatisfactory home circumstances or family difficulties militating against satisfactory treatment or a need to carry out complex physical investigations where an organic basis for mental illness is suspected.

Where in-patient admission is indicated, consideration should be given to the type of unit best suited to the patient's condition. Whereas most acutely disturbed patients can, given a sufficiency of trained staff, be treated in an 'open-door' unit, a few potentially violent patients may need treatment under secure conditions. However, the well-learned lesson that the trappings of restraint themselves promote a tendency to violence should never be forgotten.

Many patients with milder illnesses can be treated by day care from the start. Such treatment is particularly relevant in the case of those whose relatives can adequately care for them at other times. Emotionally disturbed patients unable to work on account of their symptoms are often most suitably dealt with in this way. Indeed, when admitted such patients often tend to become unduly dependent, which in itself may impede their treatment.

Many patients never need admission to hospital at any time and can be quite adequately treated as out-patients, particularly those requiring individual or group psychotherapy. There are some in whom admission to hospital is positively contraindicated. They may include certain patients who, although needing treatment, are able to continue at work; in particular those with obsessional symptoms who, if they stop work, are inclined to fill their time with increasing indulgence in obsessional rituals.

Apart from admission, consideration must be given to discharge. The day when a patient, apparently recovered, was discharged more or less abruptly and left to fend for himself is gone. For those who have spent a considerable time in hospital, gradual rather than sudden discharge may be desirable, so that following discharge they are seen at increasingly lengthening intervals in the out-patient department. Alternatively, a period of attendance at a day hospital before being referred to an out-patient clinic may be desirable. Here local authority social services often have an essential part to play. Some patients who are able to work but who have no homes to go to or are estranged from their families may, during the period of their final resettlement, spend some time in residence in a local authority hostel. Intimately bound up with discharge is rehabilitation, which of course includes placement in suitable employment where possible.

When to discharge a patient can often be as difficult a decision as when to admit. There is some truth in the saying that depressed patients tend to be prematurely discharged and schizophrenics belatedly so. Often, following appropriate treatment, depressed patients feel so much improved that they press for discharge but, if this is allowed prematurely, relapse may ensue. Under these circumstances the risk of suicide is high. Although a depressed patient *may feel* ready to leave the hospital, he *may not* be able to face the world and, in particular, to return to full-time work. This, therefore, should be delayed until lasting improvement is assured, following which former activities can be gradually resumed. This applies the more so if the patient's employment is one involving concentration, a need to take responsibility and to make decisions. Where weight has been lost, weight gain is a good guide to secure recovery.

Schizophrenic patients should not be kept in hospital for longer than necessary owing to their tendency to become institutionalized. However, the manner of their discharge should also be carefully planned. Supervision, especially where long-acting drug therapy is deemed to be desirable, must be arranged either at a specifically organized clinic or under the supervision of a general practitioner and a community-based psychiatric nurse. A *case register* is particularly useful for retaining contact and preventing relapse amongst out-patient schizophrenic patients. Thus all new cases of schizophrenia in a defined geographical area, for example a District with a population of 200 000, are registered. The type of continuing treatment is recorded so that if a patient fails to attend, the appropriate person, usually a community psychiatric nurse, is immediately informed and will seek out the patient at home. Such a system, if kept meticulously up to date, can prevent deterioration of a patient's mental stage passing unnoticed with disastrous consequences.

Return to his own family is not necessarily always in a schizophrenic patient's best interest. Where his family shows *high emotional involvement* towards him with either excessive solicitousness and anxiety or alternatively harsh scrutiny of his every activity, relapse is more likely.

Here a period in a hostel or even a placement with others who understand and can tolerate his eccentricities may be of benefit.

Those with emotional problems may also present a discharge problem in that, having become unduly dependent on the hospital, they become liable to develop a fresh crop of symptoms whenever the possibility of discharge looms. One way of overcoming this difficulty may be by carefully defining the limit of stay when first admitted, such as a period of four to six weeks duration, as appropriate. Interestingly, even though they may protest strongly about discharge, many such patients may be found, on follow-up, to have improved very much more than might have been anticipated at the time.

The therapeutic milieu

Another now well-recognized principle is greater mixing of the sexes, not merely on social occasions, but in mixed wards with separate sleeping and sanitary facilities. Those who fear that this kind of unit may lead to promiscuity should be reminded that those who run hotels have not found it necessary to segregate men and women. Likewise, the sharp division of male and female nursing staff has been swept aside so that, where accommodation is satisfactory, female nurses can work with male patients and vice versa. Such developments have called for considerable adjustment amongst those who staff mental hospitals.

Lessened authoritarianism has swept away much of the strict hierarchy which characterized the traditional mental hospital. Hence the growing practice among psychiatric nurses of no longer wearing uniform. Likewise, the day of the autocratic medical superintendent is past. Psychiatrists in mental hospitals, like other consultants, are now recognized as entirely responsible for the patients under their care. By the same token, medical administration has become a matter for committee decision and is much more democratic than it used to be.

From all this the concept of the *therapeutic community* has evolved in which patients are encouraged to identify themselves with the life of the hospital as a whole so that each unit develops its own group culture. Acting as a group, patients are encouraged to make many different kinds of decisions, some actually affecting their own treatment and that of others; technical advice being offered by the medical and nursing staff. This has met with considerable success in some places; though it can lead to difficult situations involving both patients and staff. One difficulty is that the abolition of the traditional hierarchical structure can lead to anarchical situations. Three underlying principles appear to be essential.

1. Interpersonal difficulties must be immediately aired and dissolved.
2. Communication must be maintained at all levels.

3. It must be realized that greater freedom of action involves taking a greater degree of responsibility for one's own actions.

These principles apply to staff and patients alike.

Social skills training

It is central to any claim of effective social methods of treatment that there are defects in relationships amongst psychiatric patients and that there are methods of lessening these defects. Recently, *social skills training* has become a component of treatment of the mentally ill. Patients are taught how their verbal and non-verbal behaviour influences the behaviour and feelings of others, and how to modify their behaviour to achieve worthwhile goals in social relationships.

Like other forms of behavioural modification, the first stage is the analysis of behaviour; by breaking down the desired social skill into its component parts, so that these may be achieved in sequence. It probably helps if the patient can identify with, and then *model* his behaviour upon, another person who copes satisfactorily in a particular social situation. After learning how the skill is carried out and seeing this performed by a model, the patient practises it under instruction. It is important to give him information about his performance and to reinforce positively his successes. Frequent *rehearsal* of the skill between treatment sessions is essential.

Social skills training may benefit many types of patient. A very directive form of training may assist in improving the social competence of a mentally handicapped and chronic schizophrenic. Depression impairs social competence and this in its turn causes further loss of self-esteem and lowering of mood; social skills training is an essential part of the management of those depressed patients who demonstrate *learned helplessness*. Amongst patients with neuroses there is virtually always difficulty with relationships, which social skills training may improve and consequently lessen feelings of failure and morbid mood states. Those with sensitive, schizoid and asocial personality disorders may be helped by such training; although it is, of course, a prerequisite that the subject wishes to improve his social functioning.

Some skills are especially amenable to treatment. *Assertion training* has been used to help the excessively timid and shy; in contrast, it has been attempted in excessively aggressive people to help them achieve a more socially acceptable form of behaviour. Training is also used to improve social relationships with the opposite sex and for those who have difficulties in initiating or establishing such a relationship. It is also of general use in helping to achieve a more satisfactory level of communication in ordinary conversation. While social skills training is not likely to be a wholly effective form of treatment on its own, it is a useful adjunct to other treatment.

Rehabilitation

Rehabilitation is the process of identifying and preventing or minimizing *social disablement* which causes those affected to be unable to perform at a level that could reasonably be expected. Such disablement may be due to psychiatric illness, to disadvantages such as poverty, homelessness or unemployment, and to individual reactions to symptoms. Before rehabilitation can be attempted, a thorough *assessment* in order to determine the type and severity of disability that is present must be made; also to discover what aptitudes the patient has, to agree with him what goals should be aimed for, to make a realistic treatment plan, to determine which members of staff and what treatment are most appropriate, and to monitor the progress made. Such assessment also includes an investigation of his social and family circumstances in order to determine whether further support is required. The presence of any particular problem behaviours is identified, including an assessment of his ability to carry out everyday activities of living and working.

For many patients, rehabilitation implies long-term management. Dealing with those who are mute, inaccessible, apathetic, disturbed, unhygienic or show petty delinquency, makes considerable demands upon staff treating such patients, so that a harmonious multidisciplinary professional team is necessary.

The specific techniques used in rehabilitation will include various types of behavioural therapy including *token economies* and individual methods, occupational and industrial therapy, crisis intervention and the use of appropriate drugs.

Disabled persons

The Disabled Persons (Employment) Act 1944 provides for special officers within the local offices of the Department of Employment known as disablement resettlement officers who keep a register of disabled persons and assist in their rehabilitation and re-employment. They work within a framework of industrial rehabilitation units (IRUs), government training centres and certain protected employments. The interest they show in the mentally disordered patient and the skill in placement naturally vary and depend to some extent on the amount of support and liaison they receive from the members of the psychiatric team.

Occupational, industrial and recreational therapy

The general aims of occupational therapy are to promote activity, to develop interest, self-confidence and pride in achievement and to guide morbid impulses into more desirable channels. Industrial rehabilitation is used not only to achieve these benefits, but to teach fresh skills. Much greater emphasis is now placed upon occupations in which patients are encouraged to work together on group projects, thus bringing about a greater social interaction, together with the development of social skills. Thus the borderline between occupational and social therapy has become blurred, so that the occupational therapist is now less of an expert on handicrafts and more of a social and recreational therapist. While games, gymnastics, eurhythmics, dancing, debates, musical appreciation classes, play reading and amateur theatricals may be organized primarily for exercise, relaxation and amusement, they can also be seen as activities in which patients learn to know and tolerate one another. Such encouragement towards social interaction is clearly of value to those who are friendless and isolated because of mental illness. The same process may be continued after discharge, by attendance at social clubs on one or more evenings each week at the clinic which those about to be discharged, ex-patients and their relatives are encouraged to attend, together with members of staff.

The move towards industrial therapy has brought about systematic employment in hospital on a scale never before envisaged. Many more progressive hospitals now contain factories of considerable size in which light assembly work, subcontracted from neighbouring industry, is carried out on an extensive scale. Some of these factories contain quite elaborate machinery which allows the manufacture of small parts from raw materials. Technical instructors are employed to train patients how to use these machines and acquire new skills. In industrial therapy units, activity is graded by stages towards a greater pressure of work approaching that which obtains under normal industrial conditions. It is a principle of therapy that patients shall be paid for their work, though the maximum allowable amount is controlled. 'Clocking in and out' is also desirable.

Not all patients, particularly those suffering from chronic mental disorders, or from mental handicap, can reach the maximum level of activity, though they may later be gainfully employed in sheltered workshops and other occupations, where the pace and pressure are less than on the factory floor.

A great deal of ingenuity and drive is required of those engaged in organizing programmes of industrial therapy and in obtaining subcontracts in order to keep full production going. However, as part of the process of rehabilitation, the mere organizing of work programmes has been shown not to be sufficient in itself. Without adequate social rehabilitation up to the level of coping with external environmental pressures of work, industrial rehabilitation alone is likely to fail.

The role of the social worker

The particular needs of the patient are all too easily lost in a maze of red tape, complex hierarchies and bureaucratic indifference. To offset this there came into being by the middle of this century statutory acceptance of the need for *trained social workers* to be attached to the various services under varying titles, and to ensure that legislative complexities were geared to the individual situation and vice versa, and so that clients could gain an understanding of what the social services are able to do. A social worker's prime function is to give direct help to individuals and groups with social and personal problems which they cannot otherwise handle satisfactorily. Such help may range from straightforward advice about how to use a particular social service, to skilled help with personal problems rendered by a professionally qualified social worker.

What is to be expected from social workers in the mental health field? If part of a psychiatric team, the social worker may be expected to obtain a discriminating social history from whatever source it can best be obtained, usually from the relative most concerned. By *discriminating* is meant the elucidation and selection of those social and psychological factors which throw light on the development and nature of the patient's mental disorder. Hence the importance of practical and theoretical training, the need to be able to understand psychiatric concepts and to grasp what is of particular significance in a relative's account. The occasion for history taking also provides an opportunity to develop cooperation between the family and the hospital and to deal with their anxieties, misconceptions and false hopes. It is not always appreciated how major a step it is for someone to become a psychiatric patient; referral to psychiatric care may actually increase anxiety and isolation, and hence unduly worsen a patient's situation.

Besides gathering relevant information, a social worker is able to assess the emotional climate of the patient's home, and any serious needs which may call for relief; more often than not, this may turn out to be simply the need to have someone relatively knowledgeable and sympathetic to talk to, who is not a member of the kin group and not vested with the powers of a doctor. There is often a need to interpret the meaning and implications of a patient's mental disorder to anxious or incredulous relatives, who may have listened with every outward sign of grasping what the doctor at the hospital or surgery has told them, but in fact have misunderstood or simply failed to register, bringing home with them nothing but confusion. Alternatively, under pressure of time, especially in big institutions, relatives may be told practically nothing, or told too forcibly, as a result of which they worry or become resentful or indifferent.

The emotional tangles and social crises that collect where there is mental illness, personality disorder, or mental handicap, are often protracted and difficult, and sometimes impossible to solve. When the psychiatrist feels that the limit of clinical help he can give has been reached, he may ask a social worker to try to assist either the patient himself or some member of his family or social group to reach a better understanding of the difficulties of the situation. This may constitute a task that runs on for many months of contact, at home, in the clinic or at the offices of the local authority. Needless to say, there are many enduring situations in the field of mental disorder, so that occasional contact may be had for years with some clients, such as those with paranoid schizophrenia, personality disorders, drug abuse problems, and so on, thus providing these isolated people, drifting on the borders of unreality, with a lifeline.

Social workers are often called upon to marshall the existing social services in aid of a patient under treatment; thus children may need to be taken into care, home help may be required for the schizophrenic or for the disturbed mother with a young family. Where problems of tangled finance, debt and threatened homelessness loom, the help of the disablement resettlement officer may have to be negotiated, and it may take some time of discouraging trial and error before the patient is successfully integrated into any retraining scheme and so back to work. Good plans break down because of an insufficient follow-through—the social worker has too many calls on her time or the cooperation of a patient is assumed rather than won. Other plans fail because of difficulties inherent in the problem of mental disorder itself. Much patience, a capacity to listen—particularly to the undertones—and a refusal to be exasperated by failure are all requisites for those who would do social work in the field of mental health.

Apart from all this, a social worker with some specialized training is a safeguard, both to the patient and to his relatives, in a somewhat exposed situation. While acting as mental welfare officers, they have to take their turn 'on call' by day or night, to meet emergencies caused by excited or despairing people and to help arrange compulsory admissions. The way in which these trying situations are handled may do much to reduce the fear and strain which keep alive in many people's minds the dread of any form of psychiatric care.

The psychiatric nurse

No one profession has the monopoly of treatment of the mentally ill; however, in hospital, the most contact the patient has is with nurses, who are responsible for carrying out his treatment, this having been planned jointly by a team of mental health professionals under the clinical direction of the consultant psychiatrist.

Follow-up care at home is increasingly being provided by *community psychiatric nurses*. Psychiatric nursing has thus changed its role considerably in the last few years—from an emphasis upon custodial care to more active treatment and greater involvement in rehabilitation. The psychiatric nurse of 20 years ago dealt predominantly with psychotic patients, but is now much more involved than previously with neurotic patients.

This has made a considerable impact upon the training of nurses as they now need to know much more about the social management of patients outside hospital, and about individual and group methods of psychological treatment for in-patients and day-patients. With better and more intensive training, more nurses are taking on the role of *nurse therapists* in behavioural or dynamic psychotherapy, and are having in consequence to learn about the demands and stresses that active participation in treatment makes.

The traditional skills and attitudes of nursing with considerate care and judicious kindness are very important for dealing with elderly psychiatric patients, especially those with dementia. A good nurse in this situation will put emphasis upon retaining human dignity, helping her patient to remain a distinctive individual with his own ideas and property, and upon controlling the hospital environment so that as far as possible the patient is kept in touch with reality, encouraging independence and normal coping for as long as possible.

Voluntary associations

Social concern for mental disorder expresses itself through voluntary as well as statutory organizations. Thus, earlier in this century, national and international councils of mental hygiene (later mental health) in the United States, the United Kingdom and in Europe were formed, directed towards the prevention and improved treatment of psychiatric breakdown and to ensuring adequate professional training for psychiatrists, psychologists and psychiatric social workers. The consideration of the part society and the family played in creating psychiatric disorder (and delinquent attitudes) became a major interest, and in 1927 the setting up of the Child Guidance Council in London to develop child psychiatric services in the United Kingdom bore witness to growing concern.

World War II saw the unification of the main voluntary organizations interested in mental disorder into the present National Association for Mental Health (MIND). Beginning as a Mental Health Emergency Committee, when war broke out, these bodies provided in collaboration with the Ministry of Health a network in the evacuated population and aftercare for discharged psychiatric casualties from the Services.

Since 1946, the field of statutory care for mental disorder has greatly widened—largely through pressure from voluntary bodies on the Government—but collaboration with the DHSS continues, and supporting grants are received. Experimental homes, hostels, courses and projects of all kinds have been fostered. The growth of local associations for mental health has been encouraged and regular public conferences on current issues organized. These act as a sounding-board for public opinion on government measures and a forum for the interchange of ideas between professional and lay people.

In 1948, a World Federation for Mental Health was formed, linked to the World Health Organization at Geneva, to which national associations are affiliated, and which specifically fosters the interchange of ideas between different specialist groups allied to psychiatry in different countries. This constitutes the largest organ of what has come to be known as the mental health movement. Through its international conferences, expert committees, seminars and published reports, it disseminates ideas and information in the psychiatric field between widely different cultures. A vast amount of material is being collated, compared and discussed, much of which is of sociological and anthropological as well as of purely psychiatric interest, and which is made available for public and professional consumption.

Apart from these main voluntary bodies, there are still a few small organizations serving specific ends such as the British Epilepsy Association, the Mental Aftercare Association (convalescent homes for the mentally ill), the Association of Parents of Handicapped Children, the Schizophrenia Fellowship and certain others; but the intention of forming one central body was to give strength to voluntary effort and avoid the problem of too many appeals to the private purse. In effect, MIND seems currently to be recognized as the main spokesman for the public to the Government on matters related to mental disorder.

Further reading

Wing, J. K. & Morris, B. (1981) *Handbook of Psychiatric Rehabilitation Practice.* London: Oxford University Press.

24

Treatment III: Physical

Modern physical treatments have done much to reduce morbidity, particularly in the psychoses, and have led to patients remaining in hospital for shorter periods than before. However, their action is still poorly understood. Thus, like psychological treatments, physical treatments must still be regarded as empirical procedures, although not necessarily to be despised on this account.

Physical and psychological treatments cannot be dissociated. Every physical procedure exerts a psychological effect in part derived from the nature of the treatment, from the way it is administered and from the prestige of the therapist. Of all physical treatments, this is most obvious in drug therapy. About one-third of patients are *placebo reactors* who respond favourably even though only temporarily to almost any physical or psychological procedure. Similarly, how drugs are prescribed and the belief of both patient and doctor in their efficacy may have an effect almost as profound as that of the drug itself. Although inconveniencing research, the *placebo effect* is not to be despised inasmuch as it certainly helps in treatment. It also accounts for side-effects in many cases.

General medical care

The need for careful physical examination, together with such investigations as are considered absolutely necessary, has already been stressed. Attention should be paid to the general state of physical health of those psychiatric patients who are debilitated by loss of appetite, weight, sleeplessness, and the abuse of alcohol or drugs, as well as to physical disabilities which may be only indirectly associated with the presenting psychiatric disorder but may affect its course. Thus, where anaemia etc. is present, this must be corrected. In alcoholism and in elderly patients having poor nutrition, the possibility of avitaminosis should be considered and special attention paid to diet.

Many psychiatric patients are underweight, particularly those who are depressed, tense or anxious. In these a satisfactory gain in weight during treatment may be a sign of recovery. Conversely, in depressed patients who appear to improve but who fail to gain weight, relapse is likely. Weighing should, therefore, be carried out at weekly intervals and the results carefully charted.

Drug treatment

Until the action of drugs upon the central nervous system is much better understood, only a working classification, in part based on their general clinical effects and, in part, chemical or pharmacological, is feasible. While some relationships between chemical structure and clinical effects may be apparent, this is very variable. In some cases the effect produced is uncertain, occasionally paradoxical; and may also vary according to dose and the current condition of the patient. The same is true of side-effects.

The following classification of psychotropic drugs is probably as satisfactory as any.

(*Note*. As there are now so many different preparations available, any attempt at a comprehensive catalogue is out of the question. Nor is it realistic, the position having now been reached where the wisest course of action is for the prescriber to acquaint himself as thoroughly as possible with the action of a relatively few well-tried and tested drugs as well as familiarizing himself with their toxic and other side-effects. Proprietary names are given in parentheses and should not generally be used; firstly, because they vary from one country to another and, secondly, because, even in the same country, a drug manufactured by different pharmaceutical companies may be given a different proprietary name.)

I Hypnotics and sedatives (minor tranquillizers)

1. *Benzodiazepines*, e.g. diazepam (Valium), nitrazepam (Mogadon), temazepam (Euhypnos).
2. *Barbiturates*, e.g. amylobarbitone (Amytal).
3. *Other hypnotics and sedatives*, e.g. paraldehyde, dichloralphenazone (Welldorm), chlormethiazole (Heminevrin), meprobamate (Equanil).

II Beta-blockers

Propranolol (Inderal).

III Major tranquillizers (ataraxics, neuroleptics)

1. *Phenothiazines*.
   a. With an aliphatic side-chain ending in a dimethylamine group, e.g. chlorpromazine (Largactil).
   b. With a piperazine ring on the side-chain, e.g. prochlorperazine (Stemetil), trifluoperazine (Stelazine).
   c. With a piperidine ring on the side-chain, e.g. thioridazine (Melleril).
2. *Butyrophenones*, e.g. haloperidol (Haldol, Serenace).
3. *Thioxanthenes*, e.g. flupenthixol (Depixol).

IV Stimulants and antidepressants (thymoleptics)

1. *Tricyclic antidepressants*, e.g. imipramine (Tofranil), amitriptyline (Tryptizol).
2. *Other antidepressants* such as tetracyclics, e.g. mianserin (Bolvidon, Norval).
3. *Monoamine oxidase inhibitors* (MAOI), e.g. tranylcypromine (Parnate), phenelzine (Nardil).
4. *Stimulants*, e.g. dextro- and methylamphetamine (Dexedrine, Methedrine), methylphenidate (Ritalin).
5. *Lithium carbonate*. (This could be put in a separate subcategory owing to its dual effect in controlling both elation and depression in manic–depressive psychosis.)

V Antiparkinsonian drugs

These drugs are used extensively in psychiatry, not for their psychotropic effects, but for the treatment of side-effects of major tranquillizers such as phenothiazines and butyrophenones.

VI Psychotomimetics

1. *Naturally occurring*, e.g. mescaline, psilocybin.
2. *Synthetic*, e.g. lysergic acid diethylamide (LSD 25).

VII Miscellaneous

There are also a number of other drugs which, while apparently having no direct action upon the central nervous system, may affect behaviour, for example anti-androgen drugs (e.g. Androcur) which reduce sexual desire in males and may be of value in lessening libido in those with uncontrollable antisocial tendencies (see Chapter 17), or disulfiram which, following the ingestion of alcohol, causes a build up of acetaldehyde in the body and is used in the treatment of alcoholism (see Chapter 11). Anti-epileptic drugs are also important in psychiatry and are described in Chapter 10.

Hypnotics and sedatives

Benzodiazepines

The first of the benzodiazepines to be synthesized was *chlordiazepoxide* (Librium) which was found to be a useful tranquillizer in a wide variety of anxiety and other emotional disorders. Its main disadvantage appears to be its instability in solution and unsuitability therefore for parenteral administration. Chlordiazepoxide was soon followed by other benzodiazepine drugs, of which the most popular appears to be *diazepam*

(Valium). Others include *oxazepam* (Serenid), *lorazepam* (Ativan), *medazepam* (Nobrium) and a number of others including *nitrazepam* (Mogadon), *flurazepam* (Dalmane) and *temazepam* (Euhypnos) which are marketed as sedatives for insomnia. Difference in action between these drugs is marginal; they are closely related chemically and many of them are metabolized rapidly to oxazepam and thence degraded more slowly. This means that a single dose of diazepam will have a rapid effect producing night sedation or diminishing anxiety. Repeated doses will produce a build up of metabolites which produce long-term sedation.

Most benzodiazepines are virtually free from side-effects except for producing undue sleepiness in some patients which is usually transient. (It should be noted, however, that if taken at night they may have an effect on behaviour the following day, e.g. in interfering with the ability to drive a car.) In a few persons they also appear to have the paradoxical property of promoting aggressive behaviour.

Most benzodiazepines also have a mild antidepressive action, and can usefully be given to agitated or anxious depressed patients in combination with an antidepressive drug. They also have anti-epileptic properties and may be used in disturbed epileptic patients together with anticonvulsants. This property also affects EEG findings so that, where this investigation is contemplated, they should be withdrawn at least two weeks before. Diazepam may also be given intravenously to control status epilepticus, or to control withdrawal symptoms in drug dependence. It should be noted, however, that the benzodiazepines are themselves inclined to produce dependence and that epileptic fits can occur on withdrawal. Confusional states due to chronic overdosage have also been observed. Their efficacy of action in controlling anxiety does not last more than a couple of months. However, it may be difficult to withdraw a patient who has received benzodiazepines for longer than this because withdrawal symptoms resemble those symptoms for which the drug was originally prescribed.

Barbiturates

Barbiturates at one time acquired a prominent place in psychiatric treatment both as tranquillizers and for treating insomnia. They are now rarely if ever indicated, except when administered intravenously for the occasional purpose of abreaction or narcoanalysis. In insomnia they have now been largely replaced by non-barbiturate hypnotics such as *nitrazepam* (Mogadon) or *fluorazepam* (Dalmane) which although more expensive are less liable to cause dependence and very much safer should the patient take an overdose.

Narcoanalysis is occasionally a useful short-cut method of psychological exploration, probably having its greatest application to those with emotional problems of sudden and recent onset. It may also be of value in patients who although willing to talk about their problems are prevented from doing so by undue anxiety or guilt feelings. It may also be of value in cases of genuine amnesia but, where this is feigned, as in malingering, it is useless.

Narcoanalytic abreaction may be produced in several ways. One method is to inject intravenously a 5 or 10 per cent solution of *sodium amylobarbitone* (sodium amytal) (250–500 mg) at the rate of 0.5 to 1.0 ml a minute. Alternatively, *sodium thiopentone* (Pentothal) may be used in lesser concentration. The aim is to produce a state of slight clouding of consciousness during which repressed memories may be evoked, so that the patient is able to discuss problems he could not otherwise bring himself to. Strong suggestion, even hypnosis, is a valuable adjuvant and may be used to induce the patient to relive and re-enact traumatic experiences.

Alternatively, *methylamphetamine* (Methedrine) may be injected intravenously in doses of 20–40 mg; this often promotes a press of talk and the expression of buried complexes. Some prefer a combined injection of methylamphetamine and sodium amylobarbitone, finding this more effective than either given alone. A similar state may be produced by inhaling nitrous oxide, ether, or a mixture of 30 per cent carbon dioxide and 70 per cent oxygen, a technique originally devised by von Meduna.

Other hypnotics and sedatives

Chloral hydrate is a reasonably safe hypnotic, although is best avoided in old people with cardiorespiratory disease. It is also a gastric irritant. Dependence and chronic intoxication can occur with prolonged use. *Dichloralphenazone* (Welldorm) seems a safer substitute.

Paraldehyde by mouth is safe but unpleasant, having an offensive taste and smell. Intramuscular administration should be avoided as paraldehyde cannot be sterilized. Except in a very few cases of *status epilepticus* which cannot be controlled by other means and in which intravenous paraldehyde may be effective, there is now no case to be made for its use.

No other minor tranquillizers seem so far to have achieved the same success as benzodiazepines. *Meprobamate* (Equanil, Miltown), always more popular in the United States than in the United Kingdom, has fallen largely into disuse (perhaps because of the side-effects of drowsiness and drug dependence). Major tranquillizers such as *chlorpromazine, trifluoperazine* and *haloperidol*, while all fairly effective anxiolytics when given in low dosage, never seem to have achieved great popularity, although low-dosage *flupenthixol* used as an anxiolytic agent currently appears to have found some favour.

Chlormethiazole—a somewhat difficult drug to classify—is neither a phenothiazine nor a butyrophenone. Its action lies somewhere between the major and minor tranquillizers, although it is more generally regarded as in the hypnotic–sedative class. It is useful in treating *delirium tremens* and other confusional states, particularly those affecting restless old people. In alcoholics it is useful for *short-term administration only*, owing to its addictive properties; these having also been observed in some non-alcoholic patients. Otherwise chlormethiazole appears to be a safe drug with relatively few side-effects.

Beta-blockers

Propranolol (Inderal) has been found useful in controlling the *somatic manifestations of anxiety* such as rapid pulse, palpitations, sweating and tremor. It has been used to treat neurotic patients with predominantly somatic symptoms and also to control lithium-induced tremor. It should not be used in patients with a history of bronchial asthma. Claims for its beneficial effects in the treatment of schizophrenia have not yet been substantiated.

Major tranquillizers

Phenothiazines

Chlorpromazine hydrochloride (Largactil), which remains the most popular major tranquillizer, was introduced to psychiatry in 1952 following the experience of Laborit and Huguenard who used it in the Indo-Chinese war to produce 'artificial hibernation' as a prophylactic agent against severe surgical shock. Chlorpromazine is hypothermic, hypotensive, anti-emetic and weakly antihistaminic. It has a fairly strong sedative action and potentiates the effects of other cerebral depressants, such as anaesthetics, barbiturates and alcohol. There is evidence that it acts by depressing the reticular activating system.

The main indications for the use of chlorpromazine are as follows.

1. *As a sedative.* Given at night, 50–100 mg will produce sleep in many patients. If necessary it may be used to potentiate the effect of other drugs such as nitrazepam.

2. *As a minor tranquillizer.* Small doses, for example 10–25 mg one to three times daily, may be effective. However, while controlling anxiety, chlorpromazine depresses some patients. One advantage, however, is that it appears to be non-habit forming.

3. *To control states of severe excitement and tension.* Chlorpromazine appears to be effective without regard to the basis of such states—that is, whether delirium, mania, acute agitated depression or schizophrenic excitement. In severe cases, parenteral administration may be required initially. Care should be taken as this is liable to produce a fall in blood pressure. It should also be noted that intramuscular injections of chlorpromazine are painful.

4. *As a neuroleptic or psychotropic agent.* Apart from controlling excitement, chlorpromazine has a striking effect upon certain schizophrenic symptoms such as hallucinations. Its use in doses ranging from

200 to 1500 mg daily may improve the mental state in schizophrenia such as to enable resocialization and rehabilitation. Where a satisfactory effect is obtained, long-term maintenance therapy may be required, although today this is probably better done in most cases by the use of depot injections (see p. 354).

Side-effects. Chlorpromazine occasionally induces epileptic fits, particularly in brain-damaged patients or following leucotomy. It should be used with caution in combination with ECT because of its tendency to produce confusion.

Apart from these, side-effects are of two main kinds: (1) those which are inherent in the drug's action and include dryness of the mouth, constipation, increase of appetite, gain in weight, galactorrhoea, etc.; and (2) idiosyncratic effects, notably cholestatic jaundice and agranulocytosis. The latter is extremely rare though occasional fatalities have been recorded. Chlorpromazine jaundice is usually benign, though occasionally persistent. For some, as yet unexplained, reason its incidence, which was in the region of 4–5 per cent when the drug was first used, has fallen so that it is now only rarely seen. The occurrence of jaundice is not related to dose and when it occurs does so almost invariably between 10 and 20 days after administration has begun. It is advised that chlorpromazine should not be given where there is a recent history of liver damage or in the face of abnormal liver function tests.

In larger doses, i.e. over 400–500 mg daily, extrapyramidal symptoms may occur. While parkinsonism is the commonest variety, other forms, for example *torsion spasm*, *akithisia* (restless treading of the feet) and *tasikinesia* (forced walking-about), can occur though these are seen more commonly with other phenothiazines (e.g. *trifluoperazine*) or butyrophenones (e.g. *haloperidol*). Parkinsonian symptoms usually disappear when the drug is withdrawn or the dose reduced, though in a few elderly patients with organic cerebral lesions they may persist, in particular *tardive dyskinesia* (facial movements resembling chewing). Except in such cases, parkinsonian symptoms may usually be adequately controlled by antiparkinsonian drugs, e.g. *benztropine* (Cogentin), *orphenadrine* (Disipal).

Another side-effect troublesome in subtropical or tropical climates is that of *photosensitive skin reactions*. Thus patients should be told to avoid direct exposure to sunlight and wear long sleeves and a hat. In elderly patients, chlorpromazine needs to be used cautiously owing to its tendency to produce *hypotension* and *hypothermia*.

Promazine (Sparine) is similar in its actions to chlorpromazine, although with an equipotency of about half. It is thought to be less hepatotoxic.

Trifluoperazine (Stelazine) and *prochlorperazine* (Stemetil) are much more potent than chlorpromazine. Their effects are similar, but tend to be more stimulating. Extrapyramidal symptoms are also commoner.

Trifluoperazine may be used in two ways: as a minor tranquillizer (1–2 mg thrice daily) or as a major tranquillizer (10–30 mg daily) either alone or in combination with chlorpromazine primarily in the treatment of more chronic schizophrenic illnesses; especially those of later life and in patients with fairly well-preserved personalities (paraphrenia) where it is often of value. Having a more stimulating effect, trifluoperazine may also be useful in younger withdrawn and anergic schizophrenic patients. While the drug certainly controls inconvenient psychotic symptoms such as hallucinations, it is doubtful whether it has any truly ameliorative influence on the hypothetical underlying 'process' or on passivity phenomena.

Thioridazine (Melleril) is somewhat similar in action, though is said to be effective in schizophrenia with depressive symptoms, and in calming agitation and restlessness. It is the least likely of the phenothiazines to cause parkinsonian symptoms. Retinal pigmentation has been reported.

Long-acting phenothiazines, such as *fluphenazine decanoate* (Modecate), have come into fairly wide use in recent years. Whereas the action of these drugs differs in no essential respect from other phenothiazines, they are prepared in a sesame oil vehicle and when injected are absorbed only gradually over a period of time. A single injection of 25 mg of fluphenazine decanoate may, therefore, be effective from 15 to as long as 35 days. It is, however, wise to begin treatment with a small dose to test the effect.

Long-acting phenothiazines appear to have considerable value in the maintenance treatment of chronic schizophrenia for, as schizophrenic patients are often unreliable in the manner in which they take oral medication when this is prescribed, such 'non-compliance' may lead to relapse. For this reason 'Depot Injection Clinics' have become a new feature in psychiatric out-patient departments, where patients attend for periodic injections. Alternatively, an injection may be given by a community psychiatric nurse who, acting under medical instructions, visits the patient at home.

As parkinsonian symptoms are very likely to occur following an injection of fluphenazine decanoate, an oral antiparkinsonian agent should be given at the same time. The patient is likely to cooperate if he is made aware of what may happen should he discontinue taking this.

Butyrophenones

Haloperidol (Serenace, Haldol) is at present one of the most widely used neuroleptic agents. Haloperidol is very likely to produce extrapyramidal symptoms which are usually readily controlled by antiparkinsonian drugs; however, these may develop very rapidly at any time during treatment. Haloperidol is indicated in the control of severe overactivity and excitement. As it does not have the hypothermic and hypotensive effects of chlorpromazine, it is particularly useful in elderly agitated patients, and may be used in the treatment of mania, schizophrenic excitement and in delirious states. It also controls aggression and, on this account, may be effective in certain mentally handicapped patients given to violence. It has been used in the treatment of Gilles de la Tourette syndrome in adults and children. It can also occasionally have a remarkable effect on certain paranoid states. Haloperidol may be given parenterally or orally, as indicated, in doses varying from 1.5 to 10 mg, and repeated every two hours up to 30 mg. Doses of 60–80 mg have been used orally, thus twice- or even once-daily administration is often satisfactory.

Pimozide (Orap) is sometimes used in once-daily dosage for the control of schizophrenic symptoms and is an alternative for maintenance to the depot injections. It has been recommended for the treatment of monosymptomatic somatic delusions such as those of infestation (Ekbohm's syndrome), although its value is by no means established.

Flupenthixol (Depixol), which is also available as a long-acting preparation, is a *thioxanthene* drug, chemically related to phenothiazines. While its action is similar to that of fluphenazine, it is also claimed to have an antidepressant effect and for this reason to be of value in schizophrenic patients who suffer from depressive symptoms which may sometimes be enhanced by fluphenazine.

Antidepressant and stimulant drugs

The use (and, one might add, the misuse) of antidepressant drugs presents what is perhaps currently the most controversial aspect of psychopharmacology. There are, in the United Kingdom, well over 30 tricyclic antidepressant drugs available on prescription, not including a seemingly growing number of others in different pharmacological categories.

Tricyclic antidepressants
Tricyclic antidepressants, which still appear to hold pride of place, fall into two main groups: *imipramine* (Tofranil) and *amitriptyline* (Tryptizol) and their several derivatives—*trimipramine* (Surmontil), *desipramine* (Pertofran), *clomipramine* (Anafranil), *nortriptyline* (Allegron), *protriptyline* (Concordin) etc. Imipramine has been extensively studied since its introduction in 1957. There are many reports of its use in depression, the general consensus of opinion being that *primary* (that is, endogenous) types of depressive illness are those which respond best. The same is true of amitriptyline. While both drugs are certainly reasonably effective in treating many mild or moderate states of depression, because their action does not become apparent for 14 to 21 days, or even longer in some cases, ECT is still strongly indicated in severe acute depressive illnesses, especially those accompanied by delusions and in which the suicidal risk is high. Combined treatment with antidepressive drugs and ECT seems

to produce no faster results than ECT alone, although the possibility of relapse is probably reduced thereby.

Any differences between the effects of imipramine and amitriptyline appear marginal, although some consider that the latter has more of a tranquillizing effect and is therefore more positively indicated in agitated patients, while imipramine, on the other hand, is more stimulating and may achieve better results in those who are retarded. The same can probably be said of their apparently ever-growing number of derivatives. While some appear to suit some patients better than others do, properly controlled studies usually demonstrate no more than insignificant differences.

Recently, more attention has been paid to dosage and blood concentration levels. Amitriptyline is broken down to nortriptyline which can be measured in the blood. An effective level of amitriptyline and nortriptyline of 80–200 mg/ml produces optimum therapeutic results, and the actual dosage of drug to produce this will, of course, depend upon such variables as body weight.

Once-daily administration of tricyclic antidepressant drugs is sufficient. Preferably the drugs should be administered at bedtime, owing to their tendency to produce drowsiness, at least initially. This may have the double advantage of promoting sleep and reducing drowsiness by day.

Side-effects. Side-effects are somewhat similar to those of the phenothiazines and, unlike the therapeutic action, occur quickly. Drowsiness, dry mouth, visual disturbances, postural hypotension, sweating and constipation are common in the initial stages but soon wear off. As with the phenothiazines, excessive weight gain may be a nuisance. Jaundice can also rarely occur. Night sweats, constipation, urinary retention (usually in males with enlarged prostates; rarely in females), blurring of vision and the precipitation of glaucoma are side-effects largely due to the anticholinergic action of tricyclics. More important are cardiac arrhythmias, heart block, and even ventricular fibrillation in those with pre-existing heart disease. It is wise, therefore, to avoid tricyclics when there is a recent history of myocardial infarction. Indeed, in some cases, there may be grounds for believing ECT to be safer.

Tricyclic drugs interfere with the control of blood pressure with adrenergic blocking drugs and they potentiate the action of adrenalin in local anaesthetics. They may precipitate fits in epileptic patients. Withdrawal symptoms such as insomnia, nausea and vomiting and sweating have been described when they are rapidly withdrawn.

Tricyclic antidepressants seem to have a variable effect on potency. They may sometimes assist those with premature ejaculation by causing some difficulty in ejaculation. In other instances they seem to impair potency, although how much of this is due to depression itself and how much due to treatment is often impossible to determine.

Tetracyclic antidepressants

Tetracyclic antidepressants and certain other drugs structurally resembling tricyclic antidepressants must be considered as still in an experimental stage. Some drugs, such as *mianserin, nomifensine* etc., are claimed to be effective antidepressants but with fewer side-effects than tricyclics, especially in respect of cardiotoxicity and serious anticholinergic actions.

Zimelidine, which has been introduced recently, has a more specific effect upon the 5-hydroxytryptamine system. Its therapeutic efficacy is not yet fully known.

Monoamine oxidase inhibitors

These are so called because they inhibit the action of the enzyme monoamine oxidase and thus prevent the destruction of serotonin (5HT), noradrenaline (NA), and dopamine (DA). At first it was thought that this accounted for their therapeutic effect, but this is unproven. Whatever the explanation, MAOIs appear to exert a euphoriant influence. This was observed first in the treatment of tuberculosis by *iproniazid* (Marsilid), leading to the drug being taken over into psychiatric practice, initially with encouraging results. But because of its tendency to produce liver necrosis, sometimes fatal, iproniazid and some similar drugs were soon dropped.

Despite this, it seems certain that drugs of this class, although potentially toxic, do have definite antidepressive properties. It would appear that the most effective, although possibly the most dangerous is *tranylcypromine* (Parnate). Compared with tricyclic antidepressants, tranylcypromine has a much rapider antidepressive action, having some amphetamine-like properties leading, for instance, to wakefulness. *Phenelzine* (Nardil) is also used, the indications being atypical depressive states, depression unresponsive to tricyclic drugs and phobic anxiety states.

Side-effects. These arise chiefly out of the action of MAOIs in combining with and thus inactivating the enzymes which oxidize biogenic amines. These amines may be neurotransmitters, potentially toxic substances in food or ingredients of medicines. Combination of MAOIs with such substances may produce serious and rapid action. The MAOI drugs will potentiate morphine, pethidine and other similar drugs, therefore anaesthetists and dentists need to know if a patient is taking them. Because fatalities have been recorded, the patient should carry with him a card stating that he is currently being treated with an MAOI.

Another potentially fatal side-effect is cerebral haemorrhage due to sudden severe hypertension. This is the so-called *cheese reaction*. If a patient taking a monoamine oxidase inhibitor eats foods containing tyramine, such as cheese (Cheddar cheese in particular), Marmite, yeast-containing substances, broad bean pods, red wine (Chianti notably), or takes some pressor substance such as amphetamine or ephedrine, as may be contained in a nasal decongestant, this may result in a hypertensive–hypotensive crisis resembling that produced by a phaeochromocytoma.

Some believe that MAOI drugs should not be combined with tricyclic antidepressives. Others, however, have advocated administration of the former in the morning and the latter at night. While this appears to be safe in most cases, the procedure can only be advocated with caution. In any event, and despite certain enthusiastic claims to the contrary, the combined administration of the two drugs does not seem to show any clear advantage over their being given singly. Amitriptyline is said to be safer than imipramine in combination with an MAOI in that it inhibits the absorption of tryptamine.

Amphetamines

Owing to their relatively short period of action and marked tendency towards habituation, *amphetamines* have been superseded in the treatment of depression. However, very occasionally they may be useful in 'stuck' depressions, especially in the elderly; that is, those in which a considerable degree of recovery has taken place with other treatment, but who fail to recover completely. Amphetamine is a scheduled drug (Schedule 2 of the Misuse of Drugs Act 1971) and its prescription is subject to certain restrictions on this account. The risk of other people stealing the drug from the patient should be recognized.

A combination of dextroamphetamine and stelazine in slow-release spansule form has been used in treatment of chronic monosymptomatic *depersonalization*, a condition notably intractable to most forms of treatment. Dexamphetamine has also been used in the management of hyperkinetic children and as the specific treatment for narcolepsy. Amphetamine has some anticonvulsant action and may be used in combination with barbiturates in patients who are markedly drowsy with the latter alone, for example in narcoanalysis.

Lithium

Lithium carbonate was first used by Cade in Australia to treat schizophrenic and manic excitement. A growing number of investigations by Mogens Schou and others have since shown that lithium is effective not only in controlling mania but also, by long-term administration, in preventing the recurrence of manic attacks. It has also been claimed that long-term administration will prevent the occurrence or recurrence of depressive attacks. While lithium certainly seems to control at least in part and sometimes completely, the depressive phases of manic–depressive psychosis (*bipolar depression*), its effect on *unipolar depression* appears less certain. Even in manic–depressive depression the simultaneous prescription of a small dose of tricyclic antidepressive or possibly a monoamine oxidase inhibitor may be required.

The major therapeutic use of lithium is, therefore, prophylactic, against further episodes of manic–depressive psychosis. Because of its toxicity and the fact that once prescribed it may need to be taken life-long, the decision to do so should not be undertaken lightly. Three episodes of mania or depression within five years requiring hospitalization would reasonably lead to the use of lithium, but only special circumstances would indicate its use with fewer episodes or longer intervals between attacks.

Lithium appears to work by preventing the intracellular retention of sodium which is thought to occur during some cases of affective disturbance of manic–depressive type, although there is also a suggestion that it may mobilize calcium and magnesium which may act as neurotransmitter substances.

Side-effects. The effects of lithium overdose can be serious; gastrointestinal, cardiac and renal symptoms may occur. Coarse tremor is a sign of toxicity although fine tremor may occur at therapeutic dose levels and can be controlled by propranolol. It is important, therefore, and especially so in the early stages, to check serum lithium levels at relatively frequent intervals; these are best kept between 0.5 and 1.2 m/mol, and as a general rule lower within this range nowadays, to minimize side-effects. The daily amount of lithium required to attain this level must be found by careful experiment, but usually varies between 600 and 1600 mg. Once- or twice-daily administration is generally satisfactory. As lithium works rather slowly and it may be necessary to bring manic excitement under control as soon as possible, it may be wise to give chlorpromazine or haloperidol during the first week or ten days of treatment. Haloperidol and lithium should not be given together as this is prone to cause tardive dyskinesia and confusion. Other side-effects which may occur at therapeutic dose level include tiredness, thirst and polyuria. In the long term, lithium also depresses thyroid function, particularly in women, so that this should be checked at intervals. If pregnancy occurs, lithium should be stopped as it may be teratogenic.

If the patient has poor renal function from either kidney disease, as judged by creatinine clearance and other appropriate tests, or congestive cardiac failure, or if he requires a low-salt diet, lithium should not be used. Decreased dosage and more frequent checks of blood level will be required in the elderly.

Antiparkinsonian drugs

Extrapyramidal symptoms frequently occur as side-effects of psychotropic drugs especially phenothiazines, butyrophenones and thioxanthenes. These include *acute dystonic reactions*, *opisthotonus* and *oculogyric crises*, *akathisia* ('happy feet') etc. *Tardive dyskinesia*, which may take years to develop, is usually irreversible; there is pouting and smacking of lips, protrusion of the tongue, other grimacing movements of the mouth and sometimes grunting and fidgeting.

Acute dystonic reactions may be treated by intravenous *benztropine* (Cogentin) or *procyclidine* (Kemadrin). Less acute symptoms may be controlled orally with *procyclidine*, *benztropine*, *benzhexol* (Artane) or *orphenadrine* (Disipal). Akathisia may be diminished by a benzodiazepine. Antiparkinsonian drugs should only be used in conjunction with a phenothiazine if really necessary; often dosage can be adjusted to provide good control of psychotic symptoms without side-effects.

There is no satisfactory treatment for tardive dyskinesia at the moment, although there is considerable research into the effectiveness of selective dopamine blockers. Prevention is the primary aim and the use of neuroleptic drugs should be reviewed regularly to see if they are still needed, and if so whether the dose may be reduced. In some patients, withdrawal dyskinesia will follow discontinuation of neuroleptic drugs; this may respond to diazepam as a muscle relaxant and minor tranquillizer.

Synthetic antiparkinsonian drugs such as those listed may, in larger dose, and especially in the elderly, cause an acute brain syndrome with confusion, delirium and hallucinations. Their anticholinergic effects may exacerbate glaucoma or provoke acute retention in men. Drowsiness, nausea, dry mouth and constipation may also occur.

Psychotomimetics

Psychotomimetics, sometimes called hallucinogens or *phantastica* and of which mescaline and lysergic acid diethylamide are the best known, produce 'psychotic' reactions which some believe resemble schizophrenia. However, this resemblance is much more apparent than real. They are in effect psychoses, in which clouding of consciousness may be evident. They are characterized by hallucinations, predominantly visual, mostly elementary though sometimes assuming a panoramic character. Ego disorders are characteristic, so that the subject feels his body has changed. True passivity experiences have not been observed. Although the interest of these drugs is largely experimental, they are mentioned here because they have also been employed therapeutically to encourage the abreactive release of unconscious material, although their value for this purpose is not established.

Social aspects

The social impact of new drugs calls for mention. When first introduced, their indiscriminate use, particularly in the United States, caused alarm.

The American Psychiatric Association entered a protest remarking that 'casual use of drugs in this manner is medically unsound and constitutes a public danger'. Their wholesale use in the United Kingdom has also been strongly condemned. Attention has been drawn to 'pharmacogenic disease' by Polonio, who remarks that the side-effects of most of the drugs discussed here may replace the symptoms of the original disease for which they were prescribed so that the doctor's and patient's time and attention are taken up by the management of these secondary symptoms. Regard must be paid to personality changes in the tranquillized patient, to the perseveration, retardation and limitation of activity by parkinsonian symptoms which hinder spontaneity of behaviour. This state of affairs may well be a more serious problem in other countries than in the United Kingdom. Nevertheless, it is certain that here too, drugs tend to be prescribed far too liberally and sometimes for inadequate reasons. Anxiety has a prime biological value: in some degree it accompanies the performance of every worthwhile task; only when it is excessive does it call for alleviation. The dividing line may be hard to draw. Indeed, merely suppressing anxiety does not encourage the patient or his doctor to take such measures as are necessary to try to overcome it once and for all.

A further social risk is the explosive epidemic of self-poisoning. Episodes of self-poisoning resulting in admission to hospital using drugs or other substances increased in England and Wales from about 10 000 per annum in 1955 to over 100 000 in 1978. Self-poisoning with hypnotics and sedatives has recently decreased, probably because of the diminished prescription of barbiturates and the greater safety of the benzodiazepines which have replaced them. Overdosage with aspirin and paracetamol has increased steadily, whilst the most rapid increase has occurred with psychotropic drugs, especially tricyclic antidepressants. This represents a major hazard in prescribing, as such drugs are toxic in overdose.

Special procedures

Electroplexy (ECT)

Electroconvulsive therapy is carried out by the discharge of an electric current of a few milliamps at 100–200 RMS volts from 0.5 to 2 seconds. The charge delivered is often about 200 millicoulombs and a sine wave may be used. The two standard placements of electrodes are unilateral, usually parieto-temporal, and bilateral, which is virtually always bitemporal. Given unmodified, the passage of current produces an immediate loss of consciousness followed by a typical grand mal seizure. If the latter (rarely) does not occur, this event is regarded as a subconvulsive stimulus and should be followed by a second application at a higher voltage.

Atropine is given first to dry up secretions and lessen the risk of arrhythmia. Owing to the risk of fractures and the fact that patients undergoing unmodified electroplexy tended to become increasingly anxious, treatment is now always carried out under light anaesthesia using an intravenous barbiturate together with a short-acting muscle relaxant. This should limit convulsive movements to slight twitching of the face and limbs sufficient to show that a seizure has actually occurred. A period of apnoea then follows, during which an airway should be inserted and oxygen administered under pressure via a face mask and breathing bag, until normal respiration is restored. The patient can then be safely removed to the recovery room and kept under observation until he regains consciousness, five to ten minutes later. All apparatus necessary for anaesthetic resuscitation, including suction apparatus, cardiac defibrillation and emergency drugs, should be available, though they will very rarely be required.

Electroconvulsive therapy may be given daily for a few days to the very depressed, agitated or restless patient, but is more customarily given two or three times per week. There is no such thing as a 'course' of treatment; the number of applications must be tailored to suit individual requirements. Most depressed patients respond adequately to six to eight treatments. These should be followed by an interval of seven to ten days during which, if relapse appears imminent, two or three further applications may be given as necessary. A satisfactory response may often be anticipated early during a series of treatments by transient improvement following the third or fourth application.

Preparation of the patient for ECT is very important. A full physical and psychiatric history and examination will always precede the decision to prescribe treatment. Dental treatment may need to be arranged before it is safe to proceed. The procedure, its benefits and dangers must always be explained to the patient and his written consent and cooperation obtained. Compulsorily detained patients who are prescribed ECT should also be asked to sign a form of consent for treatment. If a patient is unwilling to have treatment and ECT is considered essential, the Responsible Medical Officer (the consultant in charge) is recommended to obtain a further consultant opinion and to apply Section 26 of the Mental Health Act. This procedure should also be used if the patient requires ECT and is unable to understand what he is being told. Although relatives cannot give valid legal consent, obtaining their written approval is recommended when the patient refuses consent.

On the morning of treatment no food or drink is given; and immediately prior to treatment the patient should empty his bladder. Dentures, hair-grips, and tight clothing should be removed. Intramuscular sedation may be necessary in a few cases, but calming and encouraging words from the psychiatrist administering treatment and ensuring a humane and caring atmosphere in the treatment room should suffice.

While no one knows exactly how ECT works, there is some experimental evidence that it mobilizes certain neurotransmitter substances and possibly prevents the depletion of 5-hydroxytryptamine in the mid-brain. As this has yet to be confirmed, ECT must continue, for the time being, to be regarded as an empirical procedure. However, the convulsion is a necessary element for the therapeutic effect. Because it is liable to stimulate somewhat frightening fantasies in the minds of lay people, ECT has tended in recent years to receive rather a bad press. This is a pity for, when properly indicated, it may be remarkably effective and in many cases of depression safer and surer than drugs. Indeed, in some severe cases of depression ECT can be life saving.

Indications

The most important indication for ECT is depressive illness of endogenous type, especially if delusions are present, if there is marked agitation, if the patient is suicidal, and if there has been a failure to respond to antidepressant drugs.

While depressed patients respond best to electroplexy, particularly those with involutional depression, certain acutely ill schizophrenics may also receive considerable benefit, though a greater number of treatments may be required. Electroplexy is particularly effective in catatonic states and may also help those who are paranoid, particularly in the presence of an affective admixture. Manic states are, on the whole, less responsive and may need more vigorous treatment; however, there is some evidence that patients receiving ECT spend less time in hospital, are better on discharge and make a better social recovery than those not treated with ECT. Electroconvulsive therapy may also be used for the relief of mental depression in organic states such as occur in general paralysis and parkinsonism and occasionally in other physical conditions producing depression such as carcinoma. Although not usually advocated in epileptics, it can be employed to terminate prolonged psychomotor seizures (*epileptic twilight states*). It is of little use in emotional disorders except in certain anxiety states in which depression is a feature and where an endogenous element may be present.

Maintenance treatment

Maintenance treatment consists of the application of electroplexy over a longer period at relatively infrequent levels. While the need for this has lessened considerably since the introduction of antidepressant drugs, some advocate that a small minority of patients who have a tendency to relapse may continue to remain well if treated weekly, fortnightly and possibly thereafter at increasing intervals of time.

Contraindications

There are virtually no physical contraindications to convulsive therapy nor any real risk other than that inherent in the anaesthetic procedure.

Age is no bar. Treatment may be safely given to both old and young; to pregnant women, without fear of abortion; even to those suffering from quite severe physical illnesses including cardiovascular degeneration, though in this instance it is wise to seek the services of an experienced anaesthetist. With recent experience of myocardial infarction or cerebrovascular accident, ECT should be withheld for the time being unless there is risk of death from suicide or inanition.

Side-effects

Except for depersonalization which may be made worse and may be regarded, therefore, as a positive contraindication, the only really inconvenient side-effect of modified ECT is its effect upon memory. In younger patients this is of little importance and, in the long run, rarely extends outside the period over which the treatment is given. In those who are older with, perhaps, some degree of cerebral degeneration, the effect of ECT on memory may be more profound and, in some instances, leads to a state of confusion. It has been claimed that *unilateral* ECT, in which the electrodes are applied to one side of the head only—that containing the non-dominant cerebral hemisphere—causes less memory disturbance than the more conventional practice of bitemporal placement. This is the right side in nearly all right-handed and 70 per cent of left-handed people.

Electroplexy is compatible with drug treatment, though it is liable to produce confusional states in those who are receiving large doses of phenothiazines. There is also some risk of a fall in blood pressure in those given ECT in conjunction with chlorpromazine. Electroconvulsive therapy can safely be given together with antidepressant drugs such as imipramine or amitriptyline. Though this does not speed recovery from depression, it is thought that the combination of antidepressant drugs and ECT may help to prevent relapse.

Psychosurgery

Prefrontal leucotomy, which was first introduced by Moniz in 1935, now appears largely to be falling into disuse. The original technique has been abandoned since the operation was often followed by adverse personality changes. Many modifications have since been introduced, of which the technique of stereotactic subcaudate tractotomy probably produces the best results in terms of relief of symptoms and freedom from side-effects.

Indications

The prime indication for surgical intervention is prolonged and persistent tension and anxiety, particularly when this, as it does rarely, occurs almost in pure form. Probably, however, such operations are of greater use in patients in late middle age with chronic agitated depression who have become resistant to other forms of treatment. Although some may later relapse they may, however, then be found to be responsive once again to other forms of treatment such as ECT. Others who may respond are patients crippled by severe obsessions in whom all other methods of treatment may have been found to be useless. Even so, psychosurgery is by no means always effective. Where successful, the obsessional symptoms do not disappear, but lose their emotional investment, becoming 'blanched'. The same is true of delusional states.

It is generally agreed that surgery should only be considered after all other methods of treatment, physical, pharmacological and psychological, have been given a thorough trial. The best results, as in all forms of therapy, are obtained in those of good premorbid personality characterized by drive, activity and warm affect. Those who are flabby, inadequate or of unduly rigid outlook do not do well, neither do those with sociopathic traits.

Contraindications

Psychosurgery is contraindicated in dementia and particularly in those with cerebral arteriosclerosis who are liable to postoperative cerebral haemorrhage. It is also useless in vegetative and anergic states, as in simple schizophrenia and chronic hebephrenia, and likely even to be harmful in psychopathic and inadequate individuals in whom the operation may aggravate an existing behaviour disorder leading to aggressive behaviour and increasing lack of responsibility. It is also contraindicated in the mentally handicapped.

Complications

The operative mortality is very low indeed. Epileptic fits used to occur after the now obsolete leucotomy operations, but not with modern techniques. Similarly, temporary confusion and enuresis used to be common, but do not usually occur with more up-to-date procedures. Some changes in personality are inevitable, though once again with modern techniques and in the presence of a good premorbid personality, these are minimal. Grosser personality changes leading to tactlessness, deterioration of social behaviour and personal habits, lack of drive, initiative and interest used to occur, but very much less so nowadays. Some gain in weight is usual. This is occasionally excessive owing to the development of a ravenous appetite (*hyperphagia*).

Further reading

Clare, A. (1976) *Psychiatry in Dissent*. London: Tavistock.

Crammer, J., Barraclough, B. & Heine, B. (1978) *The Use of Drugs in Psychiatry*. London: Gaskell.

Gershon, S. & Shopsin, B. (eds) (1973) *Lithium: Its Role in Psychiatric Research and Treatment*. New York: Plenum.

Johnson, F. N. (ed.) (1975) *Lithium Research and Therapy*. London: Academic Press.

Pippard, J. & Ellam, L. (1981) *Electroconvulsive Treatment in Great Britain, 1980.* London: Gaskell.
Silverstone, T. & Turner, P. (1978) *Drug Treatment in Psychiatry*, 2nd edn. London: Routledge & Kegan Paul.

25

Psychiatry and the Law

Edited by Robert Bluglass

Legal and social reforms proceed by fits and starts, each episode following a fairly similar pattern. First, some unfortunate event comes to light leading to public outcry. If this is sufficiently clamorous and the complaints made appear to have some substance, an official enquiry is called for, both into the alleged scandal and its surrounding circumstances. The findings of the enquiry, together with recommendations designed to put matters right, are then placed before Parliament, which, if it thinks fit, passes new laws or amends old ones, so that those reforms regarded as necessary can be put into effect.

During the eighteenth century the laws governing the conditions under which the insane were kept, rather than cared for, were in a very unsatisfactory state. Thus, in 1774, an Act of Parliament was passed regulating the conduct of private madhouses run for profit. This was much needed, not only because of the appalling condition under which many of the inmates were kept but because cases of wrongful detention were by no means unknown. However, the Act was ineffective because the Lunacy Commissioners were not given adequate powers of enforcement. As a result the keepers of private madhouses continued to flout the law until 1828, when another Bill dealing specifically with these was passed. However, even this did not entirely stop cases of illegal detention occurring.

The plight of pauper lunatics was if anything even worse than that of those whose families could afford to pay for their care.

Following the Act of 1774, lunatics, in common with vagabonds, rogues and vagrants, could be apprehended and sent on a magistrate's warrant for a period of hard labour not exceeding one month. However, for those of unsound mind a special provision was made under Section 20 whereby, on the order of two or more Justices of the Peace, they could be locked up in some secure place for an indefinite period or for as long as their madness was deemed to continue; their property being distrained to pay for their maintenance. Up until 1808, when the County Asylums Act was passed, pauper lunatics were confined in gaols, bridewells, poorhouses and other unsuitable places, a situation which continued long after then because the County Asylums only came into being very gradually. Indeed, according to Kathleen Jones, 20 years after the Act was passed 9000 pauper lunatics were still in workhouses and, even as late as 1845, 4000 or so were still awaiting hospital accommodation.

The first really effective legislation governing the care of the insane was the Lunatics Act of 1845. This Act, which was very much more stringent than any previous legislation, followed an extensive report by the Commissioners in Lunacy. Prominent in carrying forward these new reforms was Anthony Ashley Cooper, later 7th Earl of Shaftesbury. In addition to being a Lunacy Commissioner and a Member of Parliament, he was the most noted social reformer of his day and also did much to improve conditions in the factories and the mines. In presenting the 1845 Bill to Parliament, Ashley stated: 'It is remarkable and very humiliating, the long and tedious process by which we have arrived at the sound practice of the treatment of the insane which now appears to be the suggestion of common sense and ordinary humanity'.

It is interesting to contrast this statement with that made 85 years later by Arthur Greenwood, the Minister of Health, in introducing the Mental Treatment Act of 1930 which for the very first time made provision for the voluntary treatment of mental patients: 'If this Act means anything at all it means we have ceased to think of mental disorder as something that is so indecent that it has to be kept in a category of its own.'

The trouble with Ashley's Act of 1845 was that it did just that. Its provisions were so stringent, particularly those covering certification, that, as Kathleen Jones again has pointed out, the only way patients could be detained without risking infringement of the liberty of the subject was to delay certification to the point where the subject was overtly insane and his illness almost certainly incurable. Early treatment, therefore, was out of the question; it might mean wrongful detention. Likewise, and despite some enlightened pleas from Samuel Gaskell and others, voluntary treatment at any stage of the illness was impossible.

Whereas Ashley's Act certainly did much to overcome the abuses to which the mentally ill were subject, as a consequence of it they were, nonetheless, shut away in the new County Asylums, more or less out of sight as well as out of mind. On this account the public also felt themselves protected. This is clearly revealed by the high walls and barred windows which were originally so much a feature of these asylums, together with, in most cases, their relative isolation, usually in rural surroundings until, during the twentieth century, many of them were gradually engulfed by suburban development.

The fact that it was so long before some form of voluntary admission to a mental hospital became possible was probably due not only to a persistent fear in the public mind of wrongful detention but to the fact that during the nineteenth century and the early part, at least, of the twentieth, treatment, even when applied early, had little to offer a mentally ill person other than custody and added discomfort, despite the progressively humane reforms brought about by the Tukes, John Conolly and others.

Following the passage of the Mental Treatment Act 1930, matters began gradually to improve. However, despite the fact that voluntary treatment became possible, certification still remained essentially a judicial procedure. Further reforms followed, of which the three most important were the National Health Service Act of 1946–8, the Mental Health Act of 1959 and the recent Mental Health Act, 1983. The National Health Service Act had the effect of removing mental hospitals from the control of the local authorities and making them, as in the case of general hospitals, the direct responsibility of the Minister of Health (later Secretary of State for Social Services). Their administration was controlled peripherally by the Regional Hospital Boards (since 1982, Regional and District Health Authorities).

The Mental Health Act 1983

The Mental Health Act of 1959 came into being following the setting-up in 1954 of a Royal Commission on the Law relating to Mental Illness, under the chairmanship of Lord Percy of Newcastle. The Commissioners' report, which was issued in 1957, made many important and radical recommendations, most of which were subsequently embodied in the Act.

In the first instance, the Act repealed all previous legislation in respect of mental disorder, largely removed all judicial measures appertaining to compulsory admission and devolved some of the provisions of the NHS Act 1946 on to the shoulders of local health authorities. Perhaps its most important reform was abolition of the provision for voluntary treatment made under the Mental Treatment Act 1930, which despite its name retained an in-built restriction in that voluntary patients had to give 72 hours' notice if they wished to discharge themselves, during which they could, of course, be subjected to certification and compulsorily detained. In lieu of this, the Act of 1959 (Section 5) made provision for informal admission whereby a patient could seek entry to a psychiatric hospital on exactly the same informal basis as any other patient suffering from some physical illness might do to a general hospital and with no in-built restrictions whatsoever. The success of this measure is clearly shown by the fact that the status of over 80 per cent of patients currently in mental hospitals is informal. Nevertheless, because a small proportion of patients lack insight, cannot cooperate or are a danger to themselves or others, some need for compulsory admission and detention remains.

The Mental Health Act 1983 becomes operational on 30 September 1983. It follows the passing of the Mental Health (Amendment) Act 1982 which made many important changes to the 1959 Act with the stated intention of improving the safeguards for patients, improving their rights, clarifying the legal position of staff looking after them and removing uncertainties in the law. A Mental Health Act Commission is to be created to have a general protective responsibility for detained patients and some concern for informal patients. The new Act also defines, for the first time, the law relating to consent to psychiatric treatment.

Terminology

The generic term *mental disorder* is used in the Act and is defined as follows (Section 1).

(1) In this Act 'mental disorder' means mental illness, arrested or incomplete development of mind, psychopathic disorder and any other disorder or disability of mind and 'mentally disordered' shall be construed accordingly.

Apart from mental illness, two subcategories of arrested or incomplete development of mind are defined: 'severe mental impairment' and 'mental impairment' together with 'psychopathic disorder'. The first two have already been defined but are repeated here for easy reference. (They replace the terms severe subnormality and subnormality used in the previous legislation.)

(2) In this Act *'Severe mental impairment'* means a state of arrested or incomplete development of mind which includes severe impairment of intelligence and social functioning and is associated with abnormally aggressive or seriously irresponsible conduct on the part of the person concerned.

(3) In this Act *'mental impairment'* means a state of arrested or incomplete development of mind (not amounting to severe mental impairment) which includes significant impairment of intelligence and social functioning and is associated with abnormally aggressive or seriously irresponsible conduct on the part of the person concerned.

(4) In this Act *'psychopathic disorder'* means a persistent disorder or disability of mind (whether or not including significant impairment of intelligence) which results in abnormally aggressive or seriously irresponsible conduct on the part of the person concerned.

(5) Nothing in this section shall be construed as implying that a person may be dealt with under this Act as suffering from mental disorder or from any form of mental disorder described in this section, by reason only of promiscuity or other immoral conduct, sexual deviancy or dependence on alcohol or drugs.

The Mental Health (Scotland) Act 1960, also amended as Mental Health (Scotland) (Amendment) Act refers to only two categories of mental disorder—mental illness and mental handicap—and does not include the category of psychopathic disorder.

Informal admission

Section 131 of the Act enables patients requiring treatment for mental disorder to enter any hospital or approved mental nursing home and certain local authority non-transferred accommodation *without legal formality*. The informal patient will be informed of his right to leave hospital if he wishes and right to refuse any particular form of treatment.

For certain designated treatments, even though he may give his consent, the treatment and the validity of his consent must be confirmed by an independent group of appointed individuals, including laymen.

Compulsory admission

Apart from cases referred by the courts, or transferred from prisons, which are dealt with elsewhere, the Act allows for compulsory admission in an emergency (Section 4), for assessment and necessary treatment (Section 2) or for treatment (Section 3) where this appears to be in a patient's own interest or that of others. In addition to these measures, if a police constable finds a person apparently suffering from mental disorder in a public place who appears to need immediate care or control, he may remove him to a place of safety (that is, a hospital or, as a last resort, police station) for a period not exceeding 72 hours in order for him to be medically examined and any necessary arrangements made for his care (Section 136). Under Section 135 a constable, following the issue of a magistrate's warrant and accompanied by a doctor and a mental welfare officer (approved social worker), is authorized to enter private premises, by force if necessary, where it is suspected that a mentally ill person is being ill-treated or not under proper control, where he is alone and unable to care for himself or where he is subject to detention under the Act and is absent without leave. This power may be used in relation to two individuals if necessary. It is rarely used.

Section 4 is used for emergency admission (for urgent assessment) and allows a patient to be detained for 72 hours. It requires an application by an approved social worker (mental welfare officer) or the *nearest relative* of the patient who must have seen the patient within the previous 24 hours, together with one medical recommendation given if practicable by a doctor who has previously known the patient. A statement that urgent admission is necessary must be made and the patient must be admitted within 24 hours of the examination.

Section 2 is for assessment (or for assessment followed by medical treatment) and allows a patient to be detained for not more than 28 days. It requires an application for admission to the managers of the hospital to which admission is sought, made by the nearest relative or an approved social worker either of whom must have seen the patient within the last 14 days. The application is founded upon two written medical recommendations on the prescribed form stating that the patient is suffering from mental disorder and that it is of a nature or degree which warrants the detention of the patient for assessment and, if necessary, treatment for at least a limited period. The patient has a right of appeal to a Mental Health Review Tribunal within 14 days, but the responsible medical officer, the hospital managers or the nearest relative may also discharge the patient.

Section 5 is used to detain an informal in-patient who has become so disturbed that he is a danger to himself or others and is threatening to take his discharge. The responsible medical officer (or his nominated deputy) may detain the patient for 72 hours. Before the doctor is found, a nurse (qualified psychiatric) may detain the patient for up to 6 hours.

Section 3 or, if made by a Court in respect of an offender, *Section 37* is for admission for treatment. It requires the same kind of application and written medical recommendations as does Section 2. It allows the patient to be detained for *six months* in the first instance, although he may be discharged before then by the responsible medical officer, the managers of the hospital (District Health Authority) or by a Mental Health Review Tribunal on appeal within six months by the patient himself or by his nearest relative. If further detention is required, this is renewable firstly for a further six months and then thereafter at annual intervals. The managers must automatically refer his case for review by a Tribunal if he has not exercised his right of appeal himself within a year or after three years.

Similar procedures required to place a patient under guardianship are laid down under Section 7. They were previously seldom used but the powers of guardians are now to be limited to 'essential' rather than unlimited powers, to require residence at a specified place, to require the patient to attend for treatment, occupation, education or training and to require that access to the patient is available to certain specified individuals.

Special provisions apply to those patients diagnosed as 'mentally impaired' or as suffering from 'psychopathic disorder' who may not be admitted compulsorily unless it is shown that the treatment is likely to alleviate or prevent a deterioration of their condition. A similar provision applies to Sections 3 and 37, and to all diagnoses on renewing an order.

Medical recommendations

Medical recommendations must be signed on or before the date of the application, and the dates of the medical examinations by the two doctors must be the same or not more than five days apart. One of the practitioners must have special psychiatric experience and be approved for the purpose by the appropriate health authority (Section 12). The other should, if possible, be the patient's general practitioner. If admission is to hospital, one of the medical recommendations should be made as far as is possible by a member of that hospital's staff and both may be on the staff of the hospital if this would prevent delay involving a serious risk to the health or safety of the patient, so long as one of the two doctors works at the hospital for less than half of the time which he is bound by contract to work in the Health Service and, where one of the doctors is a consultant the other does not work in a grade in which he is under that consultant's direction.

Neither recommending practitioner may be the applicant, nor can he benefit particularly by any fees made on the patient's account for his maintenance.

The clinical description of the patient given by the doctor must indicate the grounds for his opinion that the patient is suffering from the form of disorder specified in the recommendation and, for Section 3, that the condition is of a nature or degree which makes it appropriate for him to receive medical treatment in hospital, and that it is necessary for the health or safety of the patient or for the protection of others that he should receive such treatment and that it cannot be provided unless he is detained under the section. (Similar provisions apply in respect of hospital orders from a court.) Today, with modern methods of treatment and management, only a minority of patients should require compulsory detention in hospital.

Mental welfare officers (approved social workers)

At present, social workers carrying out the requirements of the Act are known as mental welfare officers. From October 1984, they will be replaced by 'approved social workers', officers of local social service authorities. They will be trained to have 'appropriate competence in dealing with persons who are suffering from mental disorder'.

Before making an application for admission to hospital or guardianship, a mental welfare officer is required to interview the patient in a suitable manner and satisfy himself that detention in hospital is, in all the circumstances, the most appropriate way of providing the care and medical treatment of which the patient stands in need. The application may be made outside the area of the local social services authority by whom the mental welfare officer is appointed.

It is the duty of a local social services authority, if so required by the nearest relative of a patient residing in their area, to direct a mental welfare officer as soon as practicable to consider an application to hospital and to inform the relative of his reasons if he decides not to make an application.

When a nearest relative has made the application for admission to hospital (other than an emergency application), the managers of the hospital are required to inform a local social services authority as soon as possible so that a social worker can interview the patient and provide the managers with a report on his social circumstances.

Duties of local authorities

Responsibility is put upon local authorities to provide care for the mentally sick of any description. Care comprises the provision, equipment and maintenance of residential accommodation, centres for training, occupation and education and the appointment of social workers, the exercise by the local authority of their functions as guardian and the provision of ancillary and supplementary services. The 1983 Act places a specific duty on local authorities to provide aftercare for discharged detained patients for so long as it may be required and necessary.

Removal to hospital

A properly completed application for admission is sufficient authority for the applicant, or authorized substitute, to take the patient to hospital within 14 days—with an emergency application, 24 hours—after the date the patient was last examined by the recommending doctor(s). If the patient escapes whilst being removed to hospital, he may be retaken by the person conveying him or by any social worker or constable.

Further detention in hospital

If a patient admitted under Section 2 requires detention for longer than 28 days, his admission may be prolonged by placing him under Section 3 before the expiration of the original order. Likewise, a patient admitted as an emergency under Section 4 may, following application to the managers of the hospital under Section 4(4), have his order converted to the requirements of Section 2, provided that the appropriate conditions are fulfilled.

Mental Health Review Tribunals

Each Mental Health Review Tribunal shall consist of a number of legal members, medical members and others having such experience in administration, knowledge of the social services or such other qualifications or experience as is thought suitable by the Lord Chancellor who makes the appointments. Each Tribunal must have a lawyer as its chairman and at least one member from each of the other two professional categories. Patients detained under any section other than the short-term sections, Sections 4, 135, 136, have a right to appeal at intervals against their detention. The nearest relative may appeal and, as indicated, the managers must automatically refer cases to the Tribunal at intervals when the right of appeal has not been used by the patient.

Mental Health Act Commission

The Secretary of State is required to establish a special health authority, the Mental Health Act Commission. The Commission will have about 80 members drawn from the ranks of doctors, nurses, social workers, psychologists and others. It will be divided into a number of panels to serve the Health Service regions.

The Commission will appoint doctors to provide second opinions as required by the Act and the Commission members are required to visit hospitals and mental nursing homes to interview patients and investigate complaints and undertake a general protective function for detained patients. These functions may be extended to informal patients if required by the Secretary of State. The Commission is required to publish a report every second year which must be laid before Parliament.

Consent to treatment

For the first time, the Mental Health Act 1983 defines treatments which require the patient's informed consent and/or a second medical opinion before the treatment can be given. These arrangements followed pressure from groups who were concerned about the ability of some patients to give properly informed consent to certain medical treatments considered to be irreversible, hazardous or of as yet uncertain efficacy.

The arrangements only apply to patients detained under Sections 2, 3, 36, 37, 38, 47 and 48 of the Act. Patients detained for short periods under appropriate sections of the Act may be treated as a matter of urgency in accordance with the section on urgent treatment.

Treatment requiring consent and a second opinion

This section (Section 57) applies to both detained *and* informal patients. No patient may be given: (a) any surgical operation for destroying brain tissue or for destroying the function of the brain tissue; or (b) any other form of treatment specified for the purpose of this section by the Secretary of State unless he has given his consent *and* a medical practitioner appointed by the Secretary of State (not the responsible medical officer) and two other non-medical appointed persons have certified in writing that the patient is capable of understanding the nature, purpose and likely effects of the treatment in question and has consented to it. In addition, the medical practitioner member must certify in writing that, having regard to the likelihood of the treatment alleviating or preventing a deterioration of the patient's condition, the treatment should be given. Before giving his opinion, the medical practitioner is required to consult two other persons who have been professionally concerned with the patient's medical treatment, of whom one shall be a nurse and the other be neither a nurse nor a doctor.

Treatment requiring consent or a second opinion

This section (Section 58) applies to: (a) treatments specified for the purposes of the section by the Secretary of State, initially ECT; and (b) the administration of medicine after the first three months of detention. For the first three months such treatment can be administered without any formalities. To give or continue treatment under this Section the patient must give his informed consent (recorded by the responsible medical officer or appointed doctor in writing) or a medical practitioner appointed by the Secretary of State must certify in writing that the patient is not capable of understanding the nature, purpose or likely effects of the treatment or has not consented to it but that, having regard to the likelihood of its alleviating or preventing deterioration of his condition, the treatment should be given.

Any consent or certificate under the above two sections may refer to a *plan of treatment* and the patient may withdraw his consent, but is then subject to a second opinion to review his case.

When treatment is given after three months in accordance with Section 56, the responsible medical officer must give a report on the treatment whenever the patient's order for detention is renewed (six monthly or annually as the case may be).

Urgent treatment may be given irrespective of the above restrictions: (a) if it is immediately necessary to save the patient's life; or (b) which (not being irreversible) is immediately necessary to prevent a serious deterioration of his condition; or (c) which (not being irreversible or hazardous) is immediately necessary to alleviate serious suffering by the patient; or (d) which (not being irreversible or hazardous) is immediately necessary and represents the minimum interference necessary to prevent the patient from behaving violently or being a danger to himself or others.

Any other treatments not mentioned above can be given at the responsible medical officer's discretion.

Codes of practice and regulations

The Secretary of State is required to prepare, from time to time, a code of practice for the guidance of staff in relation to the admission of patients to hospitals, or mental nursing homes, and in relation to medical treatment. This will indicate which treatments require the various forms of consent.

Regulations will also be published which will control the operation of parts of the Act, and specify treatments for the purposes of sections 57 and 58.

Forensic psychiatry

As forensic psychiatry is a large subject, and one of growing importance, no more than a brief introduction can be given here.

While there is clearly some overlap it must be emphasized that crime and mental illness are by no means synonymous. Although there are mental illnesses which may give rise to criminal behaviour—paranoid delusional states may, for example, lead to homicide, depression to shoplifting and early dementia to sexual indecency—most offenders cannot be considered as mentally abnormal, however deviant their behaviour. Likewise, most who suffer from mental illness are law abiding as are many mentally healthy citizens. Bearing this in mind, it has to be said that there remains a 'grey area', one possibly expanding, in which a decision has to be made as to just how much a person who has committed some offence can be held responsible at law on account of his or her mental condition. Such a decision is clearly necessary not only so that justice can be done but in order that disposal of the person concerned may be as appropriate as possible.

There are three aspects to be considered. Firstly, the subject may be suffering from a mental disorder at the time of committing an offence, whereupon when brought to trial the issue of criminal responsibility may be raised. Secondly, he may be found to be mentally disordered on arraignment whereupon the issue may be his fitness to plead. Thirdly, he may be found to be mentally disordered at the time of sentencing or subsequently while serving a term of imprisonment whereupon consideration will need to be given to whether he should be transferred to hospital.

Criminal responsibility

There has been much discussion of criminal responsibility without arriving at a completely satisfactory compromise between the medical and legal points of view. Interest was first aroused in 1843 when a certain Daniel McNaughton was acquitted of murder on account of suffering from delusions of persecution. After his trial the judges of the country were asked to confer and to express their opinion. This, in summary, was:

In order to plead insanity in defence of a criminal act, it must be proved that at the time of committing the act, the party accused was labouring under such defect of reason from the disease of the mind as not to know the nature and quality of the act he was doing, or, if he did know it, that he did not know he was doing what was (legally) wrong and punishable.

This is the legal test. The onus rests on the defence to raise the evidence and prove to a 'balance of probabilities' that the insanity of the defendant (usually some form of delusion) was the direct cause of the crime he committed. The defendant is not to be held responsible if he acts in a way which would be permissible if his delusions were true. Cases frequently arise in which insanity and abnormality of behaviour may be combined with a relatively high degree of reasoning power, so that the defendant, while undoubtedly *insane* at the time of the crime, both was and is able to realize the nature and quality of his act and its wrongful character, and although also capable of skilful planning, still cannot be held to be responsible by virtue of his otherwise disordered mind.

The McNaughton Rules are now relatively rarely applied; the doctrine of *diminished responsibility*, operative in Scotland for some considerable time, has now become embodied in English criminal law. Thus, under Section 2(1) of the Homicide Act 1957:

where a person kills or is a party to killing another, he shall not be convicted of murder if he was suffering from such abnormality of mind (whether arising from a condition of arrested or retarded development of mind or any inherent causes or induced by disease or injury) as substantially impaired his mental responsibility for his acts . . .

Where a defence is successful under the McNaughton Rules, the verdict will be 'not guilty by reason of insanity' leading to mandatory hospital admission with restrictions and without limit of time. In contrast, a plea of diminished responsibility is a plea which if successful reduces a charge of murder to one of manslaughter, thus avoiding a mandatory life sentence and allowing the court a greater range of disposal. In contrast to the McNaughton Rules, a defence of diminished responsibility is only raised in murder cases.

Drunkenness and responsibility
Drunkenness is not held to be an excuse for crime unless the accused was so drunk as to be incapable of forming an intent. Evidence of alcohol insanity and delirium tremens may also establish a successful defence.

Automatism
Automatism can excuse if it can be shown that at the time of his committing the offence the accused was unconscious or his actions were purely automatic, such as in a proved case of epileptic automatism. Two types of automatism have been formulated—*insane* and *non-insane*. In the former instance, there will be evidence of mental disease leading to the case being dealt with under the McNaughton Rules. In the case of non-insane automatism (for example somnambulism), this, if proved, and there being no evidence of insanity, will lead to acquittal.

Infanticide
The charge of infanticide is brought in lieu of murder in the case of a mother who due to a 'disturbance of mind' kills her child within a year and a day of its birth.

There are a large number of lesser crimes in which the mental state of the defendant may be considered in terms of mitigation of sentence. (The Butler Committee has recommended procedures which may lead to a verdict of 'not guilty on evidence of mental disorder'.)

Shoplifting
Shoplifting is occasionally associated with a variety of mental disorders, particularly in the young, the elderly and in menopausal women. These disorders are taken into account when sentencing. The defendant is

often placed on probation with or without a requirement of psychiatric treatment.

Sexual offences

Certain sexual offences result from loss of control such as may occur in epilepsy or general paralysis in other forms of dementia and sometimes depressive illness leading to sexual assaults on children and others. Middle-aged depressed patients suffering from waning potency will also sometimes commit acts of indecent exposure, although the large majority of those who do so are younger and basically sexually deviant.

Fitness to plead

A defendant should be mentally capable of instructing counsel, appreciating the nature of the charge and the significance of pleading 'guilty' or 'not guilty', challenging a juror, examining a witness and understanding and following the evidence and court procedure.

The question of his inability to do so on account of insanity may be raised on arraignment, by the defence, the prosecution or by the judge himself, or in the course of the hearing.

In the first case the following questions are put to the jury. Is the prisoner able to plead? Is he sane? And, if he fails to respond when he is asked to plead 'guilty' or 'not guilty', is he *mute of malice* or by the visitation of God?

If an accused person is found insane on arraignment, the question of whether he was insane at the time when the crime was committed is not dealt with.

In the second case, where the question of fitness to plead is raised during the course of the trial, the jury may be asked whether the accused is sane or insane.

In either case, when the prisoner is found to be unfit to plead, an order is made out for his detention in a hospital named by the Home Secretary where he is detained under conditions similar to those which pertain to Sections 37 and 41 of the Mental Health Act 1983. If his mental condition subsequently improves, the Home Secretary, after consultation with the responsible medical officer, has powers to remit him for trial. This power, however, is sparingly used owing to complications which may arise when proceeding to the prosecution of a person who has been in hospital a long time.

Admission of mentally abnormal offenders to hospital

Where a person is found guilty of an offence punishable by imprisonment but the court is satisfied on the written or oral evidence of two medical practitioners (one approved under Section 12 of the Act and one a doctor from the receiving hospital) that he is suffering from mental disorder, the court may make an order authorizing his admission to a specified hospital. The mental disorder may be mental illness, psychopathic disorder, mental impairment or severe mental impairment. The medical recommendation must state the grounds justifying admission, which are similar to those pertaining to Section 3. The order (a Hospital Order) may be renewed after six months, a further six months and then at annual intervals, and the responsible medical officer may discharge the patient at any time that he considers appropriate. The patient or his nearest relative may appeal to a Mental Health Review Tribunal within the second six months from the time that the order was made, after a further six months (and in any subsequent 12-month period). In the case of a magistrates' court, such an order can be made without recording a conviction. Such an order cannot be made in this way in a Crown Court.

In a Crown Court, the judge may, additionally, include restrictions preventing the patient's discharge or having leave of absence without the agreement of the Home Secretary. These restrictions may be applied for a fixed period of time or indeterminately. The judge must hear oral evidence and may only make an order restricting discharge (Section 41) if he is satisfied that it is necessary to protect the public from serious harm. Such patients may also have access to a Mental Health Review Tribunal after the expiry of six months.

The Court may request a regional health authority or its representative to give evidence about appropriate facilities for treatment if there is difficulty in offering a bed. Regular reports on restricted patients must be sent to the Home Secretary. The patient may be recalled or taken into custody if necessary while conditionally discharged or on leave of absence.

An offender who becomes mentally ill while on remand and awaiting trial or while serving a term of imprisonment may be transferred to a special or ordinary mental hospital by order of the Home Secretary (Sections 47 and 48) after receiving medical recommendations from two doctors (one 'approved'), the order having the same effect as a hospital order under Section 37 or Section 41. Should he still require to be in hospital after what would have been the earliest date of possible release from prison with full remission, he should then be treated as if he had been admitted under Section 37. These patients may apply to a Mental Health Review Tribunal within the first six months of transfer to hospital.

The consent to treatment requirements apply to patients under all the above sections.

Remands to hospital

The Mental Health Act 1983 allows a court to remand an accused person to hospital *for a report* to be prepared on his mental condition (an alternative to remand in custody). This applies (Section 35) *in a Crown*

Court to any person awaiting trial for an offence punishable by imprisonment or who has been arraigned before the court for such an offence and has not yet been sentenced or dealt with for the offence. It applies *in a magistrates' court* to any person who is convicted by the court of an offence punishable on summary conviction with imprisonment and any person charged with such an offence if the court is satisfied that he did the act or made the omission charged or he has agreed to the remand. Evidence, written or oral by one approved doctor, must be given indicating that there is reason to suspect that the accused is suffering from one of the categories of mental disorder and that bail would be impracticable. A bed must be available. The order may be repeated at intervals of 28 days but not for longer than 12 weeks in all. The accused person is also entitled to be examined by his own independent doctor.

The Court may also remand an accused person to hospital *for treatment* (Section 36) on the evidence, written or oral, of two medical practitioners (at least one an 'approved' doctor) that he is suffering from mental illness or severe mental impairment which makes his detention in hospital appropriate (rather than in custody). This may apply to any person awaiting trial before a Crown Court for an offence punishable by imprisonment (other than murder). One of the doctors giving evidence must be a doctor who would be responsible for the patient's treatment; a bed must be available and arrangements made for admission within seven days of the removal order being made. The order may be renewed at 28-day intervals for up to 12 weeks and the accused is entitled to obtain an independent report on his condition if he so wishes which may lead to the termination of the order.

Interim hospital order

Before a hospital order is made, as described above, an 'interim hospital order' can be made by a court (Section 38) for up to 12 weeks. This may be renewed at 28-day intervals, but for no longer than six months. The grounds are similar to a Section 37 order but the doctors must state that this is a case where a hospital order *may* be appropriate. The interim order allows the doctors to decide if a hospital order is justified and should be recommended to the court.

Note. The two forms of recommendation and the interim hospital order will be implemented at a date to be specified by the Secretary of State.

Powers of Criminal Courts Act 1973

Under Section 3 of the Powers of Criminal Courts Act, where the court is satisfied on the evidence of a qualified medical practitioner approved under Section 12 of the Mental Health Act 1983 that the mental condition of an offender is such as may require and be susceptible to treatment, but is not of such a degree as to make compulsory in-patient treatment necessary, it may, in making a probation order, include a requirement that the offender shall submit during either a part or all of his probationary period to treatment by or under the direction of a duly qualified medical practitioner with a view to bringing about an improvement in his mental condition. Various circumstances may be specified, including treatment as a resident patient in a hospital or mental nursing home, treatment as a non-resident patient in such an institution or under such other conditions as may be specified by the medical officer in the order. According to changing circumstances, some variation in these provisions can be made on the advice of the medical officer and with the consent of the probationer. A reasonable refusal by the offender to undergo surgical, electrical or other treatment may not be treated by the court as a breach of a probation order.

Juvenile courts

Juvenile offenders come before special courts in which there is considerable modification of usual law court procedure. As far as possible, the juvenile delinquent is dealt with very much as an individual problem. In many cases the magistrate will call for a medical and psychiatric report, including intelligence tests. Although it is hoped that more intensive study and treatment of the young delinquent may lead to a reduction in relapsing offenders and in juvenile crime overall, it does not so far appear that this hope is being realized. Indeed, a continuing rise in the number of juvenile crimes, particularly in those of a violent nature, is a current cause for alarm.

Writing court reports

In writing reports to the court, it should be remembered that as these are primarily addressed to laymen they should be clear, concise, comprehensible and free from all jargon. Regrettably this is not so often the case as it should be.

The report should be headed by the name of the patient interviewed, and such civil details as are needed for his further identification. The charge should also be stated. Remember that it is most unwise to prepare a psychiatric report or indeed to examine an offender without having first read the depositions or details of the offence with which the subject is charged. A short description of the person interviewed should follow together with a statement indicating his understanding of the reason and purpose of the interview. There should then follow what is, in essence, a general psychiatric report covering such topics as family and personal matters, development, educational and occupational history, previous medical and psychiatric history, sexual and marital problems and habits, including those specifically relating to alcohol and drugs.

Next, details should be obtained of present and past criminal behaviour, including also what has led up to the present charge. Factors underlying this should be fully discussed and recorded in detail. Following this, and in the light of background information, a formulation should be undertaken which should include opinion on such aspects as fitness to plead, criminal responsibility, mitigating factors, likely response to treatment of whatever psychiatric disorder may be evident, and how and where this should be carried out, together with an estimate of the likely prognosis.

Civil issues

Contracts

A contract made before the onset of mental disorder is binding. A person of unsound mind may make contracts for the necessaries of life, and such contracts are binding. However, judge and jury must decide what shall be included under the term *necessaries*.

A person of unsound mind may also make contracts for articles other than necessaries, but such contracts are not binding if they are such as would not have been made but for the insanity at the time of making the contract.

Marriage and insanity. A marriage is not valid if at the time of marriage either party was so mentally disordered as not to appreciate the nature of the contract. If such a degree of mental disorder can be proved, the marriage may be decreed null and void after application to the divorce court.

Torts. Torts are offences for which a person is liable in civil as opposed to criminal law. These include libel, slander, trespass and nuisance. A person so wronged by a person of unsound mind would probably be awarded only nominal damages in a court of law.

Receivership

The Court of Protection is an office of the Supreme Court. Its function is to manage and administer the property and affairs of those who, because of mental disorders, cannot do so themselves. The court consists of a Master, 'nominated' judges and a number of Assistant Masters. The court requires an application, usually from a relative or close friend, supported by medical evidence that the individual concerned is incapable, because of mental disorder, of managing his affairs. If the court accepts this evidence, it appoints a Receiver (in Scotland *Curator bonis*), preferably a near relative or friend willing and able to act as such, but failing this, another responsible person, most often the Official

Solicitor to the Supreme Court. The powers of the Receiver are strictly defined and limited in such a way as to safeguard absolutely the patient's estate, the administration of which is vested entirely in the court. The court has no control over the patient's person, only his property. Thus the court cannot direct where a patient shall live or that he shall enter or leave a hospital, although it is able to exercise considerable influence over matters of this kind through control of his property. The degree of mental disorder required to give the court jurisdiction is quite distinct from, and much less severe than, that which is required for compulsory detention in hospital under Sections 2 and 3 of the Mental Health Act.

Section 102 of the Act provides for the continuance of the office of *Lord Chancellor's Visitors*, of whom there are three panels: Medical, Legal and General. The Visitors are Officers of the Supreme Court and not, as is sometimes erroneously believed of the Court of Protection. The Visitors are required to visit periodically patients under the jurisdiction of the court and to report on their mental state or on any other matter, notably testamentary capacity, on which the court requires information. The Medical Visitors have the statutory right to require the production of any medical record relating to the patient; any obstruction to a Visitor in the performance of his duties is an offence punishable by imprisonment. At the present time the rules of the Court of Protection and the appointment of Visitors are under review.

The court relies greatly on the goodwill and cooperation of doctors, particularly the family doctor but also hospital doctors, particularly in respect of those patients who have been admitted, say, to the geriatric unit of a general hospital when still capable of managing their affairs but who later show intellectual deterioration. It is the duty of the doctor to advise a patient's relatives of the risks of the situation and, if they refuse to make the necessary application to the court, to do so himself. While a doctor may be reluctant to take such a step, he must fully appreciate that the responsibility of any action taken or not taken on his evidence is entirely that of the court.

Some disastrous cases, in which dissipation of sometimes substantial fortunes occurs, would be avoided if doctors fully realized their responsibility in this matter.

Testamentary capacity

Only a person with a 'sound disposing mind' can make a valid will. Compulsory detention in itself is no bar, nor is mental disorder necessarily in itself. The following points should be noted when examining a patient with regard to his testamentary capacity.

1. His ability to realize the nature of a will and its consequences.

2. His ability to recall the nature and extent of his property, but not necessarily his ability to recall details of a large estate.

3. His ability to recall the names of all near relatives and to weigh the claims of these and possibly others on his bounty.

4. Absence of a morbid state of mind which might pervert the natural feelings of the testator and influence him in his decisions. It is, however, possible for a testator to be deluded and yet to retain a sound disposing mind provided that his delusions are not of such a nature that they are likely to influence his testamentary disposition.

In the judgment delivered in *Banks v. Goodfellow* (1870) the Chief Justice stated that the testator must understand the nature and effects of the act, and the extent of the property of which he is disposing; he must be able to comprehend and appreciate the claims to which he ought to give effect. It is essential, therefore, that no disorder of his mind should poison his affections, pervert his sense of right, or prevent the exercise of his natural faculties. No insane delusion must influence his will in disposing of his property, and bring about a disposal of which, if his mind had been sound, he would not have made.

5. A testator may of course take the advice of others and have regard to their wishes about the disposition of his property, but must not be influenced by them through fear or by the threat of force. It must be said, however, that such influences are often of a subtler and more intangible kind and not always easy to assess.

6. In case of doubt, the testator should be re-examined after a period of time.

Patients under the jurisdiction of the Court of Protection are discouraged from making wills unless there is medical evidence of testamentary capacity.

Further reading

Bluglass, S. R. (1983) *A Guide to the Mental Health Act 1983*. London and Edinburgh: Churchill Livingstone.

Gostin, L. (1977) *A Human Condition: The Mental Health Act from 1959 to 1975, Observations, Analysis and Proposals for Reform*, Vol. 2. London: The National Association for Mental Health (MIND).

Hoggett, B. (1976) *Mental Health*. London: Sweet & Maxwell.

Jones, K. (1955) *Lunacy Law and Conscience 1744–1845: the Social History of the Care of the Insane*. London: Routledge & Kegan Paul.

Jones, K. (1960) *Mental Health and Social Policy 1845–1959*. London: Routledge & Kegan Paul.

Walker, N. & McCabe, S. (1973) *Crime and Insanity in England*, Vol. 2. Edinburgh: Edinburgh University Press.

Index